Childhood Pain

Childhood Pain
Current Issues, Research, and Management

Dorothea M. Ross, Ph.D.
Department of Pediatrics
University of California Medical School
San Francisco, California

Sheila A. Ross, Ph.D.
Research Institute
Palo Alto Medical Foundation
Palo Alto, California

Urban & Schwarzenberg
Baltimore-Munich • 1988

Urban & Schwarzenberg, Inc.
7 E. Redwood Street
Baltimore, Maryland 21202
USA

Urban & Schwarzenberg
Pettenkoferstrasse 18
D-8000 München 2
West Germany

NOTICES

The Editors (or Author(s)) and the Publisher of this work have made every effort to ensure that the drug dosage schedules herein are accurate and in accord with the standards accepted at the time of publication. The reader is strongly advised, however, to check the product information sheet included in the package of each drug he or she plans to administer to be certain that changes have not been made in the recommended dose or in the contraindications for administration.

The Publishers have made an extensive effort to trace original copyright holders for permission to use borrowed material. If any has been overlooked, it will be corrected at the first reprint.

Library of Congress Cataloging in Publication Data

Ross, Dorothea M.
  Childhood pain.

  Bibliography: p.
  Includes index.
  1. Pain in children. I. Ross, Sheila A. II. Title. [DNLM: 1. Pain—in infancy & childhood. WL 704 R823c]
RJ365.R67 1987   618.92   87-29567
ISBN 0-8067-1641-X

Sponsoring Editor: Charles W. Mitchell
Copy editor: Debbie Klenotic
Cover Design: Barbara Ravizza
Designed and Produced by Stony Run Publishing Services, Baltimore, MD
Typeset by Brushwood Graphics, Inc., Baltimore, MD
Manufactured in the United States of America
by R. R. Donnelley & Sons Company, Chicago, IL

ISBN 0-8067-1641-X (Baltimore)

ISBN 3-541-71641-X (Munich)

It's not good never to have pain. Pain gives you more of a lead on into life. It gives you something to think about. . . . If you never get hurt or anything you get dainty—pampered. A lot of people don't really like dainty people. What's good about pain is you learn to handle life a little better—you get a better understanding. . . . Like if you lose a job, you feel *hurt, but like if you break a leg you really think* what the word hurt or pain means.

The worst pain was the bone marrow the first time. They put in numbing medicine, you feel a lot *of pressure. . . . The doctors told me to relax for it not to hurt and it works a lot better that way. I talk to the doctor, I think about good things. I think about happy things, like I like to sail.*

When I started getting sicker in fourth and fifth grade I started coming here a couple of weeks at a time. It helped me but it didn't help the school. . . . I don't worry about flunking . . . I work hard to keep my grades up . . . the teacher helps me a lot.

I'd tell him [another boy who had just found out he had leukemia] *you have a great start on medical school. Once you get leukemia, they start doing a lot of tests, X rays. After a while you get kind of interested in the machines they use, how they work and what they do . . .*

Andrew Todd Watkins (1970–1982)

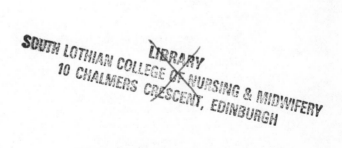

Contents

Foreword   *John J. Miller, III* ix

Preface xi

1   Pain   *An Overview* 1

2   The Child's View 35

3   Determinants of Pain 75

4   Assessment and Measurement 111

5   Management   *Physical Interventions* 167

6   Management   *Behavioral and Cognitive*
        Interventions 211

7   Pediatric Pain Problems   *Primary Dysmenorrhea,*
        Burns, Migraine, and Intrusive Procedures 251

8   Current Developments and Future Directions 293

References 313

Author Index 359

Subject Index 375

Foreword

The relief of pain and the delay of death have been the primary aims and purpose of all the shamans/priests/physicians of all societies in recorded history. Many must have been successful, at least in relieving pain. The tools were probably intuitive in nature. Only during the last two centuries has there been the logarithmic growth of technical and scientific information that has provided physicians and other health providers with the tools that prolong life and significantly alter the courses of diseases. Despite many improved ways to relieve the acute, transitory, traumatic, and surgical forms of pain, pain remains a universal human experience, one that reduces human well-being, productivity, and psychological ease far beyond the associated physical causes. Ironically, the psychosocial skills and methods used by shamans, priests, and physicians for centuries have largely been neglected and forgotten during the last hundred years as technical skills have increased. In the past two decades people have again turned their attention to pain as a specific engrossing medical problem in its own right, and attention is again returning to the nonpharmacological, nonmechanical methods of pain relief. This book represents both a theoretical and a practical approach to these methods for the control of pain in children.

The authors have extensive experience in the field of pain in children. They have worked with tools to analyze and to attempt to measure pain in different pediatric circumstances, and also have been active in exploring practical tools to provide pain relief. Those of us who have had the benefit of their teaching have been able to apply some of their techniques directly in our clinics and practices. This book brings together both their theoretical and their practical knowledge in one place, and can be read and used by all health professionals who deal with children and pain. There are practical tips for the office nurse who gives immunizations, the physical therapist who works with an arthritic child, or the physician who is planning a program for a burn patient. In addition, academicians and research workers will be able to use the sections on pain measurement for both theoretical and practical advice.

The section on methods of attempting to measure pain should be read by anyone who wants to do research in pain evaluation. All of the difficulties are discussed. The critical analyses of the various assays that have been used to date will be of great help to anyone planning a project dealing with pain measurement in children or in the efficacy of pain-relieving drugs or procedures. The explanation of the assays is clear, and the criticisms are thoughtful and helpful in understanding the usefulness and problems of each assay.

In discussing the psychology of pain in children, two important threads appear throughout the book. The first is the fact that each child is different, and that not all methods of pain control will work or be accepted by all children. Some children want specific knowledge, others do not. Some will react to one approach, and others will not. The book provides a variety of approaches to the control of pain by nonpharmaceutical means, and gives an analysis of the likely benefits of each.

The second important thread that connects many sections is the concept of "self-efficacy" versus "learned helplessness." This concept of patient psychology has become important in many areas, from general principles to health education to specific approaches taken to individual patients. It is a concept that must be considered in designing any therapeutic program, but particularly a program for the chronically ill.

Ironically, the reader will have to be wary of some of the book's descriptions of specific pharmacological or physical means of controlling pain, since these change rapidly and may be out of date within a year or two. The sections on the control of "social ecology" for pain relief and on psychosocial factors in pain control will be much more stable. I am personally convinced that the authors are describing in practical terms and in a systematic way those practices that have probably made successful shamans/priests/physicians over the centuries. The control of the environment, the development of a sense of self-control in the patient, and the use of hypnosis or other distracting mental devices are all important tools that should be available to anyone who is dealing with the therapy of pain.

John J. Miller, III, M.D., Ph.D.
Director, Rheumatic Disease Division
Children's Hospital at Stanford
Stanford, California

Preface

Despite the ubiquitous nature of childhood pain, interest in this topic has been slow to develop. It was not until the mid-1970s that the pain experience of infants, children, and adolescents began to attract clinical and research attention, albeit from a predominantly adult perspective. In the current decade a further expansion has occurred, this time to include the child's view. These two trends constitute an embryo base of information of great potential value to those in the pediatric setting. Unfortunately, much of the information is scattered throughout the medical, psychological, nursing, social work, dental, sociological, and anthropological literature, and other areas in the humanities, as well as the popular media. Our intent has been to survey, select, and consolidate this information, making it accessible to the multidisciplinary group of professionals and students who are concerned with childhood pain in either a clinical or a research capacity.

Our purpose was to provide a comprehensive overview of the current status of the available knowledge on childhood pain. The emphasis throughout is on the psychological nature of the pain experience, rather than on the neurophysiological mechanisms involved, although the latter are discussed in relation to theoretical formulations concerning the pain experience. The conceptual framework of our approach stems from social ecology theory, with the pain experience being viewed as the outcome of factors within the child functioning in a reciprocal relationship with the components of his social and nonsocial environments.

The text begins with an overview of pain that places childhood pain in the context of this complex field. A discussion of the child's view of pain and his own pain experiences follows, and this aspect is emphasized throughout the text. The theoretical and empirical bases for the determinants of pain reactivity are described. Considerable attention is focused on the assessment of pain. Following a description of the general principles of management, some of the empirically based pharmacotherapeutic, behavioral, cognitive, and psychotherapeutic interventions are presented. Special emphasis is given to the issue of prevention, a topic that has received almost no attention in contemporary texts on pain. We have tried throughout to strike a balance between the need for rigorous methodology and the value of new ideas and concepts of a speculative nature that may provide a link to innovative approaches to investigation and management. Because the book is addressed to an interdisciplinary group, we have avoided the use of jargon and have discussed most topics in such a way that specific training in any one field is not a prerequisite to using the text. The usage of the masculine pronouns throughout this book is meant to include the feminine counterparts when not referring to a specific person. This is done for simplicity and is not intended to be discriminatory in any way.

In the past two decades, basic pain research and clinical research with adults, particularly those with chronic pain, have caused the status of pain to shift from that of a symptom to be dealt with to a problem in its own right. Much of the progress that has occurred in this period can be attributed to the free and productive exchange of ideas, as well as to clinical and research collaboration across disciplinary lines. It is our hope that this book will stimulate a similar kind of exchange among professionals concerned with the problem of childhood pain.

We wish to express appreciation to our colleagues who generously sent us their prepublication materials or provided information that would not otherwise have been available to us: Martha Barnard, Kenneth Craig, Ruth Grunau, Yoon Hahn, Barbara Herman, Susan Jay, Mary Ellen Jeans, Leora Kuttner, Charles E. Lewis, Patricia McGrath, Patrick McGrath, Anne O'Leary, Don Routh, Mary Tesler, Carolynne Vair, and James Varni.

The comments and criticisms from colleagues who read chapters or sections of the manuscript were invaluable and greatly enhanced the final text. Those who undertook this time-consuming task were William Benitz, C. Richard Chapman, Kenneth Craig, Laura Jones, Patricia McGrath, Ronald Melzack, Sharon Ow-Wing, David Tatro, and Carol Whalen.

We would particularly like to thank Gerald Koocher for his support and encouragement at a critical point in the preparation of this manuscript.

Warmest thanks are extended to the children, teachers, and pediatric personnel who participated with enthusiasm and unflagging cooperation in our various studies of pediatric pain. We are particularly indebted to the children and nurses at the Children's Hospital at Stanford. The children were greatly interested in providing information about their pain problems and offered sage advice about pain management; the nursing staff were exceptionally generous in their support of all phases of the interview project. Altogether, it was a privilege to conduct research in this outstanding pediatric hospital.

The special contributions of Esther Clark, Anne Gaffney, Leonard Horowitz, Bernard Millman, and Barbara Ravizza are also gratefully acknowledged. We deeply appreciate the generous gesture of Ray Moloney, who was instrumental in drawing the proposed manuscript to the attention of Charles W. Mitchell.

Finally, it is a real pleasure to acknowledge the interest, encouragement, and support that Charles W. Mitchell, our editor at Urban & Schwarzenberg, has provided throughout the preparation and subsequent publication of this text. The lengthy task of writing this book was far more pleasant than it would otherwise have been without this help.

Dorothea M. Ross
Sheila A. Ross

Childhood Pain

1

Pain

An Overview

Pain is the most complex of human stressors (Chapman & Bonica, 1983). It is a multidimensional phenomenon that encompasses physical stimuli, autonomic changes, and sensory physiology, but also involves cognitive functions, affective states, and behavioral phenomena. A diversity of etiological factors may be implicated: Pain can occur as the result of acute or chronic illness, from psychological upset, or even spontaneously in the absence of any known cause (Melzack & Wall, 1983). Pain serves positive as well as negative functions. It can act as a warning of tissue trauma or as a diagnostic aid and treatment evaluator, but it can also become a refuge from an intolerable situation, an expiation of guilt, or a tool for manipulating others. Contributing to its complexity are a number of divergent features. The most prevalent of the major health problems, it is also the least understood (Smith, Merskey, & Gross, 1980; Smoller & Schulman, 1982). It is the most common reason for seeking professional consultation (Bonica, 1983; Bresler, 1979) as well as the most common reason for avoiding it (Weisenberg, 1977a). Although it is frequently associated with a significant drop in the overall quality of life, it may also serve as a motivating force that elicits the best from the individual. It is one of mankind's greatest enemies, yet it is a prime necessity for its survival. The hazards of life without pain are most evident in the plight of the congenital analgesic who is insensitive to pain and consequently is almost defenseless against such dangers as extreme heat and untreated wounds and infections.

Problems of Definition

In view of the wide-ranging and often conflicting characteristics encompassed in our concept of pain, it is not surprising that the problem of one definition of pain meeting with general acceptance remains unresolved. Although some investigators contend that the lack of a single commonly accepted definition has been a major impediment in understanding pain (see, for example, Bonica, 1979; Gorsky, 1981), others such as Melzack (1973, pp. 45–46) point to the drawbacks inherent in having such a definition:

> Pain is not a single quality of experience. . . . The word "pain" represents a category of experiences, signifying a multitude of different, unique events having different

causes, and characterized by different qualities varying along a number of sensory and affective dimensions.

To be clinically or empirically useful, a definition must be specific enough to be relevant to a particular event, specialty, or investigative area. Pain has applicability to many disciplines other than medicine, and within each of these its meaning changes. Consider, for example, the different meanings of pain for biology, epidemiology, theology, psychology, anthropology, and economics. Add to this diversity the fact that pain is used as a referent for such disparate and inherently unrelated events as acute and chronic discomfort, reflex adaptive behaviors, percepts, emotions, neuroanatomical entities, biochemical phenomena, and stimuli for related instrumental responses (Degenaar, 1979). It becomes clear that an adequate definition would require such generality as to be of little use to the investigator in a specific field. In an attempt to resolve this dilemma, the International Association for the Study of Pain (IASP) (Merskey, 1979, p. 250) has proposed the following definition:

> Pain [is] an unpleasant sensory and emotional experience associated with actual or potential tissue damage, or described in terms of such damage.

To this concise statement the Subcommittee on Taxonomy (Merskey, 1979, p. 250) has felt impelled to add what Wolff (1984) calls "escape clauses" and what Wall (1984) has termed "crucial notes," partially reproduced here:

> Note: Pain is always subjective. Each individual learns the application of the word through experiences related to injury in early life. Biologists recognize that those stimuli which cause pain are liable to damage tissue. Accordingly, pain is that experience which we associate with actual or potential tissue damage. It is unquestionably a sensation in a part or parts of the body but it is always unpleasant and therefore also an emotional experience. . . . Many people report pain in the absence of tissue damage or any likely pathophysiological cause; usually this happens for psychological reasons . . .

The IASP definition of pain has not gained unanimous acceptance in the scientific community. Some investigators have directly criticized it; Wolff (1984, p. 186) for example, has noted correctly that

> Not all pain is unpleasant. Furthermore, while acute pain is usually associated with tissue damage, such a correlation is much more tenuous for chronic pain.

Others have proposed definitions specific to their areas of interest, and these appear to have far greater utility than that of the IASP. Consider, for example, the value for the anatomist of Bond's definition (1984, p. 3):

> Pain is a subjective experience arising from activity within the brain in response to damage to body tissues, to changes in the function of the brain itself either as a result of damage due to injury or disease, or to changes of a more subtle nature perhaps

depending upon biochemical changes which also appear to play a role in producing mental illness.

Or compare the IASP definition with the operational clinical definition for nurses proposed by McCaffery (Meinhart & McCaffery, 1983, p. 11), that "Pain is what the patient says it is and exists when he says it does," and echoed by Noordenbos (1984, p. 2, Prologue): "Pain is what the patient tells us he feels." The essence of the definitional dilemma is contained in Degenaar's succinct comment (1979, p. 281), "I thought I knew what pain was until I was asked to say what the word pain means." His scholarly treatise (Degenaar, 1979) should be mandatory reading for those intrigued by the problem of defining pain.

Magnitude of Problem

Pain is the most prevalent of the stressors that afflict mankind (Bonica, 1983; Turk, Meichenbaum, & Genest, 1983). Pain experiences range from the common-place, transient, and relatively mild (for example, minor lacerations, simple fractures, stomachaches), to the moderate and severe pains of iatrogenic procedures (for example, dental and surgical intervention, burn debridement), to the often debilitating pains of chronic conditions (for example, arthritis, angina). Although the majority of pain experiences are neither age nor gender specific, a few are associated primarily with certain age stages, such as colic with infancy or basilar artery migraine with late adolescence and young adulthood, and there are some that are either gender specific (for example, the often severe pain of menstruation and childbirth) or almost exclusively so (for example, the predominantly masculine problem of the cluster headache).

Although the consensus is that pain is ubiquitous (Melzack & Wall, 1983; Turk et al., 1983), attempts to assess the magnitude of the pain problem have been limited to careful estimates of prevalence by experts (see, for example, Bonica, 1980). Other investigators have collected pain prevalence data by diagnostic category—Paulley and Haskell (1975) estimated that there are 25 million migraineurs in America; by body area afflicted—Clark, Gosnell, and Shapiro (1977) reported a probable 7 million victims disabled by low back pain; by symptoms reported to health professionals—Bresler (1979) estimated that 80% of all patients who consult physicians do so for pain-related problems; or by more indirect indices, such as loss of job productivity—Smoller and Schulman (1982) reported that the average American loses 2 weeks of work time per year for pain-related problems (Crook, Rideout, & Browne, 1984).

Prior to the mid-1980s, no attempts had been made to confirm these prevalence estimates independently. However, in 1985 a major breakthrough occurred when the Bristol-Myers Company commissioned a national survey of pain in the

United States. Telephone interviews were conducted with a sample of 1,254 respondents age 18 or older representing a cross section of the adult population of the continental United States. The sample was constructed statistically to permit projections to the entire adult population of 174 million, with a predicted accuracy of ± 2.3%. This survey provided quantitative data on the prevalence of seven types of pain (see Table 1-1) and data on the respondents' views of the pain's severity, cause, and impact on work and other activities as well as their demographic characteristics. Information was also obtained on the relationship between the pain experiences of the respondents and measures of stress and health locus of control, the use of medical and other professionals in pain treatment, and the efficacy of different treatments for pain relief. Published as *The Nuprin Pain Report* (Taylor & Curran, 1985), some of the major findings of this important survey have also been published elsewhere (Sternbach, 1986a, 1986b).

In the course of a year, one out of every four Americans will experience pain intense enough to prompt action (Frederickson, 1980). Some will seek qualified medical or dental consultation, but the great majority (perhaps as high as 75%) will bypass professional help (Banks, Beresford, Morrell, Waller, & Watkins, 1975; Crook et al., 1984) in favor of other alternatives such as faith healers, quacks, and a host of self-treatment procedures, including nonprescription pain medications (Americans are reported to swallow 20 tons of aspirin a day [Olson, 1985]), meditation, self-hypnosis, and prayer. A dispiriting finding in the *Nuprin Pain Report* is the fact that 18% of the respondents who rated their pain as severe or unbearable did not consult any professional because they thought that no one could help them (Sternbach, 1986a).

Despite the obvious and overwhelming importance of the problem of clinical pain, advances in the understanding of this complex phenomenon have lagged far behind other biomedical achievements (Bonica, 1984). The fundamental cause and physiology of pain are still unknown (Madden, 1985), and many experienced investigators (Bakal, 1979; Crue, Kenton, Carregal, & Pinsky, 1980; Smith et al. 1980; Smoller & Schulman, 1982) view pain as the least understood of the common health-related problems. The general consensus is that we are a long way from an understanding of pain mechanisms. In Noordenbos's words (1984, p. 2), "Our knowledge concerning the mechanisms both under normal and abnormal circumstances is deficient, incomplete, and at some levels may perhaps be faulty or altogether lacking." Furthermore, it appears unlikely that a genuine breakthrough will occur in the immediate future. Although there has been a marked increase in empirical and clinical activity, with directions for pain research clearly delineated (Bonica, 1983, 1984; Liebeskind & Paul, 1977; Ng, 1980) and accompanied by substantial advances in our knowledge and understanding of pain (Kitchell & Erickson, 1983; Noordenbos, 1984; Wall, 1984), satisfaction with such progress has been tempered by doubts concerning the significance of these achievements. As Menges (1984, p. 1257) has stated,

Table 1-1 The Types of Pain Americans Have Experienced in the Past 12 Months (Total Sampled, 1,254)

Q: Now, I'd like to read you a short list of different kinds of pain. Please say for each one, on roughly how many days—if any—in the last 12 months you have had that type of pain. How many days in the last year have you had (READ EACH ITEM)?

	Total percentage who have had pains 1 or more days (%)	Number of days have had pain (%)						
		1–5	6–10	11–30	31–100	101 or more	None	Not sure
Headaches	73	30	14	16	8	5	26	1
Backaches	56	22	7	12	6	9	43	1
Muscle pains	53	21	11	11	5	5	45	1
Joint pains	51	17	7	11	6	10	48	1
Stomach pains	46	25	8	8	2	3	52	1
Premenstrual or menstrual pains[b]	40	13	8	16	3	a	57	2
Dental pains	27	18	3	4	1	1	74	a
Other types of pain	6	2	1	1	1	1	94	a

Note. Reprinted, by permission, from Sternbach, R.A. Survey of pain in the United States: The Nuprin Pain Report. *The Clinical Journal of Pain*, 1986a, 2, 49–53.

[a]Less than 0.5%.

[b]Percentage of women with premenstrual or menstrual pains.

The question arises as to whether these developments have brought us any closer to solving the "puzzle of pain." Unfortunately the answer has to be negative: pain remains too complex; it is determined by too many factors. The expectation that the near future may bring us the answer to such a multifactorial problem seems unwarranted . . . there is still a long way to go.

Although predictions abound about the medical miracles that are expected in the 21st century (Cetron & O'Toole, 1982; Villoldo & Dychtwald, 1981), this confidence does not extend to pharmacological and other advances that could result in the conquest of pain. It appears that Freese (1975) may prove to be correct in his conjecture that 21st-century man will be plagued by the same cluster of pains that beset 20th-century man. Experts in the field have offered a variety of explanations for the gaps in our knowledge. Bonica (1983), for example, believes that the complexity of the pain problem has intimidated investigators, with a consequent reduction in the amount of research initiated. The range of the research has also been limited, focusing mainly on acute, self-controlled pain in the laboratory setting rather than on pain problems of a clinical nature. A further barrier to progress has been the interdisciplinary isolation in which research is conducted that has been engendered by the trend toward highly specialized journals and meetings. A final cause (or effect) noted by Bonica (1985a, p. xxxviii) is the fact that federal funding of basic research and clinical investigations has been miniscule:

> Analysis of the computer printout of funds expended by the various National Institutes of Health during the 1971–1974 period, on what is termed "pain and pain-related research," revealed that a total of $14.6 million was spent during that period, or an average of $3.8 million annually (12). However, when the list of projects was carefully studied, it was clear that more than one-half of the funds were supporting projects wholly unrelated to pain. Of the $1.7 million spent on pain research, only about $800,000 was spent for studies of pain mechanisms; $900,000 was spent for evaluation of narcotics and other therapeutic modalities. These figures represent 0.03% and 0.035%, respectively, of the total NIH budgets for those years. Even more impressive were the figures expended by those institutions that support research in the areas pertaining to the major causes of chronic pain—back disorders, arthritis, cancer, headaches, and cardiac pain. For those 4 years, the National Cancer Institute (NCI) expended an average of $112,000 anually, representing 0.022% of its annual budget; the National Institute of Arthritis, Metabolism and Digestive Diseases (NIAMDD) expended no funds for the study of the mechanisms of arthritis pain, and the National Heart and Lung Institute (NHLI) spent a total of $160,000 for all those 4 years for study pertaining to cardiac pain.

In discussing reasons for the slow progress in the field, Chapman (1978, p. 264) also points to the difficulties inherent in studying pain:

> . . . pain has been problematical to measure and . . . the neuroanatomy of pain has been more difficult to specify than that of some other sensory systems, such as audition or vision. Furthermore it has been hard to link pain behavior to physiological structures, because the influence of cortical factors in human perception of tissue injury is always major. In the laboratory, investigators have been forced to study care-

fully controlled experimental paradigms that bear little resemblance to pathological pain stages in order to maintain proper control over important variables. This has led to a gradual, but relatively thorough, separation of laboratory pain investigation from clinical study of pathological pain states. In recent decades, these areas have emerged as separate domains of research.

Although these explanations are unquestionably valid, they all omit any consideration of one vital element: An entire population—infants, children, and adolescents—has been virtually ignored despite evidence that this population's pain experiences have relevance for an understanding of adult pain. It is our opinion that the study of childhood pain, which in this text spans the spectrum from infancy through adolescence, must be viewed as an essential major area in the pain field. Our purpose in writing this text was to place childhood pain in its rightful place within the field. To this end, it is necessary first to look at the pain field in general and to discuss aspects and issues that apply regardless of age group. To provide a perspective for recent and current developments, the evolution of man's understanding of pain is outlined briefly, in terms of the various primitive, prescientific, and early scientific conceptualizations. Included are the historical events that are the antecedents of current pain management procedures and the concomitant theories of pain that the periods produced. Progress in the last three decades is looked at more intensively. The chapter concludes with a description of the current status of childhood pain and the influences contributing to that status.

Evolution of Man's Understanding of Pain

Although most of our knowledge of pain is the product of this century, particularly the last two decades (Menges, 1984), a brief look at the evolution of man's understanding of this phenomenon will provide a necessary perspective for the discussion of recent developments in the field. Progress from ancient times to about 1950 falls into three major periods, defined in terms of changes in the conceptualization of pain. The first two periods, the primitive and prescientific, were notable for impressive progress primarily on a nonempirical base; the subsequent early scientific period was distinguished by important theoretical advances.

Primitive Period

There is evidence from fossilized bones and tools from the period of about 40,000 B.C., and from rock paintings in Southern France and Africa dating from about 2,000 B.C., that primitive man was troubled by many of the same pains that afflict modern man and struggled against their inevitability. The headache, for example, was attributed to the presence of an evil demon in the skull and treated by trepanning, an operation in which a hole is made in the skull with a sharp instrument.

This treatment was consistent with the belief that internal pains with no obvious and visible cause were caused by the intrusion into the body of magic fluids, evil spirits, or demons. In addition to supplication to the gods, wounds inflicted by a Shaman or sorcerer allowed the evil spirits to escape through routes such as the blood, sputum, or perspiration. Trepanned skulls have been found almost everywhere that man has been known to exist. What is remarkable about these discoveries are the similarities in pain management techniques even among civilizations that geographically were widely scattered and the evidence that many patients survived the first operation (Sigerist, 1955).

Prescientific Period

The view of pain as a problem to be managed with methods other than supplications to the gods marked the onset of the prescientific period. In this period the predominant belief about the nature of pain was shaped by Aristotle in the fourth century B.C. Aristotle viewed pain as an emotion, a passion of the soul felt in the heart. He regarded the heart as the *sensorium commune,* the center of sensory perception and also the most important organ in the body. For Aristotle, pain could occur as a result of an increase in intensity of sensation. In *De Anima* (Keele, 1957) he stated, "Sensations are pleasant when their sensible extremes such as acid and sweet are brought into their proper ratio, whilst in excess they are painful and destructive." To the detriment of the pain field, Aristotle's views prevailed for almost 23 centuries despite impressive evidence to the contrary, particularly that offered by Galen and Avicenna as well as others. Galen had elaborated a complex theory on the function of the nervous system in relation to sensation in general, including pain, but it was soundly rejected as an unwarranted attack on Aristotle's scholarship.

There are well-documented records in early civilizations of a continuing and successful search for substances to alleviate pain (Bonica, 1983; Fairley, 1978; Tainter, 1948). Aspirin, alcohol, tranquilizers, narcotics, and anesthetics are not recent developments, although they do differ in form and chemical nature from those used by early medicine men to ease pain, reduce sensation, produce sleep, and induce some degree of anesthesia. The medicinal use of plants was known even to primitive man and their analgesic properties widely recognized in the ancient cultures of Europe, Asia, and Africa (Stimmel, 1983). Records of prescriptions for pain inscribed on Babylonian clay tablets date back to 2,250 B.C. One of these describes a mixture of herbane seeds and gum mastic for toothache (Tainter, 1948). The *Iliad,* which is thought to have been written during the ninth century B.C., contains references to the use of analgesic drugs in military combat, and in the *Odyssey,* Homer describes the use of a drug "to lull all pain." Avicenna, a Persian physician who practiced in the 11th century A.D., distinguished between herb/alcohol mixtures that "induce rapid unconsciousness" and those that result in "a deeply-unconscious state, so as to enable the pain to be borne" (Fairley, 1978, p. 220).

Of interest in these early accounts of analgesics is the curiously contemporary tone of much of the terminology, in particular the cautionary notes concerning their safety. In the first century A.D., for example, Pliny the Elder recommended mandragora as an analgesic that "may be used safely ynough [*sic*] . . . before]cutting, pricking or launcing any member, to take away the sence and feeling . . ." (Tainter, 1948, p. 6). Celsus described analgesic pills and their side effects in his *De Medicine* (Tainter, 1948, p. 5) as follows:

> Pills are also numerous. . . . Those which relieve pain through sleep are called *anodynes;* unless there is overwhelming necessity, it is improper to use them; for they are composed of medicaments which are very active and alien to the stomach.

Dioscoridies, a surgeon in Nero's army, cautioned against opium (Tainter, 1948, p. 6):

> A little of ye seed of the black Poppy . . . is a pain easer . . . But being drank too much, it hurts, making man lethargicall and it kills.

Categorization of Pain Experience

Primitive man had distinguished between the natural pain of injuries having obvious external causes and internal, disease-related pains for which there was no obvious and visible explanation (Fairley, 1978). This crude categorization of pain experience became increasingly refined during the prescientific period. Avicenna's *The Canon of Medicine* describes 15 different types of pain, including boring, compressing, corrosive, dull, fatigue, heavy, incisive, irritant, itching, pricking, relaxing, stabbing, tearing, tension, and throbbing. This process of refinement continued throughout the early scientific period, an example being Mitchell, Morehouse, and Keen's (1864) distinction between the posttraumatic burning pain of causalgia and peripheral somatic aching. More recently, clusters of typologies have been described relating to various facets of the pain experience such as location (cutaneous versus deep), temporal quality (continuous versus intermittent), speed of transmission (epicritic versus protopathic), functional status (adaptive versus morbid), and response mechanisms (operant versus respondent). Although most of these contemporary dichotomies are widely accepted, objections have been raised that the organic/psychogenic one is one of "the classic mischievous and meaningless dichotomies" (Steinmuller, 1979); that it represents dualistic thinking and should be discarded on the grounds that if adhered to it could adversely affect treatment (Fordyce, 1976; Liebeskind & Paul, 1977; Smith, 1984; Sternbach, 1978; Wall, 1980).

Early Scientific Period

This third period, which extends from the early 17th century to the middle of the 20th century, was most notable for the theoretical advances that were made. The first systematic physiological explanation of the pain experience, specificity theory, evolved and in turn led to alternative formulations collectively referred to as pattern theory.

Specificity Theory

The *specificity model* presented by von Frey in 1894 was essentially similar to that of Descartes (Foster, 1901), who two centuries earlier had adhered firmly to the Galenic viewpoint in attributing pain solely to sensory input. For Descartes, pain was a specific sensory modality, like vision, with its own peripheral receptors and central pain center. The transmission of pain was analogous to pulling a rope and causing a bell to ring (Feuerstein & Skjei, 1979).

The crucial assumption in the specificity model (von Frey, 1894) is the existence of modality-specific centers in the central nervous system, with independent connections to pain receptors (stimulus-specific free nerve endings) at peripheral sites. According to this model, when the pain receptors are activated by intense physical or chemical stimulation they transmit pain impulses along specific peripheral nerve tracts, A-delta (myelinated) and C (unmyelinated) fibers, which are associated with short-latency pricking pain and long-latency burning pain, respectively. These fibers synapse and ascend via the anterolateral spinothalamic tract to the thalamus and higher brain centers, where the impulses are registered as pain. The locus of this hypothetical pain center has been a source of controversy (Melzack & Wall, 1983), with some specificity theorists (see, for example, Head, 1920) positing a thalamic pain center with the cortex exerting inhibitory control over it. However, the current view (Kitchell & Erickson, 1983) is that the perception of pain depends on a functioning cerebral cortex and that no single area of the cortex is specifically necessary for the perception of pain. Instead of a "pain center," there is a complex interaction among multiple structures involving most of the brain (Melzack & Wall, 1983).

von Frey's reductionist model of pain was partially correct in that there is physiological evidence of specialization of the peripheral system, but the A-delta and C fibers do not respond exclusively to pain as he believed. Instead, the stimulation of free nerve endings is also capable of eliciting other sensations such as warmth, cold, and itch (Lele & Weddell, 1959). As one would expect, a number of other important objections have been raised. Melzack and Wall (1983, pp. 203–204) question the psychological assumption implicit in the use of the term *pain receptor:*

> To call a receptor a 'pain receptor' . . . is a psychological assumption: it implies a direct connection from the receptor to a brain centre where pain is felt, so that stimulation of the receptor must always elicit pain and only the sensation of pain. It further implies that the abstraction or selection of information concerning the stimulus occurs entirely at the receptor level and that this information is transmitted faithfully to the brain. The crux of the revolt against specificity, then, is against psychological specificity.

Dubner (1980, pp. 66–67) contends that the major defect of specificity theory is its inability to explain some of the characteristics of clinical pain:

> Referred pain produced by innocuous stimulation of normal skin, the delayed pain of posttherapeutic neuralgia produced by repeated mild stimulation, and the paroxysmal episodes of pain produced by weak mechanical stimulation of trigger zones in trigeminal neuralgia, are all examples of pains that cannot be explained by the specificity theory alone.

The theory has also been criticized for its failure to account for pain for which no noxious input can be specified, notably phantom limb, as well as for intra- and interindividual differences in reaction to apparently identical noxious stimuli; its implication of a simple invariant relationship between stimulus intensity and the magnitude of pain perception; and the failure of specificity-theory-based somatic therapies, such as nerve blocks, to eradicate pain (Melzack & Wall, 1983).

Despite these serious allegations of omission and error and the subsequent advances of other theoretical models, specificity theory still has its supporters (Iggo, 1973; Kerr & Wilson, 1978; Perl, 1971) and continues as the standard for many clinical interventions (Tursky, Jamner, & Friedman, 1982). However, specificity theory is viewed with derision by many contemporary theorists, including Weisenberg and Tursky (1976, p. 115), who have summarily dismissed it as "a simplistic S-R view of pain."

Although the criticisms that this theory has evoked are unequivocally valid, its significance in the developing pain field should be acknowledged. Descartes's formulation of pain as a sensation was the first to prevail over the firmly entrenched Aristotelian view of pain as an affective quality. As such, this unidimensional model marked an important starting point, serving as an impetus to clinical investigations as well as laboratory research (Melzack, 1973).

Pattern Theory

The shortcomings of specificity theory gave rise to a series of alternative formulations by Goldscheider (1894), Nafe (1934), Livingstone (1943), Sinclair (1955), Weddell (1955), and Noordenbos (1959), which is referred to collectively as *pattern theory*. Goldscheider's theory represented a momentous advance in our understanding of the mechanisms and nature of pain. He proposed that stimulus intensity and central summation were the critical determinants of pain. As a result, the concept of pain shifted from the simple Cartesian model of one sensation traversing one nerve from the periphery to the brain, to a beginning realization that pain is one of the most complex of the phenomena that afflict mankind.

Subsequent pattern theories shared two common assumptions. One was that pain is a sensation resulting from spatiotemporal patterns of nociceptive impulses that originate from receptor sites and summate to form the basis of a code that is interpreted centrally as pain; the other was the belief that almost any kind of stimulation can result in pain if the intensity of that stimulation exceeds a certain threshold. Pattern theories and specificity theories are similar in that they view peripheral stimulation as essential for pain perception, but they differ on how this sensory input is encoded and transmitted to the cerebral cortex. However, only pattern theory allows for the possibility of central modulation of sensory input, that is, that coding systems in the central nervous system, such as prior experience, could interact with peripheral stimulation to determine the individual's experience of pain (Noordenbos, 1959; Melzack & Wall, 1962).

Representative of the pattern theories is the sensory interaction theory of Noordenbos (1959), important for its concept of input control as well as for its explanation of clinical pain phenomena. According to this theory, two fiber systems are involved in pain, a slow-conducting, unmyelinated, small-fiber system that transmits the nerve impulses that are interpreted centrally as pain, and a rapidly conducting, myelinated, large-fiber system that under normal conditions inhibits synaptic transmission of the nociceptive signals. Under pathological conditions, the slow system establishes dominance over the fast system so that the latter is unable to inhibit the sequence of increased neural transmission, summation, and resultant pain. Noordenbos's theory is able to provide an explanation for many of the properties of clinical pain. The failure to relieve pain by spinothalamic cordotomy, for example, is attributed to the fact that the diffuse connections of the anterolateral pathways can rarely be totally eradicated, so that even after extensive surgical sectioning there may be a leak of nerve signals, with a consequent evocation of pain.

Pattern theory has made a substantial contribution to our understanding of pain. The concepts of input control and central summation have received strong empirical support (Melzack & Wall, 1983). The theory allows for the learning and retention of spatiotemporal patterns and provides a single compelling interpretation of the range of cutaneous sensation. It can account for the fact that minimal tactile stimulation of the finger causes only a feeling of touch whereas maximal tactile stimulation causes pain.

As was the case with specificity theory, pattern theory has been criticized on a number of points; it has failed to give adequate weight to the complexity of the pain experience; it cannot explain certain existing clinical evidence (as in the case of phantom limb pain) that peripheral stimulation is not necessary for pain perception; and some pattern theorists have ignored the evidence of receptor-fiber specialization, for example, A-delta and C fibers (Liebeskind & Paul, 1977). Furthermore, the theory fails to provide an adequate account of pain mechanisms, does not specify the kinds of patterns that might be related to pain, and offers no hypothesis to account for the detection of patterns by central cells (Melzack, 1973).

Despite these basic difficulties, there is little question that in terms of relative merit and impact on future developments in pain, pattern theory has outpaced specificity theory. In Melzack's summation (1984a, p. 328),

The force of history . . . lies with Goldscheider rather than with von Frey. Von Frey's theory states that pain is a simple, direct sensation while Goldscheider's concept proposes that pain is complex, dynamic, capricious, and reflects the extraordinary complexity of the central nervous system. It is particularly interesting that Goldscheider believed that the intricate networks in the dorsal horns held special secrets to the understanding of pain and all its complex clinical manifestations. Recent research has confirmed his courageous speculations (Melzack & Wall, 1983) . . . Von Frey's specificity theory lent itself to the earliest sensory neurophysiology which began with studies of receptor-fiber functions. It fit well with the concept of reflexes that began with Descartes and became an integral part of stimulus–response (S-R) theory, the most pervasive concept of psychology in this century. On the other side, Goldscheider's emphasis on neurological complexity and dynamic plasticity—on the inhibition, filtering and selection of inputs during transmission at the first synapses of the dorsal horns—gave rise to another tradition.

Current Scientific Period

Bonica's Contributions

Although the early scientific period had contributed theoretical advances, from 1850 to 1950 the field of pain could best be described as stagnant (Melzack, 1973). This state of affairs changed dramatically in the early 1950s with the publication of Bonica's (1953) text, *The Management of Pain*. This comprehensive work formalized the current status of pain knowledge and is viewed as a classic in the field of medicine; although it was written over 30 years ago, it remains valid in many respects. This singular work is consonant with the major contributions that Bonica has made as a catalyst and innovator in the study of pain, care of the pain patient, and professional development of the field. These continuing contributions have rightfully accorded him worldwide admiration and respect from his colleagues. Of particular significance was his introduction of the concept of chronic pain as an autonomous disease affecting the patient psychologically as well as physiologically. Now referred to as the *chronic pain syndrome,* its psychological effects resulted in complex changes in affect, cognitive processes, and behavioral patterns that contributed to the self-perpetuating character of chronic pain disorders. Bonica recognized that the management of these complex chronic pain problems required more knowledge and clinical expertise than any one individual could possess. His advocation of a multidisciplinary approach (Bonica, 1953) to such problems set the stage for a shift from a unidimensional to a multidimensional view of pain. This shift continued in the late 1950s in Beecher's (1956, 1959) questioning of the unidimensional concept of pain as a sensory event triggered by current or impending damage. He pointed to instances of the apparent situational discrepancy between presence of tissue damage and self-report of pain and suggested that a broader conceptualization was needed. Barber (1959) and Kolb (1962) followed this train of thought in their formulation that emphasized the psychological component in pain, particularly the importance of attention in the pain experience.

The next major event, and one having unprecedented repercussions in the field, was Melzack and Wall's somewhat tentative presentation in 1965 of a new conceptual model called the *gate-control theory*. This theory represented the culmination of an exhaustive review of the pain literature, including previous summaries of the state of the art (see, for example, Foerster, 1927; Noordenbos, 1959; Wortis, Stein & Joliffe, 1942), speculation derived from a composite view of clinical pain phenomena, and concepts from the specificity and pattern theories.

Gate-Control Theory

Melzack and Wall posited that pain is not a function of any one specific part or action of the nervous system but instead is contributed to by each specialized part of the nervous system as the peripheral input is modulated at successive synapses throughout its projection from the spinal cord to the neural areas responsible for pain experience and response. Psychological factors, far from being of secondary importance as previous theories had implied, are viewed as comparable in importance to physiological factors. The perception of pain involves a complex balance beween peripheral (physiological) and central (psychological) input. This conceptualization acknowledges the complexity of pain as well as the tenuous relationship between the character of a specific noxious stimulus at the periphery and the central perception and subsequent response to pain; that is, the pain that is perceived rarely bears an isomorphic relationship to antecedent nociceptive events.

This theory proposes that a neurophysiological mechanism located in the cells of the substantia gelatinosa of the dorsal horns of the spinal cord acts as a gate that can regulate the flow of nociceptive impulses from peripheral nerve fibers to the spinal cord transmission (T) cells that project to the brain. Pain occurs when the number of nociceptive impulses arriving at these neural areas exceeds a critical level. An important feature of the gating mechanism is that it can exert an influence on somatic input (nociceptive impulses) before it evokes pain perception and response. The degree to which the gate facilitates or inhibits nociceptive transmission is determined by two sets of factors. The first set involves mechanisms intrinsic to the spinal cord, namely, the relative activity in large (A-beta) and smaller (A-delta and C) fibers. Large-fiber activity tends to inhibit nociceptive transmission by closing the gate, whereas small-fiber activity facilitates it by activating the gate mechanism as well as the T cells that project the nociceptive information to the neural areas in the brain that are responsible for pain experience and responses. In this theory, the small fibers are of crucial importance because they activate the T cells directly and also contribute to their output.

The second set of factors influencing gate action are the powerful control influences moving centripetally from the brain downward. These autonomous descending influences are cognitive, behavioral, and affective factors that can modulate the somatic input relayed from the dorsal horn in ways not yet well understood. In other words, for this theory, central nervous system mediation is a significant factor in pain perception.

Although no gate mechanism has ever been identified, there is considerable supportive evidence for the presence of a mechanism (Nathan, 1976) for a gate opening as a result of emotional activity and closing through endorphin activity (Terenius, 1981) and peripheral electrical stimulation (Wall & Sweet, 1967). In addition, there is some evidence for the loss of large fibers in pathological conditions (Noordenbos, 1959), but this finding has been contested by Nathan (1976).

With the advent of the gate-control theory, the field of pain took a quantum leap forward, the immediate effect being a storm of controversy over the theory's worth. Recurring criticisms centered around the theme that no gate has ever been identified and that the theory is incomplete or incorrect in certain respects, particularly in regard to some of the detailed neurophysiological mechanisms (Crue et al., 1980; Nathan, 1976). Although these criticisms are not disputed as fact, the failure to provide proof that a gate exists is not a valid reason for rejecting the concept of a gate, because state-of-the-art methodology is not yet equal to the task of proving or disproving the presence of such a mechanism. In commenting on the gate concept, Noordenbos (1984, p. 4, Prologue) states

> It became extremely popular. I think for two reasons. In the first place by the use of the word *Gate* which admirably indicated the overall effect in a single term, and secondly by the use of a simple diagram which graphically illustrated the principle and made the idea understandable. As was to be expected, it was also subject to many attacks. But these were aimed at the diagram and not at the overall effect. What was meant as an illustration was taken as the true state of affairs.

It should be noted that neither Melzack nor Wall has ever stated or implied that the theory was complete and correct. In fact, from the outset they viewed it first as a tentative model (Melzack & Wall, 1965) and then as one in transition. Their reaction to criticism has reflected this position: They have been receptive to findings from others that led to modifications of the theory and diligent in pursuing refinements themselves. The gate literature contains a series of their tests of the theory (Wall & Sweet, 1967), expansions of it (Casey & Melzack, 1967; Melzack & Casey, 1968), changes in emphasis (Melzack & Dennis, 1978), major revisions (Wall, 1978, 1979a), and unequivocal statements about the gate theory's location on the path toward the ultimate truth about pain (Melzack & Wall, 1983).

There is no question that despite its omissions and flaws, the gate-control theory constitutes a major contribution to the pain field. In itself it represents a model approach for others to follow in developing theoretical formulations. Willingness to admit errors and wrong directions, active pursuit of refinements, and resilience in the face of severe criticisms are essential attributes for those engaged in the arduous task of theory development in this complex field.

The theory has generated an impressive body of basic and clinical research about the nature of pain and in so doing has helped bridge the gap, noted by Chapman (1978), between laboratory research and clinical investigations. It opened the door to many disciplines not previously an integral part of the task force attacking the problem of pain. The concept of multidisciplinary collaboration, for example, became a necessity whenever the gate-control theory was the basis for clinical investigations of complex pain problems. For the management of chronic intractable pain it prompted the reintroduction of large-fiber activation by electrical stimulation, a technique first introduced in the Socratic era but generally bypassed by the mainstream of 20th-century clinical practice (Kane & Taub, 1975). Its current use is a direct result of the gate-control theory (Bonica, 1980; Smoller & Schulman, 1982) and is one development from it that has unequivocal support from behavioral, clinical, and electrophysiological evidence (Woolf, 1984). The theory also gave credence to a scientific base for acupuncture as a therapeutic modality, provided a framework for the mediation of pain by psychological factors, and indicated the potential that psychological control techniques have for the reduction or elimination of pain (Liebeskind & Paul, 1977; Ng, 1985; Tan, 1982; Weisenberg, 1984). The heuristic value of the theory has been widely acknowledged (see, for example, Bonica, 1980; Chapman, 1984; Dubner, 1980). Representative of this reaction is Weisenberg's (1977a, p. 1012) assessment:

> . . . regardless of the accuracy of the specific wiring diagrams involved, the gate-control theory of pain has been the most influential and important current theory of pain perception. It ties together many of the puzzling aspects of pain perception and control. It has had profound influence on pain research and the clinical control of pain. It has generated new interest in pain perception, stimulating a multidisciplinary view of pain for research and treatment. It has been able to demonstrate the tremendous importance of psychological variables.

Other Developments in the 1960s

By the early 1970s, the study of pain had emerged as a field of scientific inquiry in its own right rather than as a subsidiary interest to other established domains of research. This change of status resulted in a veritable explosion of clinical and empirical interest in pain (Bonica, 1984; Liebeskind & Paul, 1977). Advances in knowledge about the scientific basis of pain mechanisms developed at an unprecedented rate (Kerr & Wilson, 1978) and have continued unabated in the 1980s (Kruger & Liebeskind, 1984a; Noordenbos, 1984). Even the most conservative assessment of the progress made between 1970 and 1985 would support the opinion that this period was associated with a greater gain in knowledge about pain mechanisms, especially those related to acute pain, than had occurred during the entire preceding century.

Some investigators (Dubner, 1980; Liebeskind & Paul, 1977) have attributed the heightened interest in pain research to the catalytic effects of the gate-control theory of pain. Without in any way derogating the enormous significance of this theory, it is our opinion that, instead, a cluster of theoretical, empirical, and clinical developments along with practical and philosophical concerns emerged in the 1960s to create a climate of readiness for a significant increase in empirical and clinical interest in the problem of pain. The gate-control theory contributed to this state of readiness but was not its sole cause. We will briefly discuss these components of readiness before moving on to the advances of the 1970s.

One component was psychologists' entry into the pain arena, their involvement prior to the 1960s having been minimal because of the widespread belief that pain was purely a sensory experience. With the growing awareness that the perception of pain involved a complex interaction among physiological, pharmacological, and psychological factors (Melzack & Wall, 1965), psychologists were prompted to develop learning theory-based treatment strategies for various problems of pain, particularly those of chronic pain. Representative of their contributions in the 1960s was the reconceptualization by Fordyce and his associates (Fordyce, Fowler, Lehmann, & DeLateur, 1968) of chronic pain in a behavioral or learning–conditioning model rather than in the previous disease model, which at that time was the only clinical model available. An offshoot of this change in orientation was the introduction of behavior modification techniques as a management tool in chronic pain problems. The precursors of biofeedback therapy were established with empirical demonstrations of changes that could be effected through learning techniques in motor (Basmajian, 1963) and autonomic, visceral, and glandular functions (Miller, 1969).

The 1960s also represented a period of transition for the medical profession, as a number of factors forced a reconsideration and reevaluation of its traditional approaches to pain management. Medically based treatments that initially had appeared highly promising in the 1940s and 1950s proved to be less effective, more hazardous, or of more limited applicability than had been expected. Sensory-based somatic treatments such as nerve blocks, analgesics, and surgical procedures often failed to alleviate pain, particularly chronic pain (Black, 1974; Halpern, 1974; Stravino, 1970; White & Sweet, 1969) and, in any case, achieved only a 50 percent success rate. Even in those patients who initially had appeared to benefit from such interventions, debilitating iatrogenic side effects and recurrences of pain, sometimes of increased severity, were a common occurrence. Then, too, confidence in the traditional pharmacological treatment of pain was undermined with the realization that the most effective analgesics, the narcotics, became progressively less effective as tolerance developed and also carried the risk of addiction. Two other factors contributed to the medical community's receptive attitude toward other treatment regimens. One was the success of the hospice movement (Saunders, 1967) in the management of pain and suffering, particularly in the terminally ill; the other was the clinical documentation of the efficacy of treatment procedures, such as hypnosis (Hilgard & Hilgard, 1975; Scott, 1973; Tinterow, 1960), that were beyond the bounds of orthodox medicine.

A third component contributing to the climate of readiness was the heightened concern in the 1960s over the prevalence and multifaceted costs of pain, particularly chronic pain (Arney & Bergen, 1984). This concern had been expressed as early as the 1920s and 1930s, when the National Health Survey collected extensive information on the personal, social, and economic impact of chronic disease (National Health Survey, 1938); and in the 1940s and 1950s, with the establishment of the National Institutes of Health for the study and control of chronic diseases (Arney & Bergen, 1984). However, by the 1960s the sharply increasing costs of health care had created a far more general and pervasive unease, in the lay and governmental sectors as well as in the medical community, that focused attention on the need to curtail increases in medical expenditures.

Part of the zeitgeist of the 1960s was an emphasis on equality, social concern, and an increased willingness to challenge arbitrary authority. Its influence spilled over to the developments described above and partially underlay events related to them. The change in values was reflected in a burgeoning sense of outrage by professionals and laymen alike regarding unnecessary suffering. Controversy raged over a diversity of pain-related issues, including abortion and the rights of the fetus to live; the moral justification for withholding vital medical treatment from defective newborn infants (see Devlin & Magrab, 1981, and Fletcher, 1973, for excellent discussions of this issue); legitimization of heroin in the management of intractable pain (see Mondzac, 1984, for an interesting account of the issues); involuntary subjection of patients to nonessential medical procedures for research purposes; inadequacy of postoperative and other acute pain management regimens (Keats, 1956; Neal, 1968, 1978); rights of the terminally ill to die peacefully (Cleland, 1968; Menefee, 1967); and rights to humane treatment for laboratory animals (American Psychological Association, 1968).

Along with this cluster of readiness factors, a development occurred in the 1960s that was to have enormous impact on subsequent events in the field of pain: the beginning recognition by both clinicians and researchers that acute and chronic pain were distinctly different entities involving different physiological mechanisms and requiring different treatment. For the first time, chronic pain was assigned the status of a medical entity, a disorder in itself rather than a symptom, and the effect of this new conceptualization of chronic pain was to pave the way for intensive empirical investigations of it as well as differential clinical treatment for it. Although Bonica (1953) had espoused this view for more than a decade, it had been ignored in the clinical and research arenas. Because acute and chronic pain disorders have many ramifications for topics throughout this book, we will discuss them here in some detail.

Acute Pain

Pain of variable duration, typically characterized by sudden onset; a demonstrable etiology such as noxious or tissue-damaging stimulation produced by trauma, disease, or treatment; and a limited and predictable course is termed *acute*. Its diagnosis is seldom difficult because the physiopathology is generally well understood. Its course is characteristically limited or predictable in that a definite endpoint to the discomfort can be anticipated, usually within days or weeks. It is often accompanied by the generalized activation pattern that Cannon (1929) called the fight or flight reaction: tachycardia, increases in pupillary diameter and blood pressure, and decreases in gut motility and salivary flow. These physiological reactions may be proportional to the intensity of the pain as well as to the patient's anxiety about its intensity or its significance (Sternbach, 1982). With anxiety-reducing measures, such as tranquilizers and reassurance concerning diagnosis and outcome, there is usually a concomitant reduction in the patient's reports of intensity. Although psychological factors are not often primary in acute pain, the immediate effect of severe trauma may be an absence of pain if survival, winning, or completion of some activity is the immediate and dominant concern. In this case, pain may not be experienced until these needs are met (Beecher, 1956; Stimmel, 1983; Wall, 1979a).

Acute pain may promote survival in that it generally serves an adaptive warning function by directing attention to injury or disease and by providing the motivating force for engaging in treatment-related behavior. Although acute pain usually functions effectively as a warning system and in its protective capacity helps defend the integrity of the body, for example, by preventing further tissue damage by limiting motion (Chapman & Bonica, 1983), it is far from infallible. The severity of the pain often has little relationship to the seriousness of the injury, thus undermining the warning function. Also, as Bonica (Ng & Bonica, 1980, p. 3) has noted, some acute pain serves no useful function:

> . . . severe acute pain in the postoperative period, or after burns or after accidental injury, has no useful function, and if not adequately relieved produces serious abnormal physiologic and psychologic reactions which often cause complications.

Chronic Pain

Definitions of *chronic* pain tend to center around duration. However, the advocation of specific temporal criteria (see, for example, Ciccone & Grzesiak, 1984; Linton, Melin, & Götestam, 1984; Meinhart & McCaffery, 1983; Roberts, 1981) has been criticized by Sternbach (1984, p. 174) as "an artificial distinction created by imposing a concept of time on a biological event." Bonica (1980) sees duration as relative, terming a pain chronic if it persists beyond the usual course of a disease or beyond a reasonable healing time for an injury. To the characteristic of long duration, Smoller and Schulman (1982) have added repeated recurrences.

Chronic pain may warn of disease and trauma in their early stages, but it generally serves no other useful protective role. Often the salient effects of the process of chronicity are to physically weaken the individual and to psychologically undermine his sense of well-being. It is this effect that has led Bonica (1977,

p. xi) to describe the process of chronicity as "a malefic force" that imposes severe and often unrelenting stresses on the patient, Smoller and Schulman (1982, p. 5) to term it "a virulent predator [that] rapidly pursues, engulfs, and incapacitates its victims," and LeShan (1964) to see similarities between the universe of the patient in chronic pain and the world of terror dreams and nightmares. The diagnosis of chronic pain is usually difficult, with even the time of onset being sometimes impossible for the patient to pinpoint (Johnson, 1977). Although it may begin as an acute pain episode (Seres & Newman, 1985), it is not simply a prolongation of acute pain (Wall, 1984). An interesting account of a behavioral analysis of such a sequence is provided by Linton et al. (1984, pp. 12–15).

Categories of Chronic Pain Patients

Chronic pain patients tend to fall into one of two categories, defined in terms of their behavior and reactions to the fact of their illness. Patients in the first category view their pain in the perspective of a symptom of the original condition. For those in the second category, the pain becomes a disease in itself and assumes a disproportionate significance in their lives and the lives of those around them.

Although the differences between the categories are diverse and marked, the two conditions are referred to in the literature indiscriminately as chronic pain or the chronic pain syndrome. Many authors use the terms interchangeably, to the detriment of clarity: Some publications entitled "Chronic Pain" refer to both categories of patients, while others are concerned with only one category. The chronic pain of the first category is sometimes referred to as *persistent pain* (Payne & Norfleet, 1986). Bonica (1980) has objected strongly to any such categorization. We contend that chronic pain patients *do* fall into two distinct groups. Accordingly, we will use the descriptor *chronic* plus the name of the specific condition (for example, "chronic arthritis") to refer to patients in the first category and will use *chronic pain syndrome* for those in the second one.

Chronic Pain Conditions   Patients with chronic pain conditions are able to accept their persistent or recurrent painful condition with equanimity even when they are partially or completely disabled. For all practical purposes, they live normal lives within the bounds of their chronic disorder, in that the pain is manageable on a therapeutic regimen that does not disrupt their daily life, family, and friendships. They generally cope surprisingly well with the resultant multifaceted problems and costs and manage to maintain a comparatively high level of activity and self-esteem (Turner & Chapman, 1982a). Typically, they comply with therapeutic regimens and benefit from them to the extent possible; their pain condition is linked with health-enhancing behavior. These patients are rarely seen in specialized pain clinics.

Chronic Pain Syndrome   For patients with the chronic pain syndrome, the chronic pain becomes a disease in itself, a distinct clinical entity rather than a symptom of the original condition. When Bonica (1953) first introduced this concept, he described the process as one that affected the patient psychologically, as well as physiologically, with the psychological effects resulting in complex changes in affect, cognitive processes, and behavioral patterns, all of which contributed to making the chronic pain disorder self-perpetuating. In contrast to those in the first category, these patients' pain condition becomes an end in itself and one that assumes a disproportionate significance in their lives. Table 1-2 describes behaviors and events that frequently occur in the chronic pain syndrome patient. It is important to note that the composite picture presented in this table is derived from descriptions by experienced clinicians (see, for example, Bresler, 1979; Fordyce, 1976; Pinsky & Crue, 1984; Roy, Bellissimo, & Tunks, 1982) of chronic pain syndrome patients in pain clinic settings. Recent epidemiological studies by Crook and her associates (Crook et al., 1984; Crook & Tunks, 1985) suggest, however, that these patients may not be representative of chronic pain syndrome patients in the general population. The pain clinic patients, for example, more frequently reported work-related accidents, pain, and pain impairment, and more often gave evidence of psychosocial and functional impairment.

Since the etiological factors that originally caused the pain in chronic pain syndrome patients are not those that subsequently serve to maintain it (Kremer, Block, & Atkinson, 1983), it is not surprising that the use of traditional pain relief procedures such as analgesic medication, destructive surgical procedures, and physical therapy, typically fails to reduce the pain and in fact may exacerbate it (Chapman, 1984). Often there is an extraordinary stability about the problem, with the patient showing neither progressive improvement nor deterioration while

Table 1-2   Chronic Pain Syndrome

Primary Characteristics

Persistent and stable pain of long duration
No causal relationship to existing physical problems or illness
Multiple pain complaints
History of multiple physician contacts, ineffective medical and surgical interventions, and iatrogenic complications
Excessive preoccupation with pain problem on part of patient and family
Failure to complete therapeutic regimens that require sustained effort and active participation from the patient

Secondary Problems

Significant physical changes including escalating physical incapacity, chronic fatigue, loss of appetite, constipation, and loss of libido
Significant psychological changes including decreased ability to enjoy life, loss of confidence and self-esteem, increasing depression and anxiety, and feelings of helplessness and hopelessness
Disturbed psychosocial functioning: deteriorating family relationships, decreased social interaction, discontinuance of normal recreational pursuits, and conflicts and disagreements with medical personnel
Multiple, inappropriate drug use
Drug abuse with resultant substance-use disorders

continuing to make regular and usually excessive use of health care delivery systems; the longer the pain persists without effective interventions, the greater the likelihood that environmental operants will come into play.

With the introduction of psychological mechanisms as mediators of the chronic pain in addition to the physiological mechanisms, behavioral intervention and psychotherapy become of critical importance to the treatment regimen. It is of crucial importance that such intervention be initiated in the early stages, a point that is underscored by the dispiriting findings of a recent study by Swanson, Maruta, and Wolff (1986) of patients whose chronic pain had persisted for 25 years or more. Swanson et al. found that patients in this category, termed "ancient pain," were "treatment resistant" after 6 years of pain: By this time the pattern of chronicity was well entrenched and subsequent change was limited, despite the fact that the patients actively continued to search for pain relief.

Bonica (1953) recognized that the management of these complex chronic pain problems required more knowledge and clinical expertise than any one individual could possess. Accordingly, he advocated a multidisciplinary approach within a *pain clinic* setting and in 1961 founded such a clinic at the University of Washington that subsequently became a model for other clinics in the chronic pain field. Although these clinics have generally provided help for the chronic pain syndrome patient that is far superior to the care that the individual practitioner is equipped to provide, they are not a panacea (Boyd, Merskey, & Nielson, 1980), in that all too often they achieve only limited long-term results (Painter, Seres, & Newman, 1980). For reviews relevant to this topic, see Aronoff, Evans, and Enders (1985), Latimer (1982), Linton (1986), and particularly the response by Fordyce, Roberts, and Sternbach (1985) to critics of behavioral management.

The chronic pain syndrome phenomenon with its complex puzzle attributes has aroused considerable interest in the possibility of deriving a theoretical explanation from which to develop a model as a basis for treatment. In view of the complexity of this syndrome, the formulation of a single model seems neither probable nor desirable. It would be preferable to have a variety of models from which to select the one, as a basis for treatment, that best reflects the configuration of causative factors descriptive of the specific patient.

Whether by design or necessity, most of the models that have been proposed are limited to selected clusters of chronic pain syndrome patients. Engel (1959), for example, approaches the problem from a *psychoanalytic model* and describes a group of pain-prone patients whose entire lives have been marked by painful conditions and events. For these patients pain functions as a prime regulator of their psychic economy, with guilt playing a central role in their symptom choice. They cannot tolerate happiness and success so they use pain symptoms to combat these events.

Fordyce (1976) has proposed an *operant conditioning model* to explain the occurrence of the chronic pain syndrome when changes in the status of an individual's pain are clearly elicited, maintained, and strengthened by powerful reinforcing consequences such as money, attention from others, and avoidance of threatening situations.

The *systems theory model* (Engelbart & Vrancken, 1984) views the chronic pain syndrome as a pathological state resulting from the reaction of an already psychologically unhealthy person to painful conditions. Closely aligned with this view is the *intrapsychic model* (Pinsky, 1978), in which the chronic pain syndrome is seen as a primarily psychological disorder that represents the patient's attempt to cope with intrapsychic conflicts.

Newman, Painter, and Seres (1978) have presented a *psychophysiological model* that assumes that chronic pain often leads to a set of physiological responses that result in an increase in the intensity and duration of the pain. Finally, Lethem and his colleagues (Lethem, Slade, Troup, & Bentley, 1983; Slade, Troup, Lethem, & Bentley, 1983) are formulating a *fear-avoidance model* to explain why some patients develop a more substantial overlay to their pain problems than others do.

While these and other hypotheses (Swanson, 1984; Violon & Giurgea, 1984) are promising, the overall prognosis is not promising (Engelbart & Vrancken, 1984, p. 1384):

> . . . the presence of chronic pain . . . is . . . a problem to which appropriate answers are still lacking and to which any final answer seems remote.

This state of affairs is particularly sobering in view of the pervasiveness of both chronic pain and the chronic pain syndrome. Together they constitute the third leading cause of disability in this country, ranking just below cancer and heart disease (Smoller & Schulman, 1982). In the case of the chronic pain syndrome, the costs to the individual are incalculable in terms of social and emotional impairment and economic stresses (Roy et al., 1982); many of the families of these patients also pay a heavy price in emotional wear and tear and other forms of psychological distress (Bonica, 1980; Hendler, 1982; Payne & Norfleet, 1986; Rowat & Knafl, 1985). All together, the cumulative costs to society are formidable (Cataldo, Russo, Bird, & Varni, 1980) and the financial costs horrendous. For 1983 the latter were projected at $90 billion (Chapman & Bonica, 1983) a figure that includes all medical costs, loss of job productivity and income, disability payments, and litigation settlements.

Advances of the 1970s and 1980s

The 1970s were characterized by a vigor and productivity in the study of pain far beyond that of any previous period. This heightened activity, which has continued in the 1980s, stemmed in part from the climate of readiness that had evolved in the 1960s and set the stage for action in the pain arena. It was also causally related to two disparate and important developments. One was a new awareness of the advantages of multidisciplinary teams in research as well as in treatment of pain. Basic scientists honed in on the mechanisms of acute pain and the chronic pain syndrome and collaborated with clinical investigators on some of the major clinical problems (Bonica, 1980). Psychiatrists and psychologists worked together on research that focused on the influence on the patient's pain behavior of personality and culture (Weisenberg, 1977b) and the immediate social environment (Fordyce, 1976). With the multidisciplinary approach came recognition of the need for interdisciplinary communication, resulting in 1974, in the founding of the International Association for the Study of Pain (IASP) and, a year later, the publication of the first journal, *Pain,* devoted exclusively to this topic. In addition, there was a series of well-attended and highly productive triennial world congresses on pain, sponsored by the IASP.

The other important development involved the sharp increase in funding provided by the National Institutes of Health for research, interdisciplinary meetings, and development of long-range plans for the study of pain. Early in the 1970s, a blueprint for pain research over a 10-year period was charted under the sponsorship of the National Institute of Neurological and Communicative Diseases and Stroke. Comprehensive research programs were launched on dental pain mechanisms by the National Institute of Dental Research and on cancer pain and therapy by the National Cancer Institute. The National Institute of Drug Abuse was active in obtaining support for research on the endorphins and for the evaluation of analgesics. Research funding by the various institutes for the 1977–78 period totalled more than $2.5 million (Report of the Interagency Committee, 1978), a significant increase over the amounts spent earlier in the decade. The amount of federal funding is obviously important for its immediate effect on pain research, but such support also constitutes an endorsement that could serve as a stimulus to funding by other federal, state, and municipal agencies as well as the phamaceutical industry and private foundations.

The advances of the '70s and '80s far exceed the confines of this chapter. We therefore limit our discussion to five of the advances, selected on the basis of their importance to progress in the field of pain and relevance to the topics in this text. The first of these was the discovery of the endorphins.

Endorphins

A quantum leap forward occurred in the 1970s with the discovery of an endogenous analgesic system. In 1973, stereospecific opiate receptors were identified in the central nervous system, and in 1978 endogenous compounds with pharmacological properties virtually identical to those of morphine were isolated from the brain.

Although this discovery transformed thinking in the pain field in a manner that could not have been anticipated even as little as a decade earlier (Kerr & Wilson, 1978), the chain of events leading to it began early in the century with an hypothesis of modulatory influences on pain (Head & Holmes, 1911). Several decades later, the centrifugal control of sensory transmission was demonstrated empirically (Carpenter, Engberg, & Lundberg, 1965; Hagbarth & Kerr, 1954). In 1965, Melzack and Wall made a clear theoretical statement of a specific pain-control system. Their gate-control theory, in turn, received strong support from the work of Reynolds (1969) and subsequently from that of Mayer, Wolfle, Akil, Carder, and Liebeskind (1971) in their reports of stimulation-produced analgesia. This important development was followed by the discovery of opiate receptors in the mouse brain (Goldstein, Lowney, & Pal, 1971) which acted as a catalyst for research on the fundamental mechanisms of action of the opiate narcotics and also provided the requisite methodological procedure (Goldstein, 1973). In 1973, three teams of investigators (Pert & Snyder, 1973; Simon, Hiller, & Edelman, 1973; Terenius, 1973) working independently and using refinements of Goldstein's (1973) paradigm, confirmed the presence of stereospecific opiate receptors in mammalian brains, particularly in the limbic system and the substantia gelatinosa of the spinal cord, which was one of the lamina identified in the gate-control theory (Melzack & Wall, 1965). The next step was the isolation of the natural ligands of these opiate receptor systems, that is, the short-chain enkephalins (Hughes, Smith, Kosterlitz, Fothergill, Morgan, & Morris, 1975) and long-chain endorphins (Li, Chung, & Doneen, 1976). Subsequently another neuropeptide that is found throughout the nervous system, substance P, was identified as important and perhaps crucial in the transmission of pain signals throughout the spinal cord and in the regulation of their strength (Morley, 1985).

Research in the area of the endogenous opioid peptides increased sharply as investigators sought answers to such problems as the role of the endorphins in chronic pain (Terenius & Wahlstrom, 1979). Terenius and his associates (Terenius, 1981) reported low endorphin levels in the cerebrospinal fluid of patients with chronic organic pain, with the lowest levels occurring in patients with chronic painful neuropathic syndromes. This finding suggested that patients with chronic pain, particularly neurogenic pain, might be using up their available endorphins. An alternate possibility is that chronic pain is associated with changes in opiate receptor binding affinity. Of particular interest was the finding of normal or above-normal cerebrospinal fluid endorphin levels in patients with psychogenic pain. Another problem that intrigued investigators concerned the function of the endorphins in congenital analgesia. A study by Dehen, Willer, Prier, Boureau, and Cambier (1978) presented some evidence of a continuum of endorphin sufficiency with congenital analgesia representing an excess of endorphin that may temporarily be modified with naloxone, with a consequent lowering of the pain threshold.

Chronic Pain and Pain Clinics

A second major advance during the 1970s was the formal acknowledgment, finally, of the validity of a recommendation proposed two decades earlier by Bonica (1953) that chronic pain should be viewed as a complex autonomous disease requiring a multidisciplinary approach to its management. The acceptance of Bonica's idea of pain clinics followed logically, with the establishment in the early 1970s of a small cluster of such clinics for the diagnosis and treatment of chronic pain in adults. By the end of the decade their number had increased to more than 800 in the United States alone (American Pain Society, 1980). Some of these clinics were patterned on Bonica's *major comprehensive model,* which accepted all pain syndromes and used all treatment modalities with multidisciplinary collaboration on patient care, teaching, and research (Murphy & Anderson, 1984). Others were *modality-oriented,* that is, they used a limited number of treatment methods for a wide range of clinical conditions. Still others were *symptom-oriented* and focused entirely on the treatment of specific symptoms such as headache or low back pain (Boyd et al., 1980). For a comprehensive critical review of multidisciplinary pain clinics and pain centers, see Ng (1981).

Theoretical Developments

On the theoretical front, the gate-control theory (Melzack & Wall, 1965) continued to stir up productive controversy (Iggo, 1972; Kerr & Wilson, 1978; Liebeskind & Paul, 1977; Nathan, 1976; Schmidt, 1972) and stimulate new approaches to pain management, particularly those based on behavioral and cognitive interventions (Melzack & Wall, 1983; Tan, 1982; Turk, 1978).

Consequently, there was an increase in empirical assessment of the efficacy of these approaches for the attenuation of clinical pain as well as experimentally induced pain. Melzack and Wall continued their own revisions and evaluations of their theory. The most important of these later refinements was Wall's (1979a) proposal that pain be viewed as a *drive* to promote recovery from injury. In these terms, pain becomes a need state, such as hunger, which the organism strives to satisfy or reduce. Its phases are divided into immediate, acute, and chronic. In the immediate phase, pain may not be perceived because it is overridden by the higher priority drives associated with fight or flight activities. Once the immediate danger to the organism has passed, the organism becomes aware of the acute pain and focuses on it. At this time, the attendant components of anxiety and fear come into play. In this acute phase the pain functions as an aid in promoting tissue recovery and preventing further damage. If the injury is under the direct control of the organism or if it is neither anxiety producing nor life threatening, the immediate phase may be skipped and the acute phase experienced at once.

Support for the concept of a "pain-free" immediate phase can be found in interview data (Beales, 1983) from 14 children and adolescents whose burn injuries had resulted from their clothing catching fire. Only two of the children reported experiencing pain at the time of the incident or immediately after it, while nine children reported extinguishing the flames with their hands and running a substantial distance home without significant pain. Similarly, adult patients interviewed in an emergency department (Melzack, Wall, & Ty, 1982) in a study of minor and moderate trauma emphasized the latency of onset of pain. The response data showed that many injuries, particularly those at skin level as opposed to deep tissue injuries, were followed by a pain-free period that surprised the patients to the extent that they reported waiting for the onset of pain.

Although the concept of pain as a drive is not new, Hull (1952) having treated pain as the paradigm for other drives and others having posited drive qualities in pain (see, for example, Hannington-Kiff, 1976; Izard, 1977; Melzack, 1973; Weisenberg, 1977a), Wall's formulation represents an important advance. His conceptualization of pain as an aversive drive rather than as a sensory modality leads to a different view of pain and its management, the latter having particular relevance for the clinician. There is no question that the drive model represents an important contribution having the potential for increasing our understanding of pain, particularly acute pain, and for improving pain management. Despite certain criticisms, Bonica (1979) described Wall's drive model as one of the most thought-provoking papers ever presented by a pain scientist. For further informative comments on this innovative theoretical model, see the Ciba Foundation Symposium papers by Wall (1979b) along with the commentary (Wikler, 1979) and general discussion.

Reevaluation of Traditional Views

The fourth advance, primarily a product of the 1980s, consisted of taking a closer look at well-entrenched beliefs about various facets of pain conditions and in the process cast sufficient doubt upon them to compel a reevaluation of traditional views. Two examples of this trend will be discussed here, with others appearing in subsequent chapters.

In developing a new empirically based conceptual framework for understanding chronic headaches, Bakal and his associates (Bakal, Demjen, & Kaganov, 1981, 1984; Bakal & Kaganov, 1977) have raised serious and convincing doubts about the validity of certain headache-related "facts." They contend that the etiological processes underlying tension and migraine headaches are more similar than dissimilar, thus discounting the belief that these two types of headache differ in etiology as well as prevention and management interventions. Further, they question the role of specific physical or psychological triggers in precipitating these headaches and, instead, attribute them to intraindividual psychobiological processes. Within this framework, psychological variables function as components of the headache syndrome rather than as antecedents of it. There is empirical evidence in support of Bakal et al.'s beliefs with adults as well as children (Bakal et al., 1984; Joffe, Bakal, & Kaganov, 1983).

A second common belief that has been questioned (see, for example, Leavitt, Garron, McNeill, & Whisler, 1982; Mendelson, 1982, 1984) is the idea that chronic pain patients who receive or are applying for workman's compensation frequently are neurotics or malingerers who are exaggerating their pain for financial benefits (see, for example, Sternbach, Wolf, Murphy, & Akeson, 1973; Weighill, 1983). A review by Melzack, Katz, and Jeans (1985) of recent research on this topic has shown unequivocally that there is no evidence to support this belief. Additional evidence against the neurotic malingerer attribute for chronic pain patients was provided from an assessment of 145 compensation and noncompensation cases by Melzack et al. (1985), who concluded that neurotics and malingerers appear to be relatively rare among chronic pain patients on disability pay.

Childhood Pain

The last of the advances of the 1970s to be discussed here occurred in the latter part of the decade when the focus of interest in human pain broadened to include childhood pain. In this text, *childhood* spans the spectrum from infancy through adolescence.

Prior to the mid-1970s, the focus of clinical and empirical interest had been limited almost entirely to pain in adults. Pain in infants, children, and adolescents was virtually ignored, a state of affairs reflected in the absence of information about the pediatric pain experience in the journal, conference, and textbook literature. A search of the relevant journal literature from 1970 to 1975 (Eland & Anderson, 1977) yielded 1,380 articles on pain, of which only 33 dealt with pediatric pain. The term *pain* did not even appear in the indexes of many of the major medical and nursing pediatric texts of the 1970s (see, for example, Barnett, 1977; Marlow, 1977), and in the few instances when it did appear the discussion dealt mainly with specific disease conditions rather than with topics such as pain management. Generally, pediatric pain was viewed as a diagnostic aid rather than as a symptom that required management, a clinical entity in its own right, or an accepted topic for research.

The reasons for the almost total lack of interest in the pain problems and experiences of children ranged from unsubstantiated or erroneous beliefs, probably adhered to in good faith, to ethical concerns. Conviction was widespread that the younger the child, the less likely it was that he would sense pain neurologically, interpret noxious stimulation as pain, or experience the negative effect of severe pain as adults do (Schechter, 1984). This belief was based in part on the unsubstantiated assumption that the incomplete myelinization characteristic of infancy precludes pain perception. It was supported by the interpretation of equivocal findings from methodologically flawed research on responsivity to aversive stimulation as evidence that newborns and young infants do not experience pain (for reviews see Owens, 1984; Rosenblith & Sims-Knight, 1985).

A third cluster of "support" rested on the inference from empirical findings of elevated pain thresholds in animals reared under conditions of sensory deprivation (Melzack, 1965; Melzack & Scott, 1957; Nissen, Chow, & Semmes, 1951) that the ability to discriminate pain is learned and that this learning has not yet occurred in infancy. It was also believed that an absence of verbal speech or even the presence of a low level of speech performance formed an insurmountable barrier to communication about pain experiences. The final point in justifying disinterest in research on children's pain concerned the potential ethical difficulties in research with this age group.

Opposition to these firmly entrenched but unsubstantiated beliefs first appeared in the late 1960s and early 1970s and has accelerated ever since in the form of an increasingly vigorous attack from multiple and disparate sources. Because of the importance of this cluster of beliefs as a deterrent to progress in the field of childhood pain, we will discuss in some detail the rebuttals and disclaimers that by 1985 had succeeded in reducing the beliefs to an archaic status.

The idea that infants and young children do not feel pain was largely discounted by evidence that myelinization, although incomplete at birth, may be more intact than originally assumed (Smith, 1980; Volpe, 1981) and that the process may proceed rapidly during the first weeks of life (Gross & Gardner, 1980). Quite apart from the myelinization question, the weight of clinical (Barr, 1982; Hahn & McLone, 1984; Poznanski, 1976; Robertson, 1981; Swafford & Allen, 1968) and investigative expertise provided support that the neonate perceives pain not only during circumcision (Kirya & Werthmann, 1978; Williamson & Williamson, 1983) but also in other moderately (Craig, McMahon, Morrison, & Zaskow, 1984; Dale, 1986; Grunau & Craig, 1987a; Izard, Hembree, Dougherty, & Spizzirri, 1983) to severely painful clinical (Merskey, 1975) and experimental procedures (Fisichelli, Karelitz, Fisichelli, & Cooper, 1974; Fisichelli, Karelitz, & Haber, 1968). The consensus of some investigators was that neonates and infants do experience pain (Hazinski, 1984; Owens, 1984; Schechter, 1984), although to what degree remains unknown. Others took the more conservative view that there was no evidence that newborns are impervious to pain (Beyer, DeGood, Ashley, & Russell, 1983; Rosenblith & Sims-Knight, 1985).

Alternate explanations were proposed for the findings from animal studies on the role of learning in pain discrimination. The fact that puppies reared in a restricted environment were, at maturity, unable to respond normally to a variety of noxious stimuli including flame and electric shocks (Melzack & Scott, 1957) could also be interpreted as neurotic behavior (Sternbach, 1978), as a failure of an inborn mechanism concerned with maturation (Merskey, 1970), or as a strong need for stimulation consequent to a restricted environment (Hebb, 1949; Merskey, 1975; Petrie, 1967). Furthermore, as Hahn and McLone (1984) have commented, the fact that young children have to learn that a certain unpleasant feeling in a part of their body indicates they should draw back from tactual contact with a noxious stimulus or terminate their ongoing activity is not evidence that this learned association must take place before they are able to perceive pain. Children do not have to know the meaning of the experience in order to have the experience.

The absence of speech in infants and the limited verbal ability of young children were no longer viewed as deterrents to pain research with these age groups. It is extraordinarily naive to continue to equate verbal capacity with the ability to communicate about pain, in view of the wealth of scientifically acceptable information about pain in infancy that has been obtained through the medium of nonverbal responses and from measures of autonomic activity in naturalistic settings (Craig et al., 1984; Owens, 1984; Owens & Todt, 1984; Taylor, 1983). In their study of infants' reactions to immunization in a clinic setting Craig et al. (1984) documented a transformation in pain expression from reflective, diffuse reactions in infants 2 to 12 months of age to localized, protective, and socially responsive patterns of behavior in those between 13 and 25 months of age, a progression that has been noted by other investigators. Trevarthen (1979, p. 325) has commented that "babies . . . are initially capable of projecting a general state of pain very powerfully. Quite soon they can indicate what part is hurting." In addition, Hahn and McLone (1984) have presented impressive clinical evidence supporting the ability of infants and children age 3 and younger to communicate effectively about their pain. This developmental sequence is described (Hahn & McLone, 1984, p. 37) as typically showing "a classic evolution starting with nonverbal responses and/or infantile pain talk and moving on before the age of three to verbal pain descriptors."

Ethical difficulties and other constraints of an external nature were no longer seen as an insurmountable barrier to research and clinical investigations with children. It became apparent that some kinds of research were possible. There are, in fact, three options available to the researcher in pediatric pain. Although they differ in the extent of intrusiveness involved, all entail the obligation of adhering to the general ethical principles that have been so carefully spelled out by professional organizations (American Psychological Association, 1982), federal agencies (National Commission for the Protection of Human Subjects of Biomedical and Behavioral Research, 1977; U.S. Department of Health and Human Services, 1983), and concerned professionals (Keith-Spiegel & Koocher, 1985; Nicholson, 1986).

The first option is to study events of a noxious nature that occur in the clinical setting, for example, burn debridement, circumcision, dental and orthodontic procedures, and venipuncture. There is no barrier to the study of these naturally occurring pain events if the dependent measures are purely observational and are obtained so unobtrusively that the ongoing interventions are not modified in any way for research purposes. These guidelines were followed by Craig et al. (1984), for example, in collecting observational data on the reactions of infants and toddlers to immunization shots.

A second option involves the introduction of painless autonomic and other measures, such as pain ratings and interview responses, not ordinarily used in the ongoing treatment intervention and therefore categorized as intrusive. To evaluate the use of new pain assessment instruments, for example, children's assessments of naturally occurring ongoing or recent pain could be obtained in the clinical setting, as LeBaron and Zeltzer (1984) did with children and adolescents who were undergoing bone marrow aspirations. Problems of an ethical nature should not arise here if the task is presented properly, without arousing fear or imposing restraints.

The remaining option involves the study of experimentally induced pain in children in clinical settings, that is, pain that children are undergoing purely for research purposes. The investigator who pursues this approach faces two problems of an ethical nature. One is that he is obligated to ensure that the child and his or her parents clearly understand what is involved in the child's participation, a task that is more difficult to accomplish than one might expect. In a study of children and adolescents' concepts of research involving hospitalization, Schwartz (1972), for example, reported that despite careful preparation of the children and their parents, subsequent interviews revealed that those children under age 11 were not aware of the research nature of their hospitalization, and of the older children who were aware of it, all but one had overwhelming anxiety concerning the research aspect. Schwartz's procedure involved having a child psychiatrist interview each child twice, which gave the children ample opportunity to express their fears and uncertainties. This finding puts the facile explanation that is usually given to children concerning their participation in research projects in a new light. Inflicting pain on a child, particularly one who already suffers some degree of pain, raises the second ethical problem: It is unlikely that the experimentally induced pain is of either therapeutic or diagnostic value. The use of experimentally induced pain has other shortcomings. Feuerstein and his colleagues (Feuerstein, Barr, Francoeur, Houle, & Rafman, 1982) used a cold pressor stimulus to test the hypothesis that children and adolescents with recurrent abdominal pain (RAP) would exhibit a deficit in autonomic nervous system recovery to stress and/or an enhanced behavioral and subjective response to induced pain. In a discussion of their negative findings they noted several limitations of the laboratory approach, including the difficulty of ensuring that the pain stimulus used was sufficiently analogous to naturally occurring pain episodes to differentiate between RAP subjects and controls. Clearly, the use of experimentally induced pain should be weighed carefully before proceeding with it. Melzack (1980, p. 186) has cautioned,

> I think it's useful to have experimental methods for the study of pain, but I think we ought to make a lot more use of patients who are in pain. It seems to me wrong to go about inducing pain in people when we have a huge population already in pain, and we have techniques that we can use to measure clinical pain in human beings.

As the barriers to progress in the field of childhood pain fell or were pushed aside in the absence of supportive evidence, a sudden influx of clinical and research papers appeared on childhood pain, but from a predominantly adult perspective. This increase was dramatic, but only in relation to previous levels of interest shown in the topic. When compared to the volume of output on adult pain, it represented a mere trickle.

The primary focus of this surge of interest centered on management. Since an empirical base for the management of pediatric pain was virtually nonexistent, many clinicians had simply proceeded as they would with adults, often to the detriment of the child (Jeans, 1983a). The clinicians and researchers laid down ground rules for a diversity of topics ranging from general guidelines on the care of the child and young adolescent in pain in the pediatric clinical setting (Ack, 1976; Azarnoff, 1976; Beuf, 1979; McCaffery, 1969; Neal, 1978) and dental setting (DeFee & Himelstein, 1969; Melamed, 1979; Wright & Alpern, 1971) to the management of specific pain events such as burns (Bailey, 1979; Leavitt, 1979; Nover, 1973; Quinby & Bernstein, 1971), certain chronic pain conditions (Alexander, 1972; Apley, 1975; Dodge, 1976; La Greca & Ottinger, 1979; Travis, 1969; Zeltzer, Dash & Holland, 1979), and life-threatening and terminal pain (Beales, 1979; Mennie, 1974; Travis, 1969). Cutting across this spectrum were the specifications of other pediatric investigators concerning optimal procedures in preparing children and adolescents for an impending pain experience (Fassler, 1978; Ferguson, 1979; Siegel, 1976; Visintainer & Wolfer, 1975; Wolfer & Visintainer, 1979) or, in the case of ongoing pain in children, therapeutic pain reduction techniques that adults could use (Johnson, Kirchhoff, & Endress, 1975; Sank & Biglan, 1974) or that children could be taught to use themselves (Ferguson, 1979; Gardner, 1976; Setterlind & Uneståhl, 1978).

Pursuing a line of investigation that could be described as more clearly psychologically oriented, others wrote knowledgeably and thoughtfully on children's communication of pain (Eland, 1974), pain analysis (Boehncke, 1970), aspects of the development of pain awareness in children (Poznanski, 1976; Schultz, 1971; Smith, 1976; Vernon, 1974), the pain "games" and other maneuvers that children employ (Chapman, 1971; Friedman, 1972), and the symbolic meaning of children's pain (Szasz, 1975). An overview of the field in terms of the state of the art in childhood pain was the focus of the landmark review paper by Eland and Anderson (1977).

In the 1980s, interest in childhood pain continued to increase sharply. At the time this text went to press, there were two other books on childhood pain in preparation (P. A. McGrath, 1987b; P. J. McGrath & Unruh, 1987). In the journal *Pain*, for example, articles on pediatric pain appeared in 1982 for the first time since the journal's inception in 1975. For almost the first time there were chapters on pain in children and adolescents in texts (Barr, 1982; Craig, 1980; Gross & Gardner, 1980; Jeans, 1983a, 1983b; Lavigne, Schulein, Hannan, & Hahn, 1987; McGrath, P. A., 1987a; McGrath, P. J., 1983) and year books (McGrath, de Veber, & Hearn, 1985; McGrath et al., 1985), and whole sections of journals (*American Journal of Maternal/Child Nursing*, 1984; *Issues in Comprehensive Pediatric Nursing*, 1984) were devoted to this topic. Comprehensive articles also appeared on a variety of facets of it (Beyer & Byers, 1985; Lavigne, Schulein, & Hahn, 1986a, 1986b; Passo, 1982; Schechter, 1984; Thompson & Varni, 1986) including pain in infancy (Owens, 1984). However, when viewed en masse, it gradually became apparent that the impact and potential value of this work, all of which was from an adult perspective, was weakened by the omission of input from a crucial source, the children themselves. The realization grew that the children and adolescents' perspectives of pain were an indispensable facet of the field as a whole and an essential element in the specialized study of childhood pain. There was an increasing awareness, for example, of the potential importance of information about childhood pain for theoretical advances at the adult level.

It was also clear that childhood pain should be viewed from a number of different perspectives, an essential one being a developmental viewpoint. Very little was known about the normal development of pain perception and response, or the conceptual meaning of pain for the child and adolescent. A description of the unfolding patterns of pain expression, perception, and cognitive awareness of pain across developmental stages was seen as an indispensable component in the establishment of a sound base of information about pain. By enhancing an understanding of the pain process, such information could lead to the refinement of existing theories of pain and the addition of new theoretical views of pediatric pain. An offshoot of these insights was a relatively small but influential cluster of interview studies and clinical reports of children and adolescents' view of pain and of their own pain experiences, a cluster that will be discussed in Chapter 2.

The purpose of this text is to place childhood pain in its rightful place as an important facet in the pain field. The focus will be primarily on the psychological nature of the pain experience in the preschool and school-age child and young adolescent and the social and cultural milieu in which it occurs, rather than on the neurophysiological mechanisms involved. To this end, the conceptual framework that has been chosen is a transactional one in which the pain experienced is viewed as the outcome of the conglomerate of characteristics and attributes of the child in a reciprocal relationship with the components of his social and nonsocial environments.

Following a discussion of children's views of their pain experiences and the theoretical and empirical bases for their development, we describe the most commonly used pain assessment procedures and offer a critical appraisal of the current status of pediatric pain assessment. The treatment modalities that are emphasized are those having a strong psychological component. For some of these, adult monitoring is mandatory; for others, the child can initiate them independently. In either case, a basic assumption here is that most school-age children and adolescents have the capacity to take some responsibility for the management of their pain and that they benefit psychologically from doing so. Along the way current issues relevant to the aforementioned topics are discussed and areas that should be investigated are specified; the implications for childhood pain research of research on topics other than pain are considered; and speculations about future developments and directions in this emerging field are offered.

2
The Child's View

Although there is widespread agreement about the importance of the subjective report of pain in adults (Hilgard, 1969; Jacox, 1980; Syrjala & Chapman, 1984), it is only in the current decade that the child and adolescent's view of pain and their pain experiences have attracted clinical and empirical interest. Information on this topic stems from a diversity of sources. One of these is a cluster of interview and questionnaire studies ranging from major and comprehensive projects concerned with the broad spectrum of the pain experiences of childhood to small-scale studies concerned mainly with specific groups of children or pain events. As Table 2-1 shows, the studies in this cluster vary markedly in amount and quality of information yield, methodology, subject characteristics, locus of study, and recency of the pain experience. Other sources of information are generally less structured, but are important nonetheless. Included here are children's spontaneous discussions of their pain experiences during their participation in pain instructional programs in school settings (Ross & Ross, 1985, 1986), videotapes of their comments during pediatric consultations (University of California Medical Center, 1975), case studies (Beuf, 1979; Hahn & McLone, 1984; Remen, 1980), reports from pediatric personnel (Eland & Anderson, 1977; Hahn, 1986; Hilgard & LeBaron, 1984; Lewis, 1978), and biographical (Ross, M., & Ross, A. P., 1980; Tucker, 1982) and autobiographical accounts (Bruce, 1983; Rosenbaum, 1984).

The information from these sources constitutes a comprehensive and well-documented account of children's cognitions about pain as opposed to adults' interpretations of these cognitions. This information makes it possible now to begin to construct a composite picture of children's understanding of pain, that is, their reasoning about what it is and how it happens; how they talk about it, use it, and cope with it; and their sources of information about it. The salient characteristic of the accumulated data is the finding that children pass through distinct stages in their understanding of the many facets of pain. Their thoughts and perceptions for the most part develop in an orderly and hierarchical sequence of stages, each characterized by a distinct, formal structure of thought that parallels the developmental sequence of other health-related concepts, such as health and illness (Bibace & Walsh, 1980; Feldman & Varni, 1985), hospitalization and related procedures (Redpath & Rogers, 1984), and death (Lonetto, 1980). In the period from preschool through adolescence, thoughts about pain change from simple to com-

Table 2-1 Interview Studies on Childhood Pain

Author(s)	N	Age	Ethnic Group	Geographic location	Condition	Site	Procedure
Abu-Saad (1984a)	24	9–12	Asian-American	California	Healthy	Home, play area, school	Taped oral interview, semistructured
Abu-Saad (1984b)	27	8–12	Arab-American	California	Healthy	Home, play area, school	Taped oral interview, semistructured
Abu-Saad (1984c)	24	9–12	Latin-American	California	Healthy	Home, play area, school	Taped oral interview, semistructured
Bibace & Walsh (1980)	237	4–14	—	Massachusetts	Healthy	School	Oral interview, 5 questions
Gaffney (1983)	680	5–14	Caucasian	Ireland	Healthy	School	Oral interview (young), written questionnaire (Older), 10 incomplete sentences
Glick & Nakayama (1985)	45	5–13	—	Kentucky	Healthy	School	Taped oral interview, 5 questions
Gordon (1981)	54	5–13	Caucasian	Montreal, Canada	Healthy	School	Taped oral interview after drawing of pain
Jerrett (1985)	40	5–9	—	Ontario, Canada	Acute health problem	Outpatient ENT clinic	Taped oral interview after drawing of pain

Study	N	Age	Ethnicity	Location	Health status	Setting	Method
Lollar et al. (1982)	240	4–19	—	Georgia	Healthy	—	Oral interview using Pediatric Pain Inventory
Reissland (1983)	58	4–13	Caucasian	London, England	Surgery	Pre-op in hospital	Oral interview, 11 open-ended questions
Ross & Ross (1982a, 1984b)	994	5–12	Caucasian, Mexican-American, Oriental, Black	California	Healthy, chronic illness	School, hospital, clinic	Taped oral interview, 9 interview forms, open-ended questions
Savedra et al. (1982)	214	9–12	Primarily Caucasian	California	Healthy, post-op, injury, diagnostic	School, hospital	Written questionnaire, semi-structured
Savedra et al. (1985)	156	13–17	Caucasian, Black, Latin, other	California	Healthy, acute/chronic illness	School, hospital	Written questionnaire, semi-structured
Schultz (1971)	74	10–11	—	New York	Healthy	School	Written questionniare, semi-structured
Scott (1978)	58	4–10	—	Ohio	Healthy, unspecified clinic	School, clinic	Taped interviews, projective test with 2 cartoon pictures
Vair (1981)	32	7–12	Caucasian	Ottawa, Canada	Acute post-op abdominal pain	Hospital	Oral interview, open-ended questions, pain map, visual analogue scale (VAS)

plex, egocentric to less egocentric, concrete to more abstract, subjective to more objective, and prelogical to logical. These changes occur gradually and at varying rates, with the child moving on in some areas but clinging to old beliefs in others.

Although Piaget did not specifically discuss the topic of pain, the conceptual framework that best fits many of the findings on children's knowledge of pain is the Piagetian model (Piaget, 1973). According to Piaget, children's thoughts, perceptions, and reasoning are generally qualitatively different from those of adults. Children see the world differently, but the differences are not based on misunderstandings or lack of information; rather, they reflect the fact that children have their own interpretations of events in their world, and these change gradually in orderly and predictable ways until in mid- to late adolescence they become very similar or identical to those of adults. Piaget (1973) has divided this cognitive process into three major periods linked with increasing chronological age. Cognitive activity in the *sensorimotor period* (birth to 2 years) consists of sensory and motor actions that become established as behavioral sequences forming the foundation for later intellectual structure and function. In this period language development is limited, although there is well-documented clinical evidence (Hahn, 1986; Hahn & McLone, 1984) that some children at this period can generate pain descriptors. By the end of the sensorimotor period, the child has a vocabulary of approximately 300 words. During this time, he learns to differentiate himself from the environment, and pain experiences facilitate this differentiation process. The child has no concept of reality, and Piaget also believes that no conscious thinking occurs. Bower (1974) and Gratch (1977) are among those who have debated this latter position.

The *concrete operations period* is subdivided into two stages. In the *preoperational thought stage,* or early childhood period of 2 to 7 years, the child is egocentric: he does not grasp the idea that his perception of an event may be different from that of others; for example, he thinks his pain is as obvious to others as it is to him. McCaffery (1977, p. 12) cites as an example of this egocentrism a 2-year-old girl with a stomachache who, when asked where she hurt, disgustedly raised her skirt and said, "There. Can't you see it?" The child is unable to reason beyond his immediate experience and interprets events in terms of immediate perceptions. Magic and animism are a part of his world; cause and effect are not understood; and pain is often viewed as punishment. The child has little ability for abstract thinking and, although competence in language is increasing, his thought processes remain empirical rather than logical and are associated with static characteristics of direct experiences.

By the time the child reaches the *concrete operations stage* of middle childhood (age 7 to 11 or 12) the move away from egocentric orientation has begun and he has become aware of the subjectivity of his own ideas and thoughts. He is capable now of understanding the cause of pain and has the verbal skills to express pain. Although his thinking has become logical, he is more concerned with the concrete rather than the abstract; wherever possible, reasoning is based on direct observation.

The final period, of *formal operations,* carries the child from age 12 through adolescence and into early adulthood. During this period he begins to achieve his full intellectual capacity and can generalize, reason deductively, and deal with abstract ideas.

Fletcher and Johnson (1982) contend that the concept of formal operations has little clinical explanatory power and advocate a broader perspective on adolescent thinking in clinical contexts. It should be noted that relating periods and stages for any attribute to specific ages must always be viewed as an approximation in the case of a specific child. However, the framework that these approximations provide has some value as a starting point for the interpretation of children's responses, in this case, their information about specific aspects of pain.

The fact that most of the children's reports presented in this chapter are of a retrospective nature raises the issue of recall versus learned response. Are the children's responses first hand, that is, recall, or are they learned—mere repetition of their parents' accounts of the pain events? There is clinical (Hahn & McLone, 1984; Hawley, 1984; Peterschmidt, 1984; Travis, 1969) and empirical (Kassowitz, 1958; Levy, 1960; Ross & Ross, 1982a) evidence that infants as young as six months can remember noxious events and that toddlers and older children can recall such events, sometimes in surprising detail. Kassowitz (1958), for example, found that there was little or no evidence of apprehension in the reactions to injections during the first six months of life, but toward the end of the first year and continuing through the fourth year a high incidence of intense fear was exhibited. An explanation for this memory pattern can be found in the research on the influence of attention on learning. Pain, whether spontaneous or treatment induced, is almost always an attention-directing event. Unless the infant or child is effectively distracted, he will focus on the pain, encode it along with the associated affect and relevant contextual cues (Pennebaker, 1982), and store the pain experience. Furthermore, several kinds of information from the Ross and Ross (1982a) study support the validity of the response data as recall. No child described a pain event that occurred prior to age 4, and a number ($n = 28$) spontaneously distinguished between pain events that they could clearly remember and those of a hearsay nature:

> I know it [herniectomy at age 4] hurt a lot and and I screamed all the time because my Mom said so, but I can't remember it at all. (Boy, CA 6)

In addition, the parents to whom Ross and Ross talked rarely agreed with their child's choice of "worst pain ever" and sometimes barely remembered the event, which suggests that the child's account was not learned recall. However, the most powerful support for confidence that the responses represent true recall data comes from the children's descriptions of specific pain experiences. In these accounts childlike imagery set within a child-appropriate frame of reference was the predominant characteristic. As can be seen from the following representative responses, the imagery differs markedly from that typically used by adults.

> It was like a hundred red-hot monsters all biting my arm hard. (Boy, CA 8, second degree burns)

> Like there's a big bomb in my stomach, it feels like it's going to explode. (Girl, CA 7, stomachache)

Similarly, the finding in Gaffney's (1983) study of age-linked patterns for thematic elaboration suggests that the children were presenting their own views of their pain experiences rather than those of their parents. Had the latter been the case, the themes would have tended to appear in random order rather than age-related patterns.

In the following sections, the response data from the studies listed in Table 2-1 and the other previously cited sources are discussed in terms of the children's definitions of pain, their pain descriptors, views on causality, opinions concerning the value of pain, and maladaptive pain usage. Also included are their ideas on the worst things about pain, their worst pain experiences, their opinion of what helps most when they are in pain, and the coping strategies that they use. The children's accounts of specific pain experiences, including acute, chronic, and treatment-related pain, are described in some detail.

Definitions of Pain

The often expressed belief that *pain* is too abstract a term for preschool children to understand (Eland & Anderson, 1977; McCaffery, 1969; Molsberry, 1979) and the sporadic clinical support for that belief (see, for example, Eland, 1974) are strongly refuted by the findings of the major interview studies (Gaffney, 1983; Ross & Ross, 1982a). Most of the four- and five-year-old children and almost all of those over age 6 possessed an accurate, though often limited, understanding of the word *pain*. Gaffney (1983) has documented developmental transitions in children's definitions of pain that correspond to the three major Piagetian stages. For purposes of data analysis, she has defined these in terms of age as preoperational (5–7 years), concrete operations (8–10 years), and early formal operations (11–14 years) and refers to them as the younger, middle, and oldest groups, respectively. In her data (Gaffney, 1983) there was a significant shift from concrete, perceptually dominated perspectives in the younger children to a semiabstract perspective in the middle age group, to a more abstract, generalized, and psychologically oriented view in the oldest group. When asked to complete the sentence "Pain is . . . ," the youngest said, "a sore thing," "a thing that hurts," and "when you fall you get it." The middle age group's responses were "a hurting sensation" and "a feeling that is sore." The oldest children responded, "an attacking of the nerves," "something physical or psychological that hurts a person," and "mental, when we are not hurt physically but our feelings are hurt, when someone is rude and inconsiderate."

A second significant trend in the Gaffney (1983) data, that of increasing thematic elaboration with age, reflected a growing awareness of the more abstract aspects of the pain experience. At the oldest level there was evidence of a beginning understanding of the neurological process involved: Pain was described by one boy (CA 13) as "the damage or band of a bone, etc., which sets off the nerves and which is registered in the brain. It is a feeling." Another boy (CA 14) described it, "When the nerves on my body are disrupted in some way it causes discomfort." The older children also showed a grasp of the biological purpose of pain: A pain is sometimes "to warn one he is in the danger zone of overdoing any particular thing" (Boy, CA 13).

The same general trends were apparent but did not approach significance in the studies of Bibace and Walsh (1980) and Glick and Nakayama (1985). The small sample in the latter study coupled with the interviewers' use of "probes and rephrasing" renders the results almost meaningless in that it would be pointless to attempt cross-study comparisons and virtually impossible to replicate the procedures.

In marked contrast to the findings of Gaffney (1983) are those of Ross and Ross (1984b). In their sample of children age 5 to 12, the definitions of pain tended to be brief and unidimensional, that is, they emphasized the sensory dimension of the pain, with no apparent age trends: 80.9% of the respondents emphasized general discomfort ("Pain is when it hurts"), and 12.2% focused on specific pain events ("Pain is a squeezing headache"); only 1.8% of the definitions mentioned either the process of pain ("It's a signal sent by a nerve") or its functions ("It tells you something is wrong someplace"). Some children at all ages gave more detailed answers, but there was no trend toward increased thematic elaboration with increased age.

The divergence in results on the definition of pain question cannot be attributed, as Gaffney and Dunne (1986) have speculated, to the differences in age range among the three studies. Even when the analysis was limited to the data on the 5- to 12-year-old children, the same developmental transitions were present in Gaffney's (1983) data. The differences in results could be a function of the ubiquitous problem of method variance and consequent differences in response set in the subjects. The incomplete sentences used by Gaffney (1983) were of a very general nature, for example, "Pain is . . . " and "A pain is sometimes . . .," whereas those of Ross and Ross (1982a) were very specific: "What would you tell your best friend if he/she was going to the dentist for the first time?" It is our opinion that if the subjects in Ross and Ross (1982a) had been given Gaffney's (1983) questions, the same developmental transitions would have been documented. To this end a replication of the Gaffney (1983) study is presently under-way (Ross & Ross, 1987) with children in Northern California. Preliminary results show the same Piagetian developmental transitions that were documented by Gaffney.

Pain Descriptors

The belief that young children lack the ability to provide information about their pain experiences has received no support whatsoever. Children as young as 3 years have described their pain as shooting and hurting (Hahn, 1986), and in the studies listed in Table 2-1 many children age 5 and older generated descriptors that appear on the McGill Pain Questionnaire in the sensory ("burning," "dull," "not stabbing"), affective ("exhausting," "tiring"), and miscellaneous ("agony," "tight") categories. From these data there was no evidence that for children dif-ferent types of pain have unique qualities that can be described by distinctive clus-ters of words, as Dubuisson and Melzack (1976) have reported for adults. There were only occasional instances of an association between single pain descriptors and specific pain events, for example, tension headaches were often described as "squeezing." These findings do not rule out the possibility that children might use clusters of descriptors specific to certain pain conditions. As Craig (1986) has pointed out, the lack of data may reflect only the relative disinterest in the topic as a target for research.

Some children made discriminative comparisons. A boy (CA 11) dis-tinguished between pain that "stings" and "dull" pain (Bibace & Walsh, 1980), another boy (CA 8) differentiated between the "rough" pain of a sore throat and the "smooth" pain of an earache, and a girl (CA 9) described her stomachaches as sometimes "kinky, like a lot of knives poking me one after the other and just when one is stopping the next one starts" and other times a "long smooth pain" (Ross & Ross, 1982). Other children used ordering—"It's [a burn] worse than scraping your knee but not as bad as a broken elbow" (Boy, CA 7); equating with other pain—"An ear ache is equal in pain to a strep throat" (Boy, CA 11); and quantifica-tion—"It [a stomachache] feels like a thousand bee stings inside" (Girl, CA 11) (Ross & Ross, 1982a) and "like inside you is cracking up and splitting into millions of pieces" (Boy, CA 10) (Gaffney, 1983). In an occasional case, the child's descrip-tion implied a ratio scale: "The spinal tap hurted an inch less than the bone mar-row" (Boy, CA 7) (Ross & Ross, 1982a). From the children's descriptors it is diffi-cult to believe that they are relatively insensitive to pain or that their pain intensity level is not comparable to that of adults. Table 2-2 presents a comparison between some representative descriptors of different pain events used by children (Ross & Ross, 1982a) and those commonly used by adults.

Table 2-2 Descriptors Used by Children and Adults for Specific Pain Experiences

Pain	Child's descriptor	Adult's descriptor[a]
Migraine headache	"like somebody has a hammer or something and they are banging on me from the outside or trying to get out from the inside" (Girl, CA 10)	"pounding"
Tension headache	"feels like someone is pushing my head in from the outside" (Girl, CA 10)	"terrible pressure"
Stomachache	"like someone is inside your stomach with a blunt knife trying to cut his way out" (Boy, CA 11)	"like a cramp that stabs"
Burn	"like millions of needles stabbing into a red hot sunburn" (Boy, CA 9)	"a terrible hot stinging feeling"
Runner's cramp in legs	"like a giant has your leg in a vise and he's tightening it up and then doing a corkscrew" (Boy, CA 8)	"a twisting squeezing pain"

[a]From clinical reports and articles.

Use of Analogies

In response to the item "A pain can feel like . . .," Gaffney (1983) reported a significant increase in the use of analogies with increasing age. The fact that only 5.7% of her youngest group used analogies and this increased to 42.1% for the middle group and 70.1% for the oldest caused Gaffney (1983, pp. 269, 273) to conclude that

> prior to the development of concrete operations children are unable to use analogies in their description of pain. . . . The ability to use analogies to describe pain begins to be evident at age 8.

Gaffney's finding that few of the youngest group used analogies received some support from findings of Bibace and Walsh (1980), who asked, "What is pain?" and then, "What does it feel like?" Although analogies did occur—pain was described as "like a knife" (Girl, CA 4) and "like your heart, but it beats, but it's like a needle" (Girl, CA 8)—they were rare until Grade 6 (equivalent in age to Gaffney's oldest group), when 50.9% of the children used an analogy, for example, "like sharp arrows beating the inside of my stomach" (Boy, CA 11).

However, when Ross and Ross (1982a) asked children to describe their pre-viously reported specific pain experiences, many younger children used analogies, for example,

> like a rock was bouncing round in my chest hitting the sides hard. (Boy, CA 6, irregu-lar painful heart beat)

> like someone is biting your ear . . . like a big volcano in your ear. (Girl, CA 7, earache)

On an abstract–concrete continuum, Gaffney's and Bibace and Walsh's ques-tions would lie well toward the abstract end, whereas Ross and Ross's question was more concrete in that it referred to a specific pain event that the child had spon-taneously mentioned. These differences suggest that whether children use analo-gies or not may depend less on developmental stage than on the content of the question. It appears that contrary to Gaffney's conclusion that analogies do not occur until the period of concrete operations, children 5 or 6 years old are able to use analogies to describe specific pain events but either are unable to use them for pain in general or choose not to do so.

Reports of Causality of Pain

Causality refers to the child's opinion of why a specific pain event happened. Ac-curacy is not the issue here; rather, it is the child's view of the event that is of interest. For example, a child in an emergency room reported that he fell "because the Devil pushed me." Causality has been investigated in respect to both pain in general and pain from specific events, with questions that vary greatly across stud-ies. Gaffney (1983) used the incomplete sentence "A person gets a pain be-cause . . .," and Bibace and Walsh (1980) asked, "Why does pain come?" In the Northern California studies, Abu-Saad (1984a, 1984b, 1984c) and Savedra et al. requested children (Savedra, Gibbons, Tesler, Ward, & Wegner, 1982) and adoles-cents (Savedra, Tesler, Ward, & Wegner, 1985) to "list three things that have caused you pain." Ross and Ross (1982a) were interested in the causality of spe-cific pain events: Following a question about the child's "worst pain ever," he was asked, "Why do you think that happened to you?" In all of these studies illness-related pain, malfunctioning of some part of the body, and accidental or induced trauma were cited most often as the cause of pain, with these responses occurring significantly more often in Bibace and Walsh's (71.8%) and Ross and Ross's (69.7%) studies than in Gaffney's study (55.9%).

Psychological causes of pain were also reported in all these studies: Children attributed pain to feeling tension, being under pressure that they could not handle, being teased, and experiencing sadness at a relative's leaving. In a study of adoles-cents (Savedra et al., 1985), psychological causes of pain included deaths of family and friends, disruption of heterosexual relationships, and feelings associated with athletic incompetence. In respect to age and sex differences, Gaffney (1983) reported significant differences in the direction of increased citing of psychological causes with increasing age, with girls citing these causes more often than boys. These trends were apparent but not statistically significant in the other studies.

Although the causality responses from children and adolescents fell clearly into either the physiological or the psychological category, it was not clear from the data whether the respondents had the concept of these two different kinds of pain. One 10-year-old boy (Ross & Ross, 1982a) stated, "You can have pain in your body or in your mind—a miserable feeling," but such discriminations were rare.

Pain-as-punishment reponses were infrequent in the Bibace and Walsh (1980) and Ross and Ross (1982a) studies, even when the pain experiences were clearly the result of disobedience:

> Boy (CA 6): I went down the big slide . . . which I am not allowed to go on and I was gonna shoot through the barrel real fast. But I got too far to one side and I hit the edge and cut my head open.
> Interviewer: Why do you think that happened to you?
> Boy: I need to practice more on real steep slides before I shoot the barrel. (Ross & Ross, 1982a)

Instead, in both studies pain in general as well as specific pain experiences were attributed in a logical and matter-of-fact way to clearly associated and immediate causes such as accidents, environmental nonsocial factors such as heat and noise, illness, surgery, and the aggressive actions of others.

In contrast, in the Gaffney (1983) study there was unequivocal evidence of a pain-as-punishment belief: 43.9% of the children cited explanations involving transgressions or carelessness, self-causality, particularly in respect to eating ("He ate too much sweets"—Boy, CA 5); other excesses ("He runs too far"—Boy, CA 9); and failure to comply with rules ("They open their jumper and their things are not tied and tucked in"—Boy, CA 7). Some of the older children described direct punishment by God: "God cutting bad pieces of us and making sure that we're ourselves again" (Girl, CA 10); "They offend God and he makes them suffer" (Boy, CA 11); and "Sometimes he might be disobedient and God makes him suffer" (Boy, CA 12). Gaffney (1983) interprets the persistence of transgression-type responses in these older children within a Piagetian framework as evidence of adherence to precausal thinking. It could also reflect the religious teaching that Roman Catholic children typically are exposed to at this age level. Another possibility is that by fixing the blame on himself, the child feels in control of his pain. In this situation being in control is very reassuring because it implies that having caused his pain, he may also be able to alleviate it. Preliminary findings from the ongoing replication (Ross & Ross, 1987) of the Gaffney (1983) study show many of the same trends documented by Gaffney. One notable exception is the finding that pain as punishment for transgressions involving eating was seldom mentioned.

Only rarely did any sense of immanent justice (Piaget, 1973), that is, instances of punishment for misbehavior totally unrelated to the pain event, occur in the Bibace and Walsh (1980) study. The only such explanation in the Ross and Ross (1982a) study came from a boy (CA 6) who stated, "I forgot to take out the trash on Friday and that's why I broke my leg" (at school the following Monday). On the basis of research on illness causality (Perrin & Gerrity, 1981) and death (Lonetto, 1980; Travis, 1969), some of the large contingent of children in the 4- to 6-year-old range might have been expected to invoke an immanent justice explanation. However, the overall empirical evidence on immanent justice suggests that this explanation occurs more often in hospitalized children (see, for example, Bergmann, 1965; Brewster, 1982; Remen, 1980; Richter, 1943) rather than those in nonclinical (see, for example, Haight, Black, & DiMatteo, 1985) settings.

Value of Pain

It was clear from the cluster of Northern California interview studies (Abu-Saad, 1984a, 1984b, 1984c; Ross & Ross, 1982a; Savedra et al., 1982, 1985) that concepts of pain held by children and young adolescents seldom included any awareness of the positive aspects of pain, such as its warning function, diagnostic value, or treatment evaluation role. This finding stands in the face of wide variations in methodology (type of question, mode of interview presentation) and subject characteristics (cultural group, hospitalized versus nonhospitalized). In the light of the barrage of negative information about pain that most children in our society experience, it is not surprising. From their early years on, children hear detailed and often fear-arousing descriptions of adults' pain experiences, particularly of postoperative, chronic, and terminal pain; they are bombarded with television commercials depicting the agony of pain; and the threat of pain is used to promote appropriate dental care and discourage forbidden activities.

The question "We can all think of *bad* things about pain. Can you think of anything *good* about pain?" (Ross & Ross, 1982a) elicited emphatic and often surprised negatives from 88.7% of the children, with secondary gains ("You can get out of giving your book report") cited by 5.3%. Only 4.9% identified true benefits. A subsequent study (Ross & Ross, 1985) obtained similar results. In a study of hospitalized and nonhospitalized children age 9 to 12, Savedra, Tesler, Ward, Wegner, and Gibbons (1981) found that two thirds of the group could not identify positive values of pain when asked, "What is good about pain?" Data on the remaining third are not provided other than to say that some (number not given) cited secondary gains and others saw pain as a warning that something was wrong. Abu-Saad asked the same question and obtained the same findings in a series of studies of children age 8 to 12 from different cultural backgrounds: Arab-American (1984b), Asian-American (1984a), and Latin-American (1984c). In a study of adolescents (Savedra et al., 1985), only 18% of the respondents cited positive values of pain.

In the small group of children and adolescents who recognized that pain could be of value, various facets were mentioned. In describing the restraining function, one boy (CA 9) said, "Pain is a way of telling you *not* to do it in a way that you don't like. If something in your head just said, 'Don't do it,' you would just say, 'Aw, shut up!'" (Ross & Ross, 1984b). An adolescent (Savedra et al., 1985) pointed to both the warning and diagnostic functions: "lets you know something is wrong, or you're getting better." The cathartic function was presented as "pain is good because it lets your feelings out and makes you feel better" (Boy, CA 10, Abu-Saad, 1984a). Some children and adolescents viewed pain as a preparation for life: "It toughens you up and gets you ready to stand other things when you're older" (Boy, CA 9, Ross & Ross, 1982a); "It hardens you . . . and it gets you ready for life" (Boy, CA 11, Abu-Saad, 1984b); and "you'll be better prepared if you have the same kind again" (adolescent, Savedra et al., 1985). One value mentioned only by the adolescents concerned the idea that pain puts things in perspective. As one respondent said, "It makes you realize how lucky you are when not in pain and realize how often people overlook their blessings" (Savedra et al., 1985).

Maladaptive Pain Usage

Children in our society learn through the process of direct reinforcement and observational learning that a complaint of pain may elicit sympathy and attention from others. Often these positive consequences are coupled with secondary gains such as preferential treatment and avoidance of disliked activities. For children who crave more attention than they are able to elicit through more socially acceptable channels and for those whose ineptitude makes certain school-related and other activities psychologically painful, it is a short step to the intentional use of existing pain in the service of secondary gains such as attention from others. The next phase in this sequence is the logical one of pretending pain when no pain exists. In both instances, this use of pain is considered maladaptive because the child should achieve these goals and cope with difficulties by other, more acceptable, means. If the pattern of maladaptive pain usage is rewarded, it may persist into adulthood where it continues to absolve the user from disliked activities and to elicit sympathy from others (Black, 1980; Bresler, 1979). It is one of the cornerstones of the costly chronic pain syndrome (Bonica, 1953, 1980; Sternbach, 1984).

In the early school years, intentional maladaptive pain usage takes two forms. One is the use of existing pain for secondary gains. Often the pain is quite mild and the individual exaggerates its severity, for example, "You can be running around holding your finger while it's bleeding or you could do other things. Some people want sympathy so they hang on other people yelling, 'Oh, I hurt all over'" (fifth-grade child, Glick & Nakayama, 1985). Young children, particularly those with chronic or recurring pain problems, sometimes use this mode to control other members of the family. Wilkinson (1984) reported the case of a much-indulged nine-year-old girl with arthritis who had learned how to use her pain to control her mother. Often the child called her mother several times during the night to move her arm to relieve the pain. When the child was in the hospital, however, she slept through the night.

The other type of maladaptive pain usage is malingering, the deliberate pretense of pain in an individual who is pain free. Lewis (1982) has found that the prevalence of malingering increases with age and is more common among children from families with higher socioeconomic backgrounds. One possible explanation for this latter finding is that children in affluent families have more adult-directed activities that they would like to avoid. Ross and Ross (1982a) assessed the use of malingering by first asking children to name some activities that they disliked and then following up with this question:

> Sometimes when a boy [girl] doesn't want to go somewhere like school or a music lesson or do something, he [she] says he [she] has a pain or doesn't feel well, when he [she] really feels fine. Do you ever do anything like that?

Of the 740 respondents, more than one-third reported one or more instances of using nonexistent pain for secondary gains (mainly for increased parental attention, avoidance of school and of athletic training activities). Typical of these responses was that of a girl, age 8, who was enrolled in a championship swimming program:

> Whenever I don't want to go to swimming practice I grab my stomach and moan and make a face like eating a lemon and I say, "Gee, Mom, I *hope* I don't have to miss *swimming* . . ."

Although Ross and Ross (1982a) did not directly ask about the use of existing pain for secondary gains, 9% of the children spontaneously reported this behavior. Some went to great lengths in establishing the necessary background:

> See it [stomach] just hurt a little from gymnastics and just like that [snaps fingers] I thought, "There goes the book report." So in church I made sure to sit next to Mom and I like grabbed it a couple of times, you know? And when she whispered was I O.K., I said, "Sure, Mom," but I tried to *sound* not O.K. Then at dinner I was real picky and didn't have no dessert and I went to bed early even though I missed [favorite TV program]. My Mom felt my head, "No school for you tomorrow." I just argued a little bit . . . " (Boy, CA 10)

Others were more straightforward:

> I mostly just moan and say I don't feel very well. I say it's both my head and my stomach and usually my stomach hurts before I say I have it—it hurts a little bit, I think, but I will blow it up. (Girl, CA 10)

Mothers were not always taken in by these gambits:

> Sometimes I say I'm tired or I have a bad headache when it's only a small one but they never believe me. I used to always tell lies about headaches, now they never believe me even when I have a bad headache. (Girl, CA 9)

Perceptions of Worst Thing About Pain

In response to the incomplete sentence "The worst thing about pain is . . . ," children most frequently mentioned the unpleasant physical concomitants of pain. Gaffney (1983), who has the only data on this point, reported a curvilinear relationship between age and reports of unpleasant physical qualities, with the youngest and oldest children citing these qualities significantly less often than did children in the middle age group. The following are representative of their responses:

> It keeps going sore. (Girl, CA 5)

> The sting. (Boy, CA 8)

> You can be in agony. (Boy, CA 10)

> Its sharp, killing-like sting. (Girl, CA 12)

> Its hurtfulness. Pain can be most excruciating. (Boy, CA 14)

The category, immobilization and disruption of activity patterns, occurred more frequently in the responses of the middle and older age groups. Concern about the general unpredictability of the duration of pain emerged at age 8 and increased markedly by age 11 in girls and by age 13 in boys. Representative responses are those of a girl (CA 9) who thought that the worst thing about pain was that "it might never go away" and a boy (CA 13) who wrote, "it can last for any amount of time."

Psychological effects of pain were also of concern, primarily in the oldest group. The children were quite perceptive about the effects of pain on mood, with girls mentioning this relationship significantly more often than did boys: "It puts you in a bad mood and makes everything around seem noisy and annoying" (Girl, CA 11). The effects of pain on interpersonal relationships were also noted: A boy age 12 commented that "it prevents enjoyment and when you're miserable you make others miserable," and one of 13 noted "the losing of your temper which hurts others." Less frequently mentioned as the worst thing about pain were responses that indicated a beginning awareness of the subjectivity of pain and the feeling of psychological isolation engendered by it, for example, "that people do not know how bad it is" (Girl, CA 9) and "that nobody seems to understand it . . . they don't know what torture the person is going through" (Boy, CA 14).

Reported Worst Pain Ever

The pain experiences most often perceived by children as their "worst pain ever" varied with locus of interview, with the reponses of hospitalized children differing from those of children who were interviewed in clinic and school settings. Hospitalized children and adolescents most frequently reported their worst pain to be either the disease/trauma reason for their hospitalization or a medical/surgical treatment procedure such as suction:

> It's hard to describe, gagging, can't breathe, trapped like a torture treatment. (CA and sex not provided, Savedra et al., 1981)

For young hospitalized children, needle procedures figured prominently among the "worst pains": Almost two thirds of a group of children ages 4 to 8 mentioned a shot or other needle procedure as their worst pain experience (Eland, 1974). Of particular interest was the finding that the worst-pain status of needle procedures appears to diminish rapidly with increasing distance from the hospital setting. Only 15% of a group of children in a clinic setting (Jerrett, 1985) chose needle procedures, and this figure dropped to 8% for a group of nonhospitalized children in the Eland study. When healthy, nonhospitalized children and adolescents (n = 240, CA 4–19) rated 24 pictures of pain-evoking situations of a medical, psychosocial, recreational, or daily-living nature in terms of intensity, the picture of a child being given a shot ranked 17th (Lollar, Smits, & Patterson, 1982).

For nonhospitalized children, the choices most frequently cited (30.4%) as "worst" were dramatic, isolated, but medically relatively minor incidents such as cutting a knee open on the curb of a sidewalk or having hot wax spilled on a small part of the body while making candles (Ross & Ross, 1982a). For these children, the surprise/shock element, in the form of a sharp contrast beween an enjoyable ongoing activity and its abrupt halt by a sudden, intense, and unexpected pain, appeared to contribute heavily to the heightened pain experience. The surprise/ shock element was also clearly apparent in children's reports of their worst pain in other studies:

> A hole in my head, felt like biting, itching, horrible and unbearable. (CA 8–12, Abu-Saad, 1984b)

> Hit in the head with a stone. Stunning, sore, and shocking. (CA 9–12, Savedra et al., 1981)

> I was cutting fabric and I cut the tip of my thumb off. It hurt so bad that I screamed. . . . It was *terrible!* (CA 9–12, Savedra et al., 1981)

No data are available on the surprise/shock aspect of the worst pain at the adolescent level. In their descriptive account of the pain experiences of hospitalized and nonhospitalized adolescents, Savedra et al. (1985) combined the responses about "worst" and "most recent" pain experiences, thus effectively rendering the data useless.

The foregoing findings represent the first step in investigating children's worst pain experiences. The utility of the data is limited, however, by the generality of the questions. The logical next step in investigating this phenomenon would be to conduct more fine-grained analyses of children's worst pain experiences by first identifying worst pains in multiple settings (hospital, doctor's and dentist's office, school, athletic training center) and then by determining the facet of pain that is so distressing for the child. From the data presented here, one such source of distress was the surprise/shock element. It would be of great value for pediatric personnel concerned with pain management to identify other distressing facets, by setting. In the case of the hospitalized child, for example, possible sources of acute distress include the fear that the pain will not end, the meaning of the pain, and the lack of information about its source or an excess of such information (Ross, S.A., 1984).

What Helps Most When in Pain

An important aspect of the child's pain experience is what the child thinks would help him to bear ongoing pain. Several investigations (Abu-Saad, 1984a, 1984b, 1984c; Gaffney, 1983; Glick & Nakayama, 1985; Jerrett, 1985; Savedra et al., 1981, 1982, 1985; Tesler, Wegner, Savedra, Gibbons, & Ward, 1981) have included this question, but in only one of these were the data reported in a form adequate for the drawing of conclusions. Gaffney (1983) found that the younger children were dependent on such passive external treatment-related factors as medicine, medical personnel, and hospitals. With increasing age, a significant shift occurred toward self-generated behaviors (for example, physical strategies like rubbing the sore spot, cognitive strategies like positive thinking) involving the child in a more active role in his own treatment. At around age 8, children reported resting, relaxation, and other similar remedies that were self-initiated, a trend that increased significantly in the 11- to 14-year-old age group. Also increasing in the latter group, particularly in girls, was the need for psychological forms of comfort, the presence of family and friends for sympathy and comfort as well as for distraction. Findings of the other investigations all appear to support those of Gaffney, but the procedural inadequacies of these studies generally limit their value.

As far as preferred treatment for specific pain is concerned, only one study (Ross & Ross, 1982a) has data on this topic. The question "What would have helped most when in [child's report of his worst pain ever]?" yielded the most consistent finding in the entire data set of this study: 99.2% of the children felt that the "thing that helped most" regardless of the kind of pain was to have one or both parents present. In answer to a specific question about what actions of the parents would help, the children freely acknowledged that often there was nothing that the parents could actually do but emphasized that having them there helped. This finding is consistent with the *direct social support model* of Cohen and Wills (1985), which states that an increase in support should result in a concomitant increase in well-being irrespective of the actual amount of concrete support given, as opposed to their *buffering model,* which attributes the need for the parents' presence to the perception of them as allies who might, or could, protect the child from adverse events likely to occur in the treatment setting. No child's responses could be interpreted in terms of the latter model.

Coping Strategies

Within the children's responses to the question on what would help during pain, one cluster could be categorized as coping strategies, that is, cognitive or behavioral actions initiated by the child to modify his pain. Before moving on to the specific strategies reported in the various studies, we shall briefly discuss the general topic of coping.

Pain is a stressor that disrupts the child's equilibrium. Stressors of any kind generally elicit efforts to restore equilibrium. The characteristic way in which a child deals with stressors in general is called his *coping style.* Coping styles evolve from a diversity of intrapersonal sources, such as developmental level or personality, and from the child's experiential background of early social experiences and relationships, previous stressful experiences, and history of success or failure in dealing with them (Lazarus & Folkman, 1984). The specific techniques that he uses to defuse the stressor's effects are called *coping strategies.*

A child's coping strategies may be externally or internally directed. Lazarus, Averill, and Opton (1974) categorize the externally directed strategies as *direct actions* on the self or environment that include behaviours such as making active preparations against harm, devising an escape plan, or exhibiting avoidance behavior. Their internally directed category is labeled *intrapsychic coping processes* and includes forms of coping such as attention deployment, reappraisal, and wish-fulfilling fantasy that are characterized by cognitive activity designed to help the child maintain or achieve internal equilibrium. Other researchers (see, for example, Murphy, 1974; Rose, 1972; White, 1974) have developed similar categories: For example, Murphy's (1974) Coping I is defined as the capacity for dealing with obstacles and opportunities in the environment, and Coping II is the capacity to maintain internal equilibrium, an example being a coping strategy that allows the child to contemplate an approaching dental appointment without undue anxiety.

When seeking information on the child's coping strategies, it is essential that the question format clearly distinguish between self-help and others' help. Most of the information on strategies that hospitalized and nonhospitalized children and adolescents have used to minimize pain comes from the small group of studies in which this distinction was made clear to the respondents (Jeans & Gordon, 1981;

Reissland, 1983; Ross & Ross, 1982a). In these studies, children were first asked questions exploring possible external sources of pain relief, such as parents and pediatric personnel, from whom the child could seek help. The purpose of these preliminary questions was to make it easier for the child to respond to the critical question about self-help (for example, "When you had the pain was there anything you tried to do *yourself* so that it wouldn't hurt so much? If so, what?" [Ross & Ross, 1982a]) without referring to help from external sources.

When this distinction is not made, considerable information may be lost and faulty conclusions drawn. In answer to more general questions about what would help a child feel better when he is in pain, Abu-Saad (1984a, 1984b, 1984c), Gaffney (1983), and Savedra et al. (1981, 1982), among others, reported only the occasional use of self-help coping strategies such as distraction, with the great majority of responses focusing on other-generated solutions. The fact that few children in these studies reported the use of self-help coping strategies does not mean that they did not use them. Rather, it reflects the problem of method variance, that is, the fact that the wording of a question may create a certain response set and the set in these studies apparently was toward others' help, whereas the set created by the wording of Jeans and Gordon (1981), Reissland (1983), and Ross and Ross (1982a) emphasized self-help. To create the latter set, the question should be spelled out in no uncertain terms, as Reissland (1983), for example, has done: "What could *you* do to make the pain not hurt so much? What could *you* think about to make the pain not hurt so much?" The two main categories of coping strategies to be discussed here are direct actions (externally directed) and cognitive strategies (internally directed attempts by the child to modify his thought processes in order to attenuate ongoing pain).

Direct Action

Children frequently use direct action modes to cope with experiences known or thought to be painful. When confronted with new, potentially aversive experiences, children in the Ross and Ross (1982a) study reported the use of a variety of direct action strategies that could be described as *escape:*

> I heard my mom say we soon had to go to the doctor and I'd heard a lot of bad things about the doctor so I hid in my cupboard but she started yelling and getting real mad so I came out. (Boy, CA 6)

Children with extensive hospital experience, especially those who were undergoing painful treatment procedures, frequently used *postponement/avoidance* strategies:

> When they come for me I tell them it's the kid in the other bed. (Boy, CA 6, burn dressing, Savedra, 1980)

> I ask for a drink of water even though I'm not thirsty. (Girl, CA 8, leukemia, Ross & Ross, 1982a)

Cognitive Strategies

Attention diversion was widely used by children of all ages in the Ross and Ross (1982a) study and by many older children in other studies (Gaffney, 1983; Glick & Nakayama, 1985; Hilgard & LeBaron, 1984; Reissland, 1983). Children seemed to know that strong attention to an external stimulus or an internal activity could increase their pain tolerance. As one girl (CA 11, Gaffney, 1983) observed, "When you think about it, it always seems worse." In the Ross and Ross (1982a) study, 93 children reported the use of an active attention diversion strategy (Fernandez, 1986):

> I counted the tiles on the ceiling till I couldn't count any higher, then I started over and did it again. (Girl, CA 6, having a shot)

> Our dentist has this music, see, and I say to him turn it up real loud. . . . Then I pretend that I have to really *learn* the music, like the tune, or something terrible will happen to me. And I keep telling myself to listen, listen, listen, and after a while sometimes I almost don't know I'm getting drilled. (Girl, CA 11)

Imagery in the form of transformation of context was a strategy used by 17 children (Ross & Ross, 1982a). In this strategy the child acknowledges the presence of pain but transforms the setting in which the pain is occurring:

> I pretended I was in a space ship and the pressure was making my ears hurt and I was the only one that could get it back to earth. (Girl, CA 9, painful ear procedure)

Incompatible emotive imagery involves ignoring the pain by engaging in imagery/ fantasy that is incompatible with the experience of pain:

> I look at the animals on my pillow; just think about them walking about 'cause if I don't think [about the animals] I think of my tummy, but when I'm thinking it goes away. (Girl, Reissland, 1983)

> I just think about anything, just think I'm kind of on a holiday. (Older child, Reissland, 1983)

There is some evidence for developmental changes regarding coping strategies, with older children using coping strategies more often than younger ones (Jeans & Gordon, 1981; Reissland, 1983). There are no reports of sex differences, and reports are mixed on increases in the number of different coping strategies used by a child with increasing age. Children in the Ross and Ross (1982a) study occasionally reported that if one strategy did not work, they tried another, but this was as true for the younger children as for the older ones. However, Brown, O'Keefe, Sanders, and Baker (1986) reported an increase with age in the total number of different strategies that 8- to 18-year-old children said they would use in a hypothetical dental injection situation. In most of the studies, attention deployment was the strategy most frequently used; positive self-instruction was almost never reported by children, although some of the adolescents in Savedra et al.'s study (1985) reported such strategies as "think positive," "talk to self," and "prayer and turning to God." In Brown et al.'s study (1986), however, positive self-talk ("It's not so bad," "Be brave," and "I can take this") was the strategy most frequently chosen for coping with the hypothetical dental injection, and attention deployment was the second most commonly chosen strategy.

In the Ross and Ross (1982a) study there were two subgroups of children whose coping responses formed a pattern that represented a coping style. One group with juvenile arthritis ($n = 9$) actively confronted their pain by specifying their physical pain-free limits, keeping within them, and refusing to become depressed:

> I never do some things I'd like to do, and if I start slipping and doing them I just give myself a *terrible* lecture. And I never, ever let myself get sad about it. If I start getting sad I make myself think what are all the things I *can* do. I have to have a *lot* of talks with myself all the time. (Boy, CA 7)

The second group ($n = 89$) did not have any problem in common. They were referred to as "the Blithe Spirits" (Ross & Ross, 1984b) because of their unusual ability to take unpleasant events in their stride, view them realistically but also optimistically, and then move on. This coping ability was noticeable in their accounts of their hospitalization experiences as well as in their subsequent advice to same-age peers about to be hospitalized:

> You can make it awful or you can make it OK. (Girl, CA 9)

> Just go in there and have fun with the fun things and tell yourself it won't be long. (Boy, CA 9)

> Sure it hurts, but they help you when it does. (Boy, CA 10)

> It's [hospitalization] a whole new experience, you know, you need new things happening to you, or else you'll get in a rut. (Girl, CA 11)

A spot check with school principals showed that these children were highly regarded in the school setting while not excelling in any area. Their general psychosocial competence (Tyler, 1978) could be an antecedent of the characteristic called *hardiness* that Kobasa (1982) has identified in executives who have unusual ability to cope positively with stress. Hardiness involves three elements: a conviction that change in one's life is normal and exciting, with stress events perceived as an opportunity for personal growth; a feeling of commitment, a tendency to involve oneself fully in the many situations of life; and a sense of control over oneself and the events that happen, a tendency to believe and act as though one can influence the course of events. As one of the Blithe Spirits said, "It [hospitalization] can be awful only if you let it get you down, just remember you're in charge."

Comment

In mulling over the wealth of assorted ideas, procedures, and findings characteristic of the child-oriented approach to the search for information about the pain experience, it is possible to identify three potential sources of variation in children's responses to questions on pain, sources that are independent of the actual pain experienced by the children. The *location* of the interview causes differences in a child's response—whether it is the hospital, an ambulatory clinic, or school. The perceived *purpose* of the interview exerts an influence on his responses, as does the extent of his belief in their confidentiality. The *wording of the questions* is a prime source of variability, with seemingly minor changes having major effects. We have seen how statements such as "A pain is caused by . . ." elicit responses of quite a different nature than do statements requiring the child to "list three things that have caused you pain." Similarly, questions in the supplied format versus those in the generate format (Ross & Ross, 1984a), or oral versus written questions, all result in qualitative as well as quantitative differences in response. The interview format has the potential to be a highly useful tool in establishing a base of information about children's pain. If it is to achieve this potential, it is essential that the importance of these sources of variation be acknowledged and interview protocols be defined and standardized accordingly. If this were the case, conflicting results across studies could then be attributed with some confidence to genuine differences rather than to obvious procedural irregularities.

Specific Pain Experiences

Pain experiences can be classified in a number of different ways. Noordenbos (1984), in a description of adult pain, names four main categories: pain due to external events, pain due to internal events, pain associated with lesions of the nervous system, and pain associated with psychological, social, or environmental factors. Varni (1983) categorizes children's pain in terms of specific disease states, observable physical injury or trauma, sources difficult to identify such as recurrent abdominal pain syndrome, and medical/dental procedures. Attempts to categorize the pain experience inevitably run up against problems such as overlapping categories, single events having multiple causes, and continuum effects from degree of severity that can cut across source as a basis for placement in a category. Ross and Ross (1982a, 1985) found that the following seven categories best represented the pain experiences that were described by the children in their studies: common pain experiences, psychophysiological pain, acute pain, chronic pain, treatment-related pain, competency pain, and vicarious pain experiences. In the ensuing seven sections, all of the specific pain experiences and quotes relevant to them are from Ross and Ross (1982a) unless otherwise noted. Because of the large number of responses in several of the categories, answers representative of the range of childhood pain were selected in favor of a comprehensive report of childhood pain experiences. This selection was based on the relative frequency of pain experiences reported and has also been influenced by the extent to which the experience illustrates some particular aspect of pain as far as the child is concerned.

Although many of the responses were obtained by direct questions, for example, those concerned with treatment-related pain, a considerable number were adjuncts to questions on other topics and accounts of specific pains that occurred spontaneously in the children's answers because they were relevant. (Additional information obtained in this somewhat indirect way is one of the bonuses of open-ended interview questions with no time limit.) Very few responses were obtained about physical punishment because the wording of the questions intentionally and largely excluded this category of pain experience. Child abuse was never reported by the children nor was it suspected from their responses, but it does not necessarily follow that there were no instances of abuse in the children's past experiences.

The discussion of each of the seven categories of pain experience is based on a cluster of topics: What actual pain experiences were reported in the category? How does the child perceive the pain? How does he describe the pain? The reactive component? How well informed is the child on course, outcome, etiology, and management? Is his information accurate? What stands out about the reported pain experience?

Common Pain Experiences

Responses in this category were common pain events that were also in the mild to moderate range of pain intensity. Included here were lacerations, infections, insect bites, burns, sprains, and sore throats, as well as the moderately painful stomachaches, headaches, and earaches that many children experience but not so frequently as to categorize them as recurrent or chronic. The salient characteristic of the responses was the children's perception of these pain events as so commonplace as to be the norm. Typical of this attitude was the response of a nine-year-old girl:

> It's [earache from water in ear] a plugged-up kind of pushy feeling, you know? Like earmuffs inside my ears. Everyone gets them that goes swimming.

The perception of these pain experiences as the norm was reinforced by peer input and parental reactions. The tenor of peer comments conveyed a feeling of the inevitability of these events in the life cycle. A boy age 8 who described what appeared to be growing pains reported that his teen-age brother told him, "Don't get hypo, kid. Just live through it like the rest of us did." The perceived normality was further supported by the simplicity of the self-treatment procedures advocated by peers, for example, for earaches attributed to water in the ear, "bite down real hard on a carrot or a stick" or "stand on your head and shake all over like jelly."

Parental reaction as well as management generally conveyed further reassurance. Often the only changes in the child's routine were absence from school, nonprescription analgesics, and rest. Working parents were sometimes openly resentful about the child's being home, a reaction that further satisfied the child that there was no need to be anxious. As a girl of seven explained, "It [stomachache] wasn't anything bad 'cos my mom was *real* mad about having to stay home." There was also great confidence in the mothers' management of these pain events: A boy age 8 said, "My mom knows exactly what to do, like she's already been through this [stomachache] a zillion times with Marty and Eddie [brothers]."

The only pain descriptors used were sensory terms equivalent to those in the mild range on the McGill Pain Questionnaire (Melzack, 1975), such as "pinching," "sharp," "jumpy," and "hurting." No child expressed any anxiety about these common pains or reported the use of coping strategies. The absence of any feeling of anxiety was underscored by qualifiers that emphasized the relative unimportance of these pain events:

> It [a minor burn] only hurted like a blister from new shoes. (Girl, CA 5)

> It's [lower limb pains, probably growing pains] just a part of living. (Boy, CA 9)

Psychophysiological Pain

Pain that occurs in the absence of a detectable organic base and is more easily understood in psychological terms is often called *psychogenic* (Sternbach, 1984). Because this term may be interpreted as implying that the pain involved is imagined or inconsequential we prefer the descriptor *psychophysiological pain*. Although there is no discernible physical cause, there is no question that the pain exists. The children reported two kinds of psychophysiological stomach pain. The first kind were tension-related stomachaches that occurred irregularly, were generally associated with a specific anxiety-producing event, and disappeared as soon as the event was over. The children had a passive attitude about these pains, even in the light of obvious discomfort, and had no thoughts about how they might be prevented. One girl (CA 10) commented placidly, "I'll probably have one on my wedding day." The following quotes are representative of the children's descriptions of their discomfort:

> It really gets tight like this [clenches fist]. It feels so tight it's going to burst. (Girl, CA 6, before a piano recital)

> Agonizing like a big knot in your stomach. (Girl, CA 11, before a swimming race)

The other kind of stomach pains in this category were regularly recurring stomachaches with no known cause that appeared to meet Apley's (1975) criteria for recurrent abdominal pain (RAP). All of the children had had four or more attacks of pain over a period of three months, with most experiencing one to four episodes per month, and had seen doctors for their stomach problem. The majority reported that their symptoms were usually short lived although often severe enough to interfere with the daily routine. For reviews of the RAP phenomenon, see Apley (1975), Barr and Feuerstein (1983), and Levine and Rappaport (1984). The children generally used sensory terms in the moderate range on the McGill Pain Questionnaire (Melzack, 1975):

> It feels like a bone scratching another bone. I get this sharp pain and it kind of paralyzes me for a few seconds. (Boy, CA 9)

> It makes you want to bend over, it hurts a lot, it's there all the time. (Boy, CA 9)

The accounts of RAP were notably lacking in affect: Although the children were acutely uncomfortable, they were not anxious, afraid, or miserable. One reason was the commonality of stomachaches in general, but more important was the fact that the children were, from personal experience, well informed on course and outcome. They were secure in the knowledge that the stomachaches had always disappeared completely and that there was no evidence of organic etiological factors. While they did not know the cause, neither did their pediatricians or parents. In addition, they were well informed on management: They sought help from their mothers, and variously used rest, relaxation, heat, and sleep.

Despite these apparently desirable reactions, which were almost certain to have been rewarded by parents and others, we view the passivity characteristic of these children as cause for concern. Consider, for example, that no child attempted to impose any meaning on this puzzling condition by generating his own hypotheses in an attempt to understand it. Moreover, in response to direct questioning, no child reported using self-generated cognitive strategies or any other self-help procedure but instead relied passively on externally supplied treatment. In marked contrast to the children with arthritis or leukemia (Ross & Ross, 1982a), the RAP children made no attempt to confront the problem. Their passivity conforms in some ways to the avoidance strategy that Lethem et al. (1983) have proposed as an explanation for the process whereby some adult chronic pain patients develop a more substantial psychological overlay to their pain problem than others do, a process which may be instrumental in promoting the development of invalid status.

Acute Pain

The pain experiences described here included intense physical trauma such as severe earaches, cramps, abscessed teeth, throat infections, and appendicitis as well as accident-related injuries such as lacerations, burns, fractures, and sprains. Although many of these pain experiences overlap the category of common pains, their severity justifies their inclusion here.

The children clearly viewed these pain experiences as landmark events, with the intensity of the pain compounded by the anxiety-arousing consequences: the presence of one or both parents, their obvious concern, the immediacy of medical consultation and treatment action that in some cases required an ambulance, the tension of the emergency room, and the speed with which hospital admission was accomplished. What stood out most in their accounts were the multiple sources of anxiety, some of which underscore the divergent perceptions of child and parent of the meaning of behaviors intended to express parental concern or provide comfort.

For the homebound child, the major source of anxiety appeared to be the complete break in the normal routine: The child often lost normal social contacts, was sometimes severely restricted in terms of diet and activity, relinquished customary chores, and was exempt from all responsibilities. During the peak pain period the child was often terrified by the possible implications of such indulgence. In several instances these fears were enhanced by television-mediated fantasies in which unusual parental kindness and privileges were associated with a child dying.

For the child in the hospital, the rapid transition to an unfamiliar setting often resulted in a frightening feeling of disorientation: A 6-year-old girl described it as "like out in space, like I changed to someone else," and a boy age 7 said plaintively, "I could see the clock—it was almost dinner time—and I shoulda been watching TV—and instead I get put on a cart and all the people have creepy clothes and you can't hear them when they walk and they sorta whisper." Many of the hospitalized children reported feelings of helplessness that were often heightened by the apparent abdication of responsibility on the part of their parents in compliance with the doctors' decisions. The unpredictable character of the whole event coupled with the often sudden, intense pain apparently left the children no time to muster psychological resources. Coping strategies were seldom reported, and when they were, they usually consisted of either attempts to relax and go to sleep in the hope that it "would all be over" when the child woke up or wish-fulfilling fantasies. A girl age 7, hospitalized with second-degree burns, said:

> I just kept thinking what an awful dream this was and how real it all looked and how the burn felt just like a real burn.

The sensory descriptors used generally represented the extremes in the subclasses on the McGill Pain Questionnaire (Melzack, 1975), with words such as "pounding," "stabbing," "cutting," "stinging," "aching," and "crushing" appearing frequently. The accounts were often affect laden:

> It was a hideous, torture pain. (Boy, CA 7, broken ribs)

> It was like a terrible, ghastly nightmare that never stopped. (Girl, CA 10, burn)

> It was like a mean rat gnawing at me in a vicious way. (Girl, CA 11, abdominal injury)

This high-affect component is particularly interesting in view of Melzack, Wall, and Ty's (1982) finding that adults in an emergency room setting rarely used affective descriptors in discussing their acute trauma.

Although some children were promptly and accurately informed about the course of the pain, particularly that it was time limited and the prognosis was favorable, a number were not given this reassurance. This latter group mainly comprised those who had been unexpectedly hospitalized: Generally they were not informed because their parents did not know what to tell them and the medical staff were too involved in coping with the pain problem to spend time on explanations. For many children, this uncertainty created a near-panic state:

> Like what if they could never stop it [the pain] and it just went on and on like this and I stopped screaming inside and just went crazy. (Girl, CA 11, with multiple car accident injuries)

Chronic Pain

Of the chronic pain conditions in the Ross and Ross (1982a) study, some, such as chronic headaches, stomachaches, and earaches, occurred aperiodically, with relatively long periods in which the child was pain free and not incapacitated in any way. By comparison, children with juvenile rheumatoid arthritis (JRA) typically experience more frequent bouts of pain and are more limited physically than those in the other groups. Because JRA data are more representative of the trials of pediatric chronic pain, they are discussed in some detail here. Almost all of the 19 children interviewed were patients in a hospital/clinic (Children's Hospital at Stanford, California) noted for the excellence of its treatment regimen as well as for the superior results of its programs. A long-term follow-up study of adults who as children had been treated in this hospital (Miller, Spitz, Simpson & Williams, 1982) showed that although the condition continued into adulthood, they were, within limits (certain sports being ruled out), able to live normal lives. Consequently, the children's reactions discussed here may be representative of JRA under excellent management rather than of JRA in general.

Although children with JRA are often depicted as not complaining about pain and as having less pain than adults (Scott, Ansell, & Huskisson, 1977), there is no question that these children do experience pain (Thompson, Varni, & Hanson, 1988). In our study (Ross & Ross, 1982a) the JRA children described three distinct arthritis-related pain experiences. One of these was arthritic pain that was seen more as an annoyance than as a troubling pain, probably because it could be controlled effectively with medication. The sensory descriptors used were generally mild ones (Melzack, 1975), such as "hurt," "dull ache," an "aching feeling," or a "dull constant pain." A 7-year-old girl complained, "It's like having your hands and feet and knees all puffed up and all the things that bend hurt."

A second category of JRA pain experience included more intense pain from overexertion or from engaging in a forbidden activity. In this group of JRA children, activity limitation varied both within and between children so that sometimes a child could be quite active and at other times even a minimal amount of activity caused him pain. For some children, the limitation applied only to competitive sports; for others, the restriction was much more general, with the child almost always severely restricted, in a wheelchair, or on crutches. In this category, the pain experience was responsive to medication, heat, rest, and therapeutic exercise, and the children generally considered it to be under their own control:

> You can't do the same things other people can do because it would make my arthritis worse—I just have to be careful and if my ankles swell I know I have done too much. (Girl, CA 11)

Only occasionally did they report difficulty in striking a balance:

> When you get a flare-up it's caused from overdoing it—too much walking or exercise—but if you don't do enough exercise you get sore. If you do too much you get sore, so it's frustrating. (Girl, CA 10)

It was clear from the descriptors used that the pain of overexertion was troubling:

> Like someone hitting, hitting you. (Boy, CA 9, pain in hip)

> A burning, itching feeling; it really hurts. (Girl, 11, pain in legs)

> It's hot, shooting, stinging; it never stops. (Boy, CA 10)

In the third category of JRA pain were the spontaneous flare-ups that required medical attention and were by far the most severe of the arthritis-related pains:

> It's like sore when you move, it's like having this sharp pain all over you or just hurting you or burning you. (Girl, CA 11)

> It starts off very gradually and works its way 'til it gets to its peak. It will die down eventually but it hurts a lot. (Girl, CA 11)

> It feels like agonizing pain, like you are going to die and you can't put up with it any more. (Girl, CA 11)

How the child perceives the pain of arthritis is, to a considerable extent, a function of age, level of cognitive development, and, to a lesser extent, time since onset (Beales, Holt, Keen, & Mellor, 1983). Children eight years old and younger, who were generally at the preoperational stage (Piaget, 1973) and whose arthritis was of recent origin, were living in the present. These children seemed to view their condition as transient and were more angry and resentful about the curtailment of activities than concerned about the nature of the disease:

> It hurts, it's terrible, like the other kids don't have to stay in a wheelchair sometimes or walk on crutches or anything like that . . . but I have to do that stuff. They don't. (Girl, CA 8)

With increasing age, the children's understanding of arthritis and its implications for the future also developed (Beales, Holt, Keen, & Mellor, 1983). The older children perceived the pain as a relatively permanent state of existence. Although they were clearly aware that the pain would vary in presence and intensity, they believed, often erroneously (Miller et al., 1982), that the general arthritic condition was unlikely to improve greatly or disappear. One 10-year-old boy who felt that the pain was "always lying in wait for me to slip up," said sadly, "This is going to be my life and I just have to live with it." The older JRA children tended to attribute a more negative meaning to their pain, in part because they were more able to understand the etiological implications of their internal pathology (Beales, Keen, & Holt, 1983). Viewing the pain as a life sentence often caused them more concern than the pain itself. Although some depression is almost inevitable in a child who has experienced pain for a year or more (Masek, Russo, & Varni, 1984), the older children tended to face it squarely:

> It just hurts a lot and you get frustrated . . . and you've got to be real strong and not let it get to you. (Girl, CA 11)

> It really gets me down some days and then I get myself up, you know? I think if I just fight it I can overcome it cause like the doctors are trying to help me, like they are going to put new kneecaps in me . . . give me new hips and straighten my fingers (Girl, CA 10)

Only occasionally was there evidence in this group of the lack of confidence and feelings of inadequacy described by Morpurgo, Nobili, Leonardi, Casati, and Cacciabue (1984).

We attribute the children's psychological strength at least in part to the most striking feature of this group, that is, the way adults treated them. The children were very knowledgeable about management procedures, were actively involved members of the treatment team, regarded their input in the periodic evaluations as valuable, and had great respect for their doctors. The older children had a mature understanding of their disease that could be attributed to careful explanations appropriate for their cognitive levels. None of the environmental influences that are a force in turning an adult with chronic arthritis into a chronic pain syndrome patient (Fordyce, 1976, 1978) appeared to be present. These children generally tried to confront the problems associated with the disease and to engage in a range of acceptable physical and social activities whenever a lull occurred in the pain and related symptoms.

Wright (1960) has described the tendency of adults to add irrelevant restrictions to those that are relevant to the disease, thus creating the "spread phenomenon" that eventually leads to a devaluing of the child's self-concept. Irrelevant restrictions appeared not to have been imposed on these children, nor was there any indication of an excess of parental intrusion. Although the children's comments indicated the closeness that often typifies the family of a child with long-term illness (Ferrari, 1984), there was no suggestion of the pattern of extreme proximity and intensity in family relations that Minuchin et al. (1975) have termed *enmeshment*. Within their physical limitations they did not receive special privileges from parents, teachers, or pediatric personnel. Typically, they attended school regularly and were assigned household chores. They were not allowed to use their pain for secondary gains or encouraged to dwell on their conditions. Compliance with exercise and medication regimens, which was reportedly high, was often largely the child's responsibility. Although younger children frequently described the firmness of parents and pediatric personnel as mean and unsympathetic, the older ones saw it as tough and caring. Evidence that such firmness in adults provides immediate and potential long-term benefits is contained in a recent study (Dunn-Geier, McGrath, Rourke, Latter, & D'Astous, 1986). For a thoughtful commentary on the advantages to the child of having tough and caring adults see Beales, Holt, Keen, and Mellor (1983).

Treatment-Related Pain

Treatment-related pain refers to pain that accompanies routine therapeutic interventions. The descriptor carries with it no implication of carelessness or negligence, and although the element of professional skill may reduce the pain somewhat, it cannot eliminate it. The pain experiences included in this category range from those occurring in the treatment of life-threatening diseases, such as leukemia and sickle-cell anemia, to those associated with minimal-risk interventions in which the goals are improved functioning (joint replacement, hemodialysis) sometimes accompanied by cosmetic gains (orthodontistry, plastic surgery). The clusters of pain experiences involved in the treatment procedures used in leukemia and orthodontistry are discussed here.

Leukemia

In a recent study of the prevalence and etiology of pain in children and adolescents with leukemia and other cancers, Miser, Dothage, Wesley, and Miser (1987) reported a predominance of treatment-related over tumor-related pain. In the Ross and Ross interview study (1982a), children with leukemia reported two categories of treatment-related pain. The first of these, headaches and bone pain, occurred as side effects of the intensive multiple-drug long-term chemotherapy that constitutes the core of a treatment regimen that pushes the child to the brink of death in order to kill the leukemic cells (Hilgard & LeBaron, 1984). The second category included pain experiences resulting from the regularly occurring invasive procedures used to assess the status of the disease, that is, finger sticks, venipuncture, lumbar puncture, and bone marrow aspiration. In order to provide a base for the interpretation of the children's reports, each of these procedures is described briefly.

Finger sticks involve pricking the child's finger with a fine-gauge needle and squeezing gently to obtain a small amount of blood. For larger amounts of blood, *venipuncture* is used. The major source of pain here is the larger-gauge needle, although some discomfort also arises from the tourniquet that is fastened tightly around the arm to make the vein more prominent. *Lumbar puncture* is used to withdraw cerebrospinal fluid needed to determine the presence or absence of leukemic cells. With the child lying on his side in a fetal position with chin touching chest, novocaine is usually injected first and then a fine-gauge needle is inserted between the fourth and fifth lumbar vertebrae into the subarachnoid space containing the fluid. If all goes well there is a stinging sensation as the needle is inserted, followed by mild pressure; however, sometimes the doctor is unable to locate the right spot during the first entry and must insert the needle again. The pain may be severe if the needle is pushed against the surface of the vertebral bone. *Bone marrow aspiration* is generally regarded by patients and clinicians as the most painful of these four procedures (Schorlemer, 1984; Zeltzer, Kellerman, Ellenberg, Dash & Rigler, 1980). A large-gauge needle is pushed into the hipbone in order to withdraw a sample of marrow for examination. With this procedure there are three sources of discomfort: a sharp stinging pain as the needle penetrates the skin, pain and heavy pressure as the needle penetrates the periosteum (covering of the bone), and finally, an intense, excruciating pain as the sample of bone marrow is sucked into the needle (see Cameron and Wallace [1983] for a child's account of this procedure). Although the suction pain may be brief and localized, it is reported by some patients to remain in the entire upper leg for 30 seconds or more. Local anesthesia can alter the degree of pain felt when the large bone marrow needle penetrates the sensitive outer tissues and possibly the periosteum, but it cannot eliminate it. Short of a general anaesthetic, there is no medication that can be counted on to make this pain more bearable (Hilgard & LeBaron, 1984).

Many children described these treatment-related pains as worse than the disease itself, a finding that is consistent with other reports (Bruce, 1983; Schorlemer, 1984; Zeltzer et al., 1980). Sensory descriptors were used almost exclusively for the headaches, bone pain, finger sticks, and venipuncture. Most of the children described the bone pain as in the heart of the bone:

> It felt like the bone in my leg had a match right in the middle of it. It burned. (Boy, CA 6)

> It was like a deep ache, like you could never get in that far. (Girl, CA 10)

Affective descriptors predominated in the accounts of the more painful and, to the child living in the shadow of remission, more threatening lumbar punctures and bone marrow aspirations. Lumbar punctures were described as "cruel," "mean," and "a terrible shock-like stab." A boy (CA 10) said, "It's like your body is giving you a vicious beating," and a girl age 12 complained that she felt "terrible, miserable." There was no question that the bone marrow aspiration was viewed as the most painful: It was variously described as "an exhausting pain," "the most hateful thing you can think of," and pain beyond description: "I don't have any words to tell how much it hurts."

Although the withdrawal of bone marrow was regarded as very painful ("It's a real aching pain, it makes you feel like you have a lot of bruises on your legs" Girl, CA 10), the general consensus was that the feeling of pain and heavy pressure as the needle penetrates the periosteum was the worst:

> You get *instant* pain like a bee stinging you. (Boy, CA 6)

> It hurt like a big giant heavy bomb was going to fall on me. Like it was going to explode in my back. (Boy, CA 9)

> When they put the main needle in—it's a real punch in the back. (Boy, CA 11)

The children were knowledgeable and accurate about the assessment procedures and why the methods used in each one were essential:

> The part that hurts the most is when they put in the numbing medicine, but if they didn't then the other part would hurt. (Boy, CA 7, bone marrow aspiration)

With the exception of very recently diagnosed cases, the children perceived the occurrence of both categories of treatment-related pain as unavoidable and the price of survival. The severity of the pain was seen as evidence that the enemy was a formidable one. That even the youngest children (CA 5 and 6) were well aware that they were engaged in a life and death struggle was evident in their drawings of fierce battles waged between the chemotherapeutic agents, depicted as "good guys," and the immature white blood cells, the "bad guys." The children rarely complained about finger sticks and venipunctures, the exceptions being the recently diagnosed cases. In the latter group, for example, a girl, age 7 said "It's [finger stick] stab, stab, stab, sometimes a lot in one day. My fingers hurt even before they do it." But as these children gradually came to view the pain event as being associated with a highly meaningful outcome, they dismissed the relatively minor pains of these procedures as unimportant:

> It's (venipuncture) so quick, it's like a cut, a sharp pain, you go like 'ouch' then it's finished. (Boy, CA 8)

This change in perception of the pain event is consistent with the conclusions of Scott and Gijsbers (1981), Thompson (1981), and others that reports of pain may decrease when the patient perceives the relevance of pain to outcome.

In this study (Ross & Ross, 1982a), no questions were asked about the course of the disease or its outcome, and the children never initiated any discussion about either topic. According to the medical personnel (Walsh, 1981) at the hospital and reports from other medical settings (Ross, M., & Ross, A. P., 1980; Schorlemer, 1984) there was no question that the children were well aware of these facets of the disease. They were also clearly well informed on the etiology of it: Neither directly nor indirectly did any child suggest that he entertained thoughts of an immanent justice link.

The most noteworthy characteristics of the leukemia group were their commitment to the life and death struggle and their confidence in the pediatric staff. In the following quote from an 11-year-old boy in his second remission, note how his personification of the disease enabled him to conceptualize the adversary in a form that he could grapple with:

> It's me against him [leukemia]. It [bone marrow aspiration] hurts a lot but I can beat him. He thinks I'll give up because it hurts so much but I won't. Just go ahead and hurt all you want, you won't get me to quit.

The children clearly believed that what was being done was in their best interest and that no matter how painful the treatment, the pediatric staff were doing their best. These beliefs should act to reduce pain or, at least, not to enhance it:

> I fairly agree with all their stuff [tests] 'cause I know they have to do it. . . . They are trying to make it as easy as possible. (Boy, CA 11)

Orthodontistry

The peak pain periods reported by children ($n = 41$) undergoing orthodontistry (Ross & Ross, 1982a) centered around the initial fitting of the braces; the periodic adjustment to them, particularly tightening; and between treatment discomfort resulting from the adjustments. The descriptors used were, in terms of the McGill Pain Questionnaire (Melzack, 1975), almost all sensory, ranging from mild ("tingling," "dull," "sharp," "pricking," "sore," "pressuring") to moderate ("hurting," "stretching," "pulling") and severe ("stinging," "knifing," "aching"). The most commonly used affective descriptors were "scared," "anxious," "glad," and "angry." The main area of focus for anger and resentment centered on the orthodontists' lack of compassion and sympathy. One-third of the children were clearly resentful about this and reported that the orthodontist either did not respond to their complaints of pain or merely agreed passively that the procedures were painful. However, it was clear that many of the orthodontists had spent time on explanations of the problem and process, because almost without exception the children were knowledgeable about them and generally perceived most of the ensuing pain as unavoidable.

In conjunction with this study (Ross & Ross, 1982a) a group of adults ($n = 23$) was questioned about their childhood orthodontic pain experiences. Most recalled mild pain during the initial fitting and adjustment sessions, with only sporadic discomfort between treatment sessions. Their accounts were in marked contrast to those of the children, for whom the treatment-related pain was seen as more severe and more frequent: More than half of the children reported moderate to severe pain during the initial fitting that sometimes persisted for a week or more. As one girl (CA 10) said, "It was like an enormous toothache that went on and on." More than half also reported considerable pain during the subsequent orthodontic sessions as well as in the interim periods:

When he's doing it [tightening the braces] it's like one big dagger after another right into my teeth. (Girl, CA 11)

It wasn't an agony pain [after he got home] but it was almost one. (Boy, CA 10)

The possibility was explored that the difference between the accounts of the two age groups could be attributed to the currently used shorter, more intensive, and consequently more painful treatment approach. Support for this explanation was provided by the reports (Ross, D. M., 1986) of 14 young adults currently undergoing orthodontistry. Twelve of this group agreed with the children that both the initial fitting and the subsequent adjustments sessions were very painful:

It's like a knife going in a long way and then he [dentist] twists it and he keeps on twisting. (Male, CA 32)

It was one of the most unpleasant pains I've ever experienced. (Female, CA 24)

The salient feature of the children's reports was their firm commitment to completing the treatment, however painful. Their sense of commitment stemmed from multiple sources: the expectation of cosmetic and dental health gains, awareness of the financial costs for their parents and appreciation of other forms of parental support throughout the treatment period, and absence of any braces-associated stigma on the part of their peer group. Furthermore, these children all believed that they had had a choice in the initial decision and subsequent treatment, a belief that is questionable, and the stamina factor was operating in their favor since in all other respects they appeared to be in good physical condition.

Competency Pain

Pains that result from sports-related and vocational training activities, such as gymnastics, tennis, dancing, and figure skating, are referred to as *competency pains*. These pains are a relatively recent phenomenon in children: prior to the late 1950s some competency pains, such as stress fractures, were virtually unheard of in this age group. However, with the advent at that time of highly organized sports training for children (Micheli, 1983), the frequency of competency pains increased sharply, a trend that has continued at an ever-increasing rate.

In the Ross and Ross studies (1982a, 1985) three general types of competency pain were reported, the first being sudden-onset injuries that occur during a specific training session or competition and usually result in acute pain such as a sprained ankle. The second type included pains from maltraining and overuse: Common here were tendinitis of the shoulder and stress fractures. The latter are most often associated with an excessive rate and intensity of training, the classic example being "Little League elbow." The third type of pains were those that appeared to be tension-related, since the temporal point of onset was precompetition rather than postexertion. These pains included headaches, stomachaches and chest pains. Although they were described in our group as precompetition pains, they can also occur as postexertion pains. Massey (1982), for example, has reported a migrainous type of effort headache in runners, and Rooke (1968) has described a vascular exertional headache in athletes. It should also be noted that the tension-related pains logically fall in the category of psychophysiological pain described earlier. However, the children's responses about tension pains related specifically to athletic activities formed such a tight cluster that we chose to discuss them here.

Injuries incurred during training and especially those that occurred during a performance were perceived with dismay unrelated to the pain when, of necessity, physical activity was terminated:

> But the worst is when you twist your ankle or something and you have to miss the whole practice . . . and the other kids are getting ahead of you. (Boy, CA 10, gymnast)

Typically, the children regarded overuse injuries as status symbols and obtained the misguided satisfaction from them that is often characteristic of older highly motivated athletes (Schollander & Savage, 1971). A boy gymnast (CA 10) with a serious stress fracture said with obvious pride, "Everyone knows you don't get one of *these* by just fooling round on the beginner bars"; a dancer (Girl, CA 12) was "thrilled" the first time her toes bled; and a boy (CA 9) enrolled in tournament tennis viewed his tendinitis as evidence that he was "going the limit." Tension-related pains, however, were viewed as commonplace and as part of the price of becoming a star:

> Boy (CA 10): Sure I get stomachaches—all the best ones [swimmers] get them, too. . . . If you aren't uptight before the race you won't do good.
> Interviewer: Does the stomachache go once you get started?
> Boy: I don't know because I just think of winning but it's mostly gone in the locker room unless I do real bad.

Although the sensory descriptors used for competency pains were among the more severe on the McGill Pain Questionnaire (Melzack, 1975) (for example, "aching," "burning," "shooting," "stabbing," "pounding," "crushing," "boiling," "tearing") the children almost invariably emphasized that "they didn't seem that bad right at the time." Affective descriptors were rarely used to describe competency-related pain experiences, but they were frequently used in the children's accounts of their frustration and anxiety over interruptions in their training schedules.

The children's reports of their competency pains serve to emphasize once again the complexity of the pain experience in general. One cluster of responses centered around pain that occurred during the ongoing activity but which the child tried or was pressured to ignore in order to continue with the activity:

> It was like a knife, you know, like stabbing and shooting way up in my shoulder and I started to sweat real heavy but you can't ever stop in a ranking competition. (Boy, CA 11, gymnast)

My chest was just a big, bursting pain and my legs felt like red-hot pokers and [coach] says, "O.K., Palmer, two more laps." The pain was so bad I wished I was dead. He does it *every* time. (Boy, CA 10, sprinter)

The ability to tolerate relatively brief periods of intense pain should not be interpreted as evidence of a generally high pain tolerance in these children. It is more likely to be a situation-specific increase in tolerance (Scott & Gijsbers, 1981) that has resulted from the contingencies in the training/performance arena. In the present study, this explanation is supported by the finding that these children expressed the same aversion to pain events, such as shots and needles, that were unrelated to training as did other children in the interview study (Ross & Ross, 1982a; 1984b). That this situation-specific increased tolerance might not generalize to other pain situations is consistent with the *radical behavioral model* of pain proposed by Jaremko, Silbert, and Mann (1981). According to this model, pain is a specific kind of self-talk or self-awareness of the physical changes that occur when an individual experiences averse stimulation (a punisher). In order for pain to be perceived, the individual must give verbal attention to the punisher, that is, he must label it as pain. Children learn through a process of differential reinforcement to label certain punishers as pain and to attach different labels to other kinds of aversive stimulation that on an objective basis appear to be equally uncomfortable. The model can therefore account for intra- and interindividual differences in pain reactivity. Because a child has learned to label many of the discomforts inherent in the competency training situation as "not pain" (or as one enthusiastic young gymnast explained, "not *real* pain"), it does not follow that the tolerance he has developed in the competency/training arena will generalize to other situations, in which his reinforcement history as well as the environmental cues are quite different.

A second cluster described experiences in which the child felt no pain at the time, although in the light of the injuries pain should have been present. The excitement of the competition or performance apparently masked the perception of it, or, in terms of the radical behavior model (Jaremko et al., 1981), absorption in the performance or the game prevented verbal attention to the punisher:

On stage, you're not aware of the pain. It's before and after. (Girl, ballet dancer, Treaster [1978])

I was coming off of the field and this other guy goes, "Hey, look at your knee," and it was all bloody and swollen and I never had felt anything in the whole game, but right when he said it, it started to hurt like crazy. (Boy, CA 11, soccer injury)

The assumption in this model that the pain must be learned in order to be perceived is contrary to a substantive body of clinical and empirical evidence, and consequently, the utility of the model is limited. It is reported here, however, because of its explanatory power in the competency pain situation.

The children were exceptionally well informed about all aspects of their injuries, particularly in respect to etiology and future prevention of recurrences. They were able to discourse knowledgeably about tendinitis, stress fractures, flexibility, shin splints, bursitis, muscle-tendon tightness, and the like. Top priority was given to recovery and compliance with all phases of the treatment regimen. Pressure to comply was exerted by trainers and parents, but the most powerful sources appeared to be top-ranked professionals in the child's field, who, in theoretical terms, became mastery models (Thelen, Fry, Fehrenbach, & Frautschi, 1979) for the children:

> Every time I did it [therapeutic exercise for severe shoulder injury] I coulda screamed. It was like a red-hot dagger plunging in but I didn't scream, not once. I just kept telling myself,"You think Jimmy Connors doesn't have pain lots worse than this? You think *he* screams? You wanna be a top rank?" (Boy, CA 10, in a tournament tennis school)

In fact, the mastery models played an incredibly important role in permeating all aspects of the child's pursuit of the goal. They were a potent force in the pattern of unreasonable dedication to one activity that many of the children exhibited to the exclusion of other childhood pleasures. They were an "inspiration" to coaches and ambitious parents who were making financial and other sacrifices. Although these latter groups emphasized display rules (Ekman & Friesen, 1969) for behavior during competitions ("Don't cry, don't give your opponent the edge by knowing you're hurt"), it was the mastery models who exerted the greatest influence. Children recounted how they closely watched stars known to be injured for any evidence of pain; how this ability to not show pain in competition, training, or treatment became their goal, along with not withdrawing from a competition because of pain. Consider, for example, the powerful modeling effect provided by Delia Peters of the New York City Ballet when she fractured her wrist during a solo (Treaster, 1978, p. 31):

> I stood up and I knew something was wrong with my hand. From the side it was the shape of an 'S'; and I couldn't lift it. Of course, all this went through my head in a split second. Then I said, 'Where am I in the music?' and I just picked it up again.

Vicarious Television-Mediated Pain Experiences

To obtain data on sources of pain information, children ($n = 844$) were asked questions about their television-mediated pain experiences (Ross & Ross, 1982a, 1985, 1986). It was clear from their responses that when they were watching television for recreational reasons their interpretations of pain events were grossly inaccurate. The children did not recognize the large majority of pain events as pain. When asked if they had seen anything about pain on television, fewer than 20 children could recall ever having seen any incident. This finding is particularly disturbing in view of the high frequency of pain-producing aggression sequences on television, such as murder, rape, and torture, combined with the high national average for number of hours per week spent by children in watching television. A further check was made by asking children ($n = 35$) age 8 and 9 who were known on the preceding day to have watched specific programs in which painful events had occurred what they could remember of a pain-related nature (Ross & Ross, 1985). Only four of the children could identify anything. When the remaining children were then asked about a specific event that had occurred in one of the programs (a child beaten up by other children on his way home from school), they conceded that it must have been painful, however, they had not on their own interpreted the event in this way. Furthermore, in both studies (Ross & Ross, 1982a, 1985) those who did report such events appeared to be totally unmoved by the experience. Their responses suggested that the pain was no more real to them than the pain in cartoons and comic strips. In fact, the children often seemed to perceive such events within an entertainment framework. Typical of these responses was that of a boy age 8 who reported enthusiastically:

> It was totally neat—they had these flame thrower things. . . . This [Vietnamese] family was all just standing there and the next second they were burned up.

In sharp contrast were their reports of pain experiences in their own lives, which showed clearly that they were capable of empathy. The boy quoted above, for example, cried when he talked about his dog being run over.

Although the responses to direct questions about pain events on television suggested that this medium's contribution to the children's concepts of pain is a negative one, it was clear from other response data that television's contribution can be positive under the following two conditions: When the program content was highly relevant to the child's interests, he assessed the pain sequence accurately and empathized with it. Those interested in sports or ballet, for example, reported in detail on how stars performed in spite of being in pain and were clearly appalled at falls and other injuries incurred during performance. When the program content was the only source of information available to the child about an impending pain event or diagnosis of illness for which he had no previous relevant first-hand experience, he retrieved "facts" from the program in an attempt to impose meaning on the fear-arousing event. The effect of television was to shape the child's expectancies about the event:

> He [doctor] said I gotta have it [appendix] taken out and I said OK. . . . I seen that on *Mister Rogers* and I know all what it's like. . . . It's OK. (Boy, CA 6)

> I never knew no person who got it but I was real scared 'cos like this old guy on TV had it [arthritis] his whole life. He couldn't bend his fingers, or hardly walk, and even when he was *real* still it hurt a lot. . . . I thought that's how I'll be. . . . I started to cry (Boy, CA 8)

With the exception of duration of specific pain events, information obtained in this way was often surprisingly accurate. Television, with its short programs, often distorts the time frame of events so that children's expectancies about the duration of the real-life pain event were highly inaccurate. For example, one child who had just been diagnosed as leukemic expected to die almost immediately, and another child with second-degree burns could not understand why he needed a series of treatments.

Comment

A base of information about children and adolescents' views of pain and their pain experiences is of critical importance to progress in understanding childhood pain. In the past decade the beginning of such an information base has emerged in a small, but highly informative, group of publications describing this age group's views of their pain experiences. The basic method of data collection has been some variant of the interview format, ranging from individual interviews to group administration of written interview questions. Overall, this approach has proved to be a productive one in terms of information yield, and there is no question that continued and further refinements should be pursued. However, in the interview situation some children were monosyllabic, no matter how skilled the interviewer (Ross & Ross, 1982a). Often the same children subsequently became almost voluble in a peer discussion group on the same topics. It follows that if the embryo base of information that we now have is to grow, it is essential that the medium used be one that enables the child to communicate freely and to the best of his ability.

Of relevance here is the concept of *fit,* that is, of harmony between the child and some social or nonsocial environmental event. This construct is assuming increasing importance in the literature: For example, Lazarus (1984) discusses stress as inharmonious individual-environment fit; Whalen and Henker (1980) have studied hyperactive children in terms of child × classroom fit; and Williams, Thompson, Haber, and Raczynski (1986) have focused on the headache patient in relation to treatment protocol fit. Of concern here is the identification of the medium best suited to the child's optimum mode of communication, that is, a child × communication medium fit. Investigators should pursue the available media with receptivity to alternatives to the standard interview format, with particular emphasis on the child's developmental level. Many young children will discourse freely with the help of a discussion prop such as a puppet, picture, or toy telephone. Jeans and Gordon (1981) obtained a wealth of descriptive data about pain by having children draw a picture of a pain experience and then talk about it. Diaries have considerable appeal, especially for girls. Taping diary entries would be particularly appropriate for children with chronic pain conditions such as JRA. These children would also enjoy reporting on their ongoing pain experience on a telephone "hot line." Classroom debates on pain issues such as the advantages and disadvantages of prior information about an impending pain event have been immensely productive (Ross & Ross, 1985). Retrospective accounts should not be overlooked here as a potentially valuable source of information. There are a number of instances (see, for example, Bruce, 1983, on leukemia, or Rosenbaum, 1984, on Legg-Perthe's disease) of an older child or adolescent remembering a pain event vividly and having the prerequisite verbal or writing skills.

All too often in the literature successful early work inadvertently has a restricting influence on subsequent investigations by focusing attention on one mode or procedure. It is essential that this narrowing of vision not occur in the burgeoning field of childhood pain.

3
Determinants of Pain

Any attempts at understanding the complexity of the pain experience must take into account the marked differences in pain reactivity that occur in situations in which the degree of aversive stimulation is apparently the same for all individuals. In routine immunizations in clinic or school settings, for example, the range of response is quite remarkable: At one extreme are the infants and children who remain calm, compliant, and appear to be almost indifferent to the noxious stimulation; at the other are those who respond with violent vocalization, physical resistance, and emotional upset, accompanied by increases in autonomic arousal indices such as cardiac rate and palmar sweat (see, for example, Craig et al., 1984; Johnston & Strada, 1986; Shapiro, 1975). This range of response is accepted as a truism by experienced clinicians and investigators (Craig, 1980; Florman, 1975; Jeans & Johnston, 1985). However, it often disconcerts the inexperienced observer, who tends to assume a direct and linear relationship between the noxious stimulation and the individual's perception of discomfort. Although many children reject this specificity view (Ross & Ross, 1984b), some accept it unquestioningly until faced with clear-cut evidence to the contrary. The following reaction is that of a child who was astonished and bewildered by the variations in behavior of his three roommates, all of whom had had the same minor surgery, a tonsillectomy, that he had undergone:

> It was really weird . . . like when you all have the same thing it must hurt the same. But it didn't. My throat was scratchy, but no big deal, like it didn't hurt when I watched TV. And the kid next to me . . . he didn't feel nothing, he goes like, "Maybe he [doctor] forgot to take them out." But the one by the window just rocked and groaned like you do when you're trying not to cry. And the kid in the other bed just cried all morning and he called the nurse five times in one [TV] program for pills or something 'cos it hurt so bad. But when we had finger sticks the first day, I *almost* cried and *he* acted like nothing even happened and, see, that was the same thing, too (Boy, CA 10, Ross & Ross, 1982a)

The related phenomenon of intraindividual variability in pain reactivity to seemingly equivalent noxious stimulation experienced at different times also poses problems. The simplistic view that how a child reacts on one occasion is predictive of how he will react on the next treats pain reactivity as a *trait*, a relatively enduring aspect of the individual's personality that enables him to withstand to some extent the pull of situational pressures. It should more accurately be viewed as a *state*, subject to a cluster of varying internal and external determinants.

Viewing pain as a state eliminates the notions that pain is a simple sensory experience, that the child is a passive recipient of impulses from the noxious stimulus, and that his attributes are the critical variables in his pain reactivity to a specific aversive event. Instead, a number of child and environmental variables are implicated. Chapman (1985) classifies these into two groups: *Predisposing factors* are variables that the child brings to the pain situation, for example, what he has learned about pain from his own and vicarious pain experiences and his age, sex, physiology, personality, and cultural background. The stability of these characteristics contributes an element of constancy to the child's pain reactivity in that their overall impact is likely to be associated with a probable range of pain response.

However, no predictions could ever be made without information about the three clusters of *situational factors* that form Chapman's second category and have relevance to the immediate pain situation. *Situation-specific child factors* are variables that are relevant to the context in which the pain is experienced, for example, the child's expectancies, state anxiety, and the significance to him of the particular pain event. *Social environmental factors* are defined as the other people who are present, their effect on the child, and his perception of them. These are generally adults, but peers and siblings can also exert an influence on the child, particularly if they serve as models (Bandura, 1969) or sources of information about the pain event (Ross & Ross, 1984b; Ross, S., 1984). *Nonsocial environmental factors* include elements of the setting, some of which are likely to be frightening or intimidating to the child, such as strange machines, high noise level, and a less tangible but nonetheless powerful atmosphere of tension or chaos.

The basic premise here is that pain reactivity is the product of factors within the child that may influence his perception of pain and complex transactions between the child and his environment. This model is consistent with Craig's (1984, p. 263) admonition that "pain occurs and must be examined in the context of complex social transactions." This thinking represents the culmination of two important theoretical developments, one of which focused directly on understanding pain, while the other concerned itself with facets of the individual–environment relationship having important implications for understanding behavioral problems.

The first of the theoretical developments was von Frey's specificity theory (Foster, 1901), the static, unidirectional, antecedent–consequent model of pain. According to this model, the perception of pain involves a sensory dimension that reflects the intensity of the noxious stimulus (see Table 3-1).

Von Frey's theory gave way to Beecher's (1959) two-component model with its sensory and reactive components, the latter including all the complex psychological processing involved in the pain experience. Beecher recognized that there was no predictable and reliable relationship between the degree of trauma and the

Table 3-1 Increasing Complexity in Models of Pain Reactivity

Model	S (Noxious stimulus)	R (Pain perceived by child)
Unidimensional	Intensity of stimulus input is ⟶ the only variable	Has sensory dimension only
Two-Component	Physiological + psychological input with environmental influence *implied* ⟶	Has sensory + reactive dimensions, with reactive possibly more important
Gate-Control	Physiological + psychological input with environmental influence clearly involved ⟶	Is multidimensional: has sensory-discriminative, motivational-affective, + cognitive-evaluative aspects
Social Ecology	Physiological, psychological, social, + nonsocial environmental components all merge as S_1 ⟶	Is multidimensional: sensory-discriminative, motivational-affective, + cognitive-evaluative aspects = R_1
	The influence of R_1 on S_1 changes it to S_2 ⟶	S_2 in turn effects changes in R_1 so that it becomes R_2
	The influence of R_2 on S_2 changes it to S_3 ⟶	S_3 in turn effects changes in R_2 so that it becomes R_3 and so on.

pain experienced. To explain inter- and intraindividual differences in pain reactivity, he invoked the reactivity component. In doing so he gave explicit recognition to the effect of the meaning of pain on pain reactivity and acknowledged the contribution of the environment to that meaning (Sternbach, 1968). The two-component model is depicted in Table 3-1.

The most important development in this sequence was the gate-control theory of pain (Melzack & Wall, 1965). According to this theory, pain reactivity is mediated by a multiplicity of factors in the individual, including cognitive, personality, learning, and cultural variables, as well as in the environment. Although gate theorists explicitly acknowledged environmental influences on pain reactivity, they assigned it a predominantly static role, with no suggestion of bidirectional and escalating environmental effects. Instead, the resultant pain equation was like a two-way analysis of variance in which child factors interact with environmental factors but each remains relatively constant within this interaction (see Table 3-1).

Theoretical development concerned with facets of the individual–environment relationship began outside the field of pain with laboratory demonstrations of the significance of environmental influences in understanding behavior. Studies of a diversity of social phenomena attested to the role of the social and nonsocial environments in determining behavior in children. Numerous laboratory investigations showed unequivocally that even relatively minor environ-

mental modifications could effect significant changes in a diversity of specific behaviors. Dissatisfaction with the limitations inherent in the laboratory setting and
the possible restrictions on generalization of findings led many investigators to
study behavioral phenomena in their natural context (Bronfenbrenner, 1979;
Willems, 1977). Prominent in this group were the social ecologists, and of particular relevance were the impressive series of studies and theoretical formulations by
Whalen, Henker and their associates (see, for example, Whalen & Henker, 1980)
of hyperactive children.

Starting with the premise that classroom settings can function either as
provocation ecologies that can accentuate the differences between hyperactive and
nonhyperactive children or as *rarefaction ecologies* that diminish such differences,
Whalen and Henker (1976) sought to identify the optimum *hyperactive child ×
environment* fit, defined as one in which the child's needs were well matched to the
social and nonsocial environmental conditions with consequent harmony between
the two. Within their conceptual framework a less than adequate match is regarded
as the manifestation of a dysfunctional system. It follows that any change process
must consider all the components of the system rather than focusing solely on the
child's behavior. The difficulty of this task is heightened by the fact that in this
theoretical framework the child × environment fit involves a dynamic, bidirectional, mutually reciprocal transactional process in which the child's behavior is
not merely a consequent of the environment, but also an influence on it. In other
words, what is a consequent at one point in time may become an antecedent at a
subsequent point (Whalen, Henker, & Dotemoto, 1980). See Table 3-1 for an application of this social ecology model to pain reactivity.

Although Whalen and Henker's (1976) formulations were developed specifically for research on hyperactive behavior in the classroom setting, their concept of
provocation and rarefaction ecologies within the environmentally oriented approach of social ecology theory extends the gains of the neurologically based gate-
control theory (Melzack & Wall, 1965) and has important implications for the
management of pediatric pain. The social ecological approach is one with great
potential for understanding inter- and intraindividual differences in pain reactivity.
From interview and discussion group data (Ross & Ross, 1984b, 1985, 1986),
clinical reports (Cowherd, 1977; Leavitt, 1979; Lewis, 1978; Stoddard, 1982), and
supporting statements (see, for example, Beuf, 1979; Eland & Anderson, 1977;
McCaffery, 1969; Neal, 1978) it is evident that as a function of differential handling, the pediatric setting can serve as a provocation ecology that mediates increased fear, anxiety, distress, and pain reactivity or as a rarefaction ecology that
minimizes these reactions. Among many strong features, the social ecological approach provides a framework for understanding the effects of differential handling
of pediatric interactions and points the way to modifications beneficial to the child.
Consider, for example, a pain-related experience such as undergoing anesthesia.
The following incidents show clearly how the fear-arousing aspects of this experi-

ence can be either sharply diminished (rarefaction ecology) or markedly enhanced (provocation ecology) as a function of differential handling:

> Six-year-old Ethan . . . listens closely as [an] anaesthesiologist, kneeling so that he is on the same level as the child, explains how he is going to ensure that it won't hurt when the surgeon fixes Ethan's ears. "We let you breathe magic air . . . out of this little mask," the anaesthesiologist says. "It will help you take a nap. When you wake up, the operation will be all over. Is that okay with you?" He waits patiently until Ethan nods. "Our masks come in six flavors." After serious thought Ethan chooses bubble gum flavor. He sits on his mother's knee while he calmly inhales the anaesthetic, and is asleep in two minutes. . . . His mother, a nurse, recalls the time her nephew had a similar operation in another hospital: "They took him wide awake and screaming to the operating room, and anesthetized him by sticking an IV needle in his arm. He never knew what was happening to him, or why." (Lobsenz, 1982, p. 80)

Traumatic experiences such as that described by this mother can have lasting effects. Remen (1980, p. 160) reported the case of a 33-year-old man whose fear of surgery was the result of two traumatic experiences in childhood:

> I know I need an operation but I don't think I could force myself even to walk through the door of a hospital. . . . When I was three, I had an operation on my left eye. And when I was seven I had a tonsillectomy. They used ether both times. The experience both times was similar; I had to be forcibly held down on the operating table, and then forced to breathe through a mask. I can remember it perfectly clearly, I was helpless and terrified. And I never really got over that. It gave me a deathly fear of the operating room and hospitals in general.

In a recent study by Dunn-Geier et al. (1986) of adolescents with chronic benign intractable pain, it was apparent that other pain-related behaviors, such as coping, may also be enhanced or diminished as a function of differential handling. In this study there was unequivocal evidence of the differential effects of maternal behavior on the adolescents' performance on a treatment-related exercise task.

In this chapter the predisposing and situational factors that contribute to pain reactivity are discussed within the framework of social ecology theory, the premise being that Whalen and Henker's (1980) construct of provocation and rarefaction ecologies has a direct application to the problem of effective management of pediatric pain. Using Chapman's (1985) categories as a framework, we begin with the predisposing factors in the child that are the result of his cumulative prior experiences and continue with the situational factors. It is apparent that many of the determinants of the predisposing factors also function as determinants of the situational factors. For example, observational learning plays an important role in establishing the child's attitudes and knowledge about pain *prior to* his subsequent participation in a specific pain event. It may also function as an important variable by shaping the child's behavior in the *immediate* pain event. The crucial difference between the two observational learning experiences is that conditions in the immediate pain event can often be modified to conform to the requirements for a rarefaction ecology.

Two other points should be noted here. In complex systems of behavioral categorization there is likely to be some overlap of categories in the form of external influences that span one or more categories, and this is the case here. In addition, a sequential description of the categories implies a temporal order in which each category forms an isolated unit. In the transactional model of pain reactivity, the basic premise is that all categories are functioning concurrently as an influence on the child's pain reactivity and effecting changes in each other that in turn set up new configurations. A methodologically sophisticated demonstration of the phenomenon of concurrent influences is contained in a study (Thompson et al., 1988) of the contributing influence of child psychosocial adjustment, family environment, and specific medical disease parameters to pain reactivity in children with JRA. A subsequent study (Varni, Wilcox, Hanson, & Brik, 1988) applied this empirical model to the investigation of functional status in children with JRA-related pain.The categories are described here one at a time only for reasons of clarity.

Predisposing Factors

Although knowledge of the child's history of pain reactivity does not permit precise predictions concerning his behavior in a specific pain event, it does make it possible to delineate the probable range within which this behavior is likely to fall. This range is determined in part by a cluster of previous learning experiences related to pain expression, including direct training; contingent social reinforcement with its offshoot, avoidant learning; and vicarious learning experiences. Each of these kinds of learning experience is discussed here.

Direct Training

Pain reactivity is the product of a combination of learning experiences. Starting early in life, a child experiences a wide variety of noxious stimulation events that may stem from external sources such as immunization shots, dental procedures, accidental falls, or physical punishment, or internal conditions such as stomachaches, earaches, and other common aches. For many of these pain experiences the child receives direct, highly explicit, and usually situation-specific instruction about how much discomfort justifies a complaint, the acceptable ways of expressing such complaints, who to approach about them, what is likely to happen as a result, and when to terminate the complaint. The distinguishing features of this direct training are that it precedes the child's response to the immediate pain experience and that the response may or may not be followed by parental action. A parent, for example, may instruct a child to sit quietly while being given an immunization shot but may or may not react overtly to how the child subsequently behaves.

Contingent Social Reinforcement

Far more pervasive than direct training and exerting a much stronger influence on the child's pain reactivity is the early shaping by his parents and others through the process of contingent social reinforcement. The distinguishing feature of this reinforcement is that it is a consequence of the child's behavior. Parental reaction to the child's pain expression covers a broad spectrum. At one end are parents who show little interest in minor pain events but, instead, are matter-of-fact and sensible about them. The child's distress signals elicit their attention and sympathy only when the magnitude of the injuries sustained clearly warrants such reactions. His reactions to minor somatic events are kept in perspective by providing him with strong corrective feedback about how to react. In this way he learns to label these events as something other than pain (Jaremko et al., 1981). The child who uses qualifiers such as "just a little blister" has learned these labels.

At the other end of the spectrum are parents who tend to overreact or be overly solicitous to even minor somatic events. At an early age their children quickly discern that crying over the most trivial accidents will elicit prompt parental attention. It is not uncommon at all to see an 18-month-old child stumble, check to see if he has elicited parental attention, and then sob piteously. Often the child will learn to "hold on" to the pain in order to prolong the parental attention; throughout the preschool years the "sustained cry" is a common phenomenon.

Typically, this oversolicitous parental behavior pattern continues as the child moves along in the early school years. As he becomes more verbal, one or both parents may urge him to describe minor pains in detail and listen attentively as he does so, thus not only giving him clear cues as to what is acceptable pain behavior but also showing him a way to get attention from others. When his minor pain experiences repeatedly elicit positive social reinforcement in the form of parental attention and proximity, and privileges, the probability is high that he will show continuing and increasing pain awareness. Consider the implications of the two hypothetical examples (Chapman, 1971, pp. 159–160) in Table 3-2 of parental response to a child's report of a headache and the cumulative effects on the child of the frequent opportunities that the daily routine would likely provide for such a sequence. The child who is rewarded for every pain event, no matter how minor, tends to build up a repertoire of pain behaviors, including nonverbal vocalizations (groaning), facial expressions (grimacing, wincing), and postural responses (hunching). These behaviors, combined with the difficulty that any parent has in assessing the seriousness of his child's pain, make it doubly hard for the overreactive parent to do so.

Table 3-2 Examples of Parental Response to a Child's Report of a Headache

Mother:	Yvonne, what's the matter?
Yvonne:	I have a headache.
Father:	Eight-year-old girls shouldn't have headaches as much as you do.
Yvonne:	I don't have so many of them.
Mother:	Where does your head hurt.
Yvonne:	I don't know. It's not too bad.
Father:	Answer your mother's question, Yvonne. Point to where your head hurts.
Yvonne:	Here and here.
Mother:	It may be sinus.
Father:	Has she been checked to see if she needs glasses?
Mother:	I'll take her to Dr. Robinson tomorrow.
Yvonne:	I'm going out to play.
Father:	I think you should stay in the house until you're better. Lie down for a while.
Mother:	I'll give you an aspirin.
Father:	How does your head feel now?
Yvonne:	I don't know. Maybe a little worse.
Father:	I'll look up headaches in the index of *The Home Medical Advisor.* Let's see now . . . Headaches, causes of . . . allergy . . . aneurysm of blood vessel, rupture of . . . brain tumor, early signs of . . . migraine . . . Does your head throb, or does it feel like there's a heavy weight pushing down, or is the pain sharp?
Yvonne:	Well, I guess it sort of throbs.
Father:	That's probably vascular. Be sure to tell Dr. Robinson that tomorrow.
Yvonne:	I'm beginning to get sick to my stomach.

Mother:	Yvonne, what's the matter?
Yvonne:	I have a headache.
Mother:	Where?
Yvonne:	In my forehead and the back of my neck.
Mother:	I have the same thing once in a while when I'm upset about something. Dr. Robinson told me that it's due to tension in the thin muscle layer in the scalp and in the thick muscles at the back of the neck. He said that 90% of the headaches people have are caused by that and it's nothing to worry about.
Father:	Many people get little headaches once in a while when they're tense about things.
Mother:	You probably got the headache because you and Harry have been fighting over that new game in the family room.
Yvonne:	Harry's a rat.
Father:	You're mad at Harry. Why don't you go next door and play with the Miller kids for a while?
Yvonne:	What about my headache?
Mother:	When you get over your upset with Harry, it will probably go away. If not, I'll give you an aspirin.

Reprinted, by permission, from Chapman, A.H., *The games children play.* Copyright 1971, Putnam's, New York.

Several lines of investigation provide some clues as to the underlying motivations of this parental behavior. In some cases, the parents obtain tertiary gains from their child's "pain" (Bokan, Ries, & Katon, 1981). The mother, for example, may find that such behavior makes her feel like a "good" mother and provides her with continuing reassurance that she is needed. A contributing factor here is that parents in our society receive considerable reward for being "caring" parents, a definition that is susceptible to marked distortion. There is also the possibility that parental overreactivity to the child's pain experiences may be consistent with a general style of overanxious and overprotective parental behavior (Apley, 1975). Sometimes the overconcern is linked to a pain condition, usually recurring or chronic, that the parents themselves suffer. Their condition causes them to focus on their own pain and this concern spills over to other family members. Craig (1978), for example, compared low back pain patients who benefited from surgery with those who did not benefit from it and found that of the two groups, the latter were more likely to report health problems in their children.

Acquired patterns of overreactivity to minor aversive stimulation often become so firmly entrenched that the responses learned as a young child persist into adolescence and adulthood (Chapman, 1971; Mechanic, 1980; Pilowsky, Bassett, Begg, & Thomas, 1982), with minor pain experiences serving an attention-getting function. A more insidious sequence occurs where the behavior pattern drops out as a result of social disapproval, particularly from peers, only to be retrieved at some point in adulthood when a pain event coincides with a strong need for attention or other secondary gains. One reason for the powerful effect of contingent social reinforcement is that learning acquired through this process is almost invariably further strengthened by observational learning experiences (Craig, 1983).

Observational Learning Experiences

Bandura (1969) believes that observational learning is the principal mode for acquiring new patterns of behavior. This form of learning occurs whenever the child voluntarily observes the behavior of others and its consequences to them and encodes the sequence. Usually he is a bystander, rather than a participant, and in all instances his observations are made without any instructions from others to attend. It is this latter criterion that distinguishes observational learning from direct training. Beginning in the preschool years there is a continuous and reciprocal interaction betwen the patterns of pain reactivity that were acquired through parental sanctions and contingent social reinforcement and those acquired through observational learning. Having a particular impact are the pain experiences of siblings and classmates, with the child seeing how they react and how adults respond to them. Because he is seldom actively involved in these pain events, the child has a certain emotional detachment. This detachment, combined with the attention-getting features of someone else's pain event, heightens the probability that the child will internalize the entire sequence, particularly if the model has high status in the peer group and is rewarded for his reaction to the pain event. The pain reactivity behavior that the child acquires becomes increasingly more specific (Craig, 1983) with age: The degree and kind of pain reactivity permissible in a preschool child is grossly inappropriate for a 10-year-old child and would likely elicit derision from peers and disapproval from adults, with a consequent weakening of the response.

Familial Models

Observing the reactions of familial models to their own pain experiences can influence the child's pattern of pain reactivity. Whether the model displays distress that is disproportionate to the degree of trauma or bears his pain in stoical silence, the effects on the child of these vicarious learning experiences again may be strengthened if the model is seen as powerful and if he is rewarded with attention and privileges or commended for his fortitude. Conversely, should the model be criticized or reprimanded, the effect would be to weaken the impact of the sequence on the child (Bandura, 1969).

There is an important and chilling body of research on the relationship between pain symptomatology in familial models and its effects on children (see, for example, Craig, 1978, 1980; Turkat, 1982; Violon & Giurgea, 1984). This research has documented the powerful role of familial models, particularly parents, in the etiology of children's pain conditions and complaints. In a study of 1,100 British school children older than age 3, Apley (1975) first identified those having chronic abdominal pain, then compared the family history of the children whose pain had a clear organic etiology with that of children whose pain had no known organic basis. In the former group, there was a positive family history of abdominal pain in approximately 13% of the children, but in the latter one this figure increased sharply to approximately 50%.

Support for the importance of observational learning in chronic abdominal pain is also provided by Hughes and Zimin (1978). They reported the frequent use of bodily sensations, physical explanations, and medical or surgical procedures to deal with psychic disturbances as a "way of life" in the families of children hospitalized for psychogenic abdominal pain. A related and disturbing finding concerns the accuracy of pain complaints acquired by children through observational processes. Two kindergarten girls whose mothers suffered severe and frequent tension headaches (Campbell, 1984) and migraine headaches (Porter, 1984), respectively, complained of headaches and described their symptoms in such explicit detail and so convincingly that they were excused from swimming lessons on several occasions before the coincidence of headaches and swimming lessons became apparent to their teachers. On being pressed, both girls admitted reluctantly that they had not had headaches and that they used their mothers' accounts as reference sources for their own symptoms. In the case of the migraine child, the pediatrician had already prescribed appropriate medication. Similarly, Craig (1978) has stated that reported complaints can simulate the characteristics of serious diseases so accurately that unnecessary surgery is then performed. Findings of familial resemblances in pain experiences inevitably raise the question of heredity versus environment. Support for the role of the environment comes from at least two studies: Christensen and Mortensen (1975) reported that the incidence of parents' abdominal disorders during childhood was unrelated to their children's complaints, whereas their concurrent problems did show such a relationship; Mohammed, Weisz, and Waring (1978) found high concordance rates in pain complaints among family members unrelated by biological bonds.

There is evidence, too, that the number of familial models is important: Children with more familial models are more likely to have pain complaints than are those with fewer models. Apley (1975) compared the families of children with and without abdominal pain and found that the families of children with abdominal pain had five to six times more pain complaints than did those of children with no abdominal pain. That the impact of multiple familial pain models extends beyond childhood is evident in a study of college students (Edwards, Zeichner, Kuczmierczyk, & Boczkowski, 1985) in which the number of familial pain models correlated positively with the number of reported current pain experiences. Similar findings have been obtained for adults with chronic pain, with prevalence of pain among family members and spouses of chronic pain patients being higher than in families of other patients (see, for example, Crook et al., 1984; Violon & Giurgea, 1984). These findings suggest that the early influence of familial pain models may play an important role in predisposing individuals to report higher frequencies of pain in later years (Edwards et al., 1985). They also support Apley's (1975) use of the label "the painful family" and Craig's (1980) more explicit descriptor, "the pain-prone family."

An offshoot of the whole problem of familial model effects on the etiology, frequency, and authenticity of children's pain complaints concerns the locus of control. Lau (1982) has found that early experiences with family illness are strongly related to current health locus of control beliefs. If the pain models' refrain is that there is nothing that they can do for their pain, that they have tried everything, and so on, continued exposure can result in the child's thinking that one's pain is not under internal control. This view sets the stage for feelings of helplessness (Seligman, 1975) and makes the child vulnerable to external locus of health control beliefs, a potentially destructive cognitive viewpoint that could have detrimental long-term effects for the child and his family.

Peer Models

Peer models are another important source of observational learning, especially in respect to pain tolerance and reactivity (Jaremko et al., 1981; Ross & Ross, 1982a). Peer models begin to be important in the elementary school years and become increasingly powerful in late middle childhood and adolescence. At any age, perceived similarity to a model enhances observational learning, but this is particularly true during these developmental periods (Bandura, 1969). Similarity may exist in relation to dimensions that are relevant to the ongoing pain experience: both the observer and the model may be undergoing routine immunization or learning how to self-inject with insulin. Or the dimensions may have little relevance: the model and observer may merely be of the same sex or attend the same school. Whatever the basis for the link between model and observer, its effects will be further enhanced if the model is seen as powerful or prestigious:

> I could stand having them [orthodontic braces] tightened, even though it was bad enough to scream, because Maxwell has them, too, and he's the star of the senior team [football], and everytime I got them tightened I'd just say to myself, "Maxwell wouldn't scream." My dentist thought I was terrific. (Boy, CA 12, Ross & Ross, 1982a).

Conflict arises when peer group standards concerning pain reactivity differ from home standards, for example, in the peer group the child may be expected to "tough it out," whereas at home, he is coddled. Rather than subsequently exhibiting one or the other of these behaviors consistently across all situations, he is likely to adapt his behavior to the demands of each situation:

> Well, my mom was real mad 'cos the school didn't send me to the hospital, or phone her when it happened [fractured arm]. But I didn't say nothing much when it happened 'cos at school it's different—like it would be the end if a guy my age cried. If it had of been at home I would have really yelled. (Boy, CA 11, Ross & Ross, 1982a)

The researcher who is interested in the transmission of pain-related responses through the medium of modeling procedures would do well to consider the impressive body of research by Craig and his associates with young adults (see, for example, Craig, 1980, 1983; Craig & Prkachin, 1980). The modification and application of some of Craig's procedures would be feasible with adolescents and would constitute an important contribution to the pain research literature on this largely neglected age group.

Avoidant Learning

Associated with the more severe pain event are certain rewards and punishments inherent in the situation. The child may enjoy staying home from school, particularly if it means missing a test or book report, even though he may also miss some high valence event such as a birthday party. For the overprotected child, the gains generally outweigh the losses. In a very short time he will learn that even mild pain enables him to avoid anxiety-arousing tasks and activities. It is a short step in this contingent reinforcement learning sequence to using pain as an excuse. It is irrelevant in this sequence that the pain now may be slight or nonexistent. What is serious is the fact that these learning sequences are almost certain to become more deeply entrenched through observational learning. Children often see their parents and peers rewarded for using real or imagined pain as an excuse, and there is no question that these models are influential in transmitting this maladaptive pain behavior. Turkat, Guise, and Carter (1983), for example, found that individuals with a parental model who avoided work unnecessarily when ill reported more avoidance of responsibility when ill than did those with no such model.

Cultural Learning

Most cultures have explicit rules about the appropriate responses to aversive events. Usually included are the behaviors the child should exhibit, the range of behavior that is considered acceptable, the kinds of pain that justify treatment and those that should be ignored, and the source of help. Within-culture variations occur in the consistency of the content of rules transmitted to a child. In cultures that are characterized by homogeneity of rule transmission across sources, the child is exposed to a steady and highly consistent barrage of direct teaching and opportunities for observational learning at home, in school, and at church, and this learning will be further consolidated by his association with the peer group, exposure to the media, and attendance at such events as sports competitions. An example of a homogeneous culture is an ethnic group in West Africa, the Bariba, who idealize stoicism in response to pain. They transmit this value to their children, particularly the boys, at about age six, using a combination of direct and highly explicit training, contingent social reinforcement, and vicarious learning experiences (Sargent, 1984). In cultures that are heterogeneous with respect to rule transmission, the same subgroups in the culture transmit information to the child, but the content often varies across sources. Behaviors that are considered acceptable at home, for example, might not be viewed as appropriate in school, and these in turn may differ markedly from those sanctioned by the peer group.

Cross-cultural variations in acceptable pain reactivity are also quite remarkable. Eskimo children learn that often the response to pain should be laughter (Christophenson, 1966); young Chinese children are taught in the early years to insert acupuncture needles and to interpret the ensuing sensation positively (Capperauld, 1972). They also learn from an early age that surgical intervention involves little discomfort and has a high rate of success. While visiting a Chinese children's hospital Brown (1972, p. 1330) witnessed

> a queue of smiling five-year-olds standing outside a room where tonsillectomies were being carried out in rapid succession. The leading child was given a quick anesthetic spray of the throat by a nurse, a few minutes before walking into the theatre unaccompanied. Each youngster in turn climbed on the table, lay back smiling at the surgeon, opened his mouth wide, and had his tonsils dissected out in the extraordinary time of less than a minute. The only instruments used were dissecting scissors and forceps. The child left the table and walked into the recovery room, spitting blood into a gauze swab.

In marked contrast are American children's behaviors and attitudes toward needle procedures and surgical intervention. Here, it is almost considered the norm that the children will cry and struggle and that the mother's presence will be needed. Hospitalization is viewed as a potentially frightening experience requiring preparation for the child in the form of prior information, reassurance, hospital orientation tours, and the like (Azarnoff & Woody, 1981; Peterson & Ridley-Johnson,

1980). It is clear that the same event may be transformed into a rarefaction or provocation ecology as a result of culturally transmitted attitudes and beliefs.

So far, the predisposing variables discussed have been associated with learned responses on the child's part. In the following sections, demographic variables as predisposing factors in pain reactivity are described briefly, as well as personality factors and diurnal variations. This cluster of variables has received little research attention. Those studies that have been done with children (or adults) have frequently presented conflicting results. The variables are discussed here because they do suggest some alternative interpretations for individual differences in pain reactivity, they may facilitate the selection of specific intervention strategies, and clinical research with children would be quite feasible in addition to being urgently needed.

Demographic Variables

Age and Sex

The empirical findings on the relationship between age and sensitivity to aversive stimulation in infants are inconclusive, with no convincing evidence that pain threshold changes during the early days of life. Although much of the research with this age group is plagued by methodological shortcomings (see Owens, 1984; Rosenblith & Sims-Knight, 1985, for reviews), a number of carefully conducted studies have failed to demonstrate clear trends (see, for example, Lipsitt & Levy, 1959). In fact, empirical findings (Craig et al., 1984; Taylor, 1983) and clinical observations (Barr, 1982; Hazinski, 1984) suggest that the behavioral changes that do occur reflect increases in efficiency, rather than in sensitivity, on the part of the infant in modulating his reaction to aversive stimulation. In the case of school-age children and adolescents, however, several studies have provided some support for an increase in pain threshold with age (Chapman & Jones, 1944; Haslam, 1969; Schluderman & Zubek, 1962), but the results must be viewed with caution. With increasing age, many psychological factors, such as cultural pressures and peer group norms, come into play. A decrease in overt pain reactivity does not necessarily mean that less pain is experienced. In a study of thermal pain with adults, Clark and Mehl (1971) found that most of the increase in pain threshold with increasing age could be attributed to a reluctance to label the aversive stimulation as pain, rather than to a change in pain sensitivity per se, and this phenomenon may also occur in older children and adolescents (Jaremko et al., 1981). It is likely that developmental level is of more importance than chronological age in understanding differences in pain reactivity since it determines how the child interprets the pain experience (Piaget & Inhelder, 1969).

The same inconclusiveness characterizes research support for evidence of sex differences in sensitivity to pain in infancy. Although Lipsitt and Levy (1959) reported weak evidence that girls were more sensitive to mild electric shock than boys, Rosenblith and Sims-Knight (1985) have contended that these differences could be artifactual: Male infants are generally heavier than females and consequently are likely to have greater deposits of subcutaneous fat, which could lessen the impact of the electric current and thus make the infant appear to be less sensitive. For older children and adolescents, experienced clinical pediatric personnel state that boys usually appear to tolerate mild to moderate pain better than do girls, presumably because of cultural and other pressures on males in our society to be brave. But here, too, there is no conclusive empirical evidence of sex differences. Studies with adults (see, for example, Notermans & Tophoff, 1967) generally fail to demonstrate sex differences for pain threshold, but often demonstrate differences for pain tolerance, with males exhibiting greater tolerance than females (Weisenberg, 1977a; Woodrow, Friedman, Siegelaub, & Collen, 1972). Wolff (1978) attributes these two sets of findings to the fact that pain threshold is more highly loaded with a physiological component. Petrie (1967) has suggested that men have greater pain tolerance because they tend to reduce the size of the incoming stimuli more than women do. The research supports the view that physiologically men are as responsive to pain as women are, but as a function of learning and attitudinal factors, they display less overt distress and upset.

Other Demographic Variables

There has been very little research on children and adolescents on sensitivity to pain in relation to ordinal position (Ernst & Angst, 1983), and findings on college students are equivocal (see, for example, Gelfand, 1963; Schachter, 1959). For those interested in this topic, Adams (1972) and Schooler (1972) are suggested authors. Findings on size of family are also equivocal (Ernst & Angst, 1983). Racial differences in adults' pain tolerance have been reported (see, for example, Wolff & Langley, 1968; Zborowski, 1952); in view of the potency of cultural transmission, it is likely that similar differences could be documented in children.

Personality

Personality characteristics in relation to pain reactivity have not been studied in children, but research with adults suggests potentially productive lines of investigation having direct application to them. Petrie (1967) has categorized adults into three categories of reactivity to aversive stimulation: *Augmenters* tend to see such stimulation as greater than it is, *moderators* neither maximize or minimize it, and *reducers* tend to diminish it. According to Petrie, reducers have a need for sensory input even when that input is of a noxious type and consequently should exhibit the highest pain tolerance. It follows that children who are reducers would find the stresses of the intensive care unit, which has frequently been viewed as a sensory deprivation experience (Carty, 1982; Cataldo, Bessman, Parker, Pearson, & Rogers, 1979), most debilitating.

Another perceptual variable of relevance here is field independence/dependence (Witkin, 1959). A child who pays no attention to the stimulus background in judging some facet of the stimulus is described as *field independent*, whereas one who takes this background into consideration is called *field dependent*. Although the evidence with adults is equivocal (Weisenberg, 1977a), one would expect that field-independent subjects would be more reactive to pain because of their narrower focus on it and that they would more frequently interpret aversive stimulation as pain. In a contact sport such as football, for example, the field-independent child would likely experience more pain under approximately similar conditions than would the field dependent one.

The strongest case for a personality variable relationship to pain lies in the construct of locus of control. Children who are in the external locus of control category interpret what happens to them as a function of external factors, such as chance or the doctors, and view events as being beyond their control. In the pain situation, external locus of control → helplessness → increased state anxiety → higher pain is a common sequence. In contrast, those in the internal locus of control category believe that their actions can influence events; consequently the "same" aversive stimulation should result in decreased pain perception in these children. However, it is conceivable that a strong internal locus of control could function to enhance pain perception if it elicited an unrealistic view of personal responsibility, guilt, or self-blame (Whalen, 1987).

In the Nuprin Pain Report study (Sternbach, 1986b), adults with high internal health locus of control scores were less likely to experience pain, reported less severe pain, and engaged in more healthful behaviors compared with those with low internal health locus of control scores.

Diurnal Variation

There is some evidence with adults that pain perception follows a diurnal variation, with pain thresholds and pain tolerance thresholds reaching maximum and minimum levels at certain times of the day. If this were the case, then there would be an optimum time for performing certain painful treatment procedures and variations in irritability, frequency of pain complaints, and requests for analgesics throughout the day might be partially explained. Some investigators (Glynn, Lloyd, & Folkard, 1976) think that diurnal variation is independent of the cause of pain, whereas others (Strempel, 1977) believe that different kinds of pain, such as epicritic and protopathic, underlie different rhythms. Circadian rhythm is often equated with diurnal variation, but Morawetz, Parth, and Pöppel (1984, p. 410) contend that this is incorrect "because it implies an underlying, self sustaining, oscillatory mechanism" for which there is no evidence. In laboratory studies, Strempel (1977) reported that the highest experimental pain threshold value occurred at 3:00 A.M. and the lowest at 11:00 A.M. for tests of needle prick pain on the finger tips. Rogers and Vilkin (1978) found the low point to be during the evening.

Other researchers (Glynn et al., 1976) have found differences in diurnal variation between males and females, between patients who stayed at home and those who went out to work, and in relation to certain personality factors. All in all, the research on diurnal variation can be characterized as ambiguous and, in terms of focus of interest, sporadic. At the same time, it appears to be a potentially productive area with direct application to management of the pain experience.

Situational Variables

Pain reactivity is determined in part by the particular combination of psychological and contextual factors that exist in a specific pain experience. Note that the effects of the individual's characteristics and of the social and nonsocial environments are all given approximately equal emphasis. Situational variables represent a unique feature of a specific transaction between the individual and the context in which the pain is experienced: Even if the pain event occurs again in the same setting, it is unlikely that these variables will have remained the same. For this reason, it is necessary to analyze the situational variables if one is to understand the puzzling and often irritating intraindividual differences in pain reactivity that occur in the face of apparently identical degrees of aversive stimulation. They also justify attention because there is unequivocal empirical and clinical evidence that pain reactivity can be significantly enhanced or attenuated by modifying one or more of these variables. Keeping in mind that each category functions concurrently with the other two, we will begin with a discussion of factors in the child, before moving on to those in the social and the nonsocial environments.

Situation-Specific Child Factors

Factors within the child include the meaning that the pain has for the child, feelings of helplessness versus control, state anxiety, the role of attention, and self-efficacy.

Meaning of Pain

The child's reactivity to aversive stimulation can be markedly influenced by the meaning that he attributes to the pain experience. Age is a particularly important variable here because the meaning that the child or adolescent attributes to pain generally varies as a function of his stage of cognitive development (Gaffney, 1983). It is irrelevant here that the meaning may be based on grossly inaccurate beliefs: If the child has the belief, then it is a valid one within this context. In any case, the meaning that the child attaches to the pain experience can serve to enhance or attenuate his pain tolerance. When having the pain and being able to tolerate it is seen as an *accomplishment,* the child can tolerate more aversive stimulation without heightened upset. When moderate to severe pain is inflicted, as part of a cultural ritual or initiation rite for example, quite young children will endure it without flinching (Sargent, 1984).

The child's priorities will take precedence over the pain when the pain occurs in the *pursuit of a goal:* If the pain occurs in the course of athletic training, a step toward vocational goals, or during an actual game or performance, the child who perceives it as "worth it" will be better able to tolerate it (Jaremko et al., 1981; Ross & Ross, 1984b). Closely related to the goal idea is pain that the child has learned to see as *essential.* Included here are most treatment-induced pains, such as burn dressing changes, bone marrow aspirations, physiotherapy, and orthodontic procedures, during which the child understands that what is being done cannot be avoided (Ross & Ross, 1984b).

When pain that happens spontaneously is seen as the *price of escape,* its effects are minimized (Beecher, 1956). The child with spontaneous pain that is severe enough to keep him home from school, with consequent avoidance of a disliked activity, will experience lessened pain reactivity.

> Sure it [sprained ankle] hurt, I guess it hurt a lot, but it was a super trade-off, like I missed the exams and being in the play so that made it not hurt so bad. (Boy, CA 11, Ross & Ross, 1982a)

On the other hand, if the child sees the pain as a *deliberate hurt,* he will be less tolerant of it, whether or not it is in fact inflicted deliberately. Young children often see pain in this light, as do children who are influenced by television-mediated distortions about events in the medical setting. Again, whether or not the doctor or dentist is being deliberately mean to the child is beside the point. What is important is the child's perceptions of the behavior in these terms. Pain that is perceived as *unnecessary* will also result in lower tolerance. Included here is pain caused by a lack of skill, which while not deliberate is certainly unnecessary, poor equipment such as a blunt needle, or treatment or tests that are not needed:

> He [doctor] looked at it [arthritic knee] and moved it like they do and it hurt, it always does, but not terrible. Then he got talking to this other doctor and he started jigging it up and down, up and down, like doodling. And he wasn't looking at my leg or me *he was just doing it!* It was terrible . . . I got so mad. (Boy, CA 10, Ross & Ross, 1982a)

A particularly strong influence on the child's pain reactivity occurs when the meaning of the pain is associated with fear, anxiety, or a combination of these emotions. The leukemic child who is anxious about the nature and source of pain might interpret the pain from a swollen gland as evidence of progression of the disease and find it more painful than it should be; by comparison, the normally healthy child would brush it aside as a petty annoyance. Among children who have rheumatoid arthritis, the younger ones see their arthritis as inconvenient and the resultant pain as a barrier to activities that they should rightfully be enjoying, whereas the older ones know all too well what the pain means, so that the "same" pain bothers them far more (Beales, Keen, & Holt, 1983).

Feelings of Helplessness versus Control

The events in some pain situations, particularly those in which the pain is treatment induced, result in the child's being in a state of learned helplessness (Seligman, 1975), in which he concludes that there is nothing that he can do to modify, terminate, or escape from the ongoing aversive stimulation. With learned helplessness, the important variable is not the occurrence of the aversive event but rather the child's perception of the relationship between his behavior and the occurrence of that event. This most distressing and anxiety-arousing experience can occur when the feedback that he gets during an ongoing pain experience is characterized by "response-outcome independence" (Miller & Norman, 1979), that is, the feedback is completely unrelated to his complaints, questions, or pleas for relief from pain. Note the forlorn quality of the following comments:

> It's like we don't speak the same language—I coulda said anything, it wouldn't have changed what he [orthodontist] said. (Boy, CA 10, Ross & Ross, 1982a)

> I told him [dentist] it hurt a lot and he just asked the nurse to give him something and then he said to open wider. (Girl, CA 7, Ross & Ross, 1982a)

It is heightened when the pediatric personnel behave as though the child is not there. A common example of this thoughtlessness is that of a doctor or dentist verbalizing decisions with another professional in front of the child, but without informing him first, soliciting information from him, or acknowledging his presence or role as a patient/participant:

> It was like there was just a broken leg but not me, like there was a leg and me on the table and they only were interested in the leg. (Girl, CA 10, in emergency room, Ross & Ross, 1982a)

Regardless of the source of learned helplessness, its usual effect is to have the child give up in despair, not because of the severity of the pain but rather because he concludes that he has no influence of any kind on what will happen. These feelings lead to increased state anxiety relative to the situation, which in turn heightens attentional focus on the pain events; this combination intensifies the child's pain reactivity.

The antithesis of learned helplessness is the feeling of having some control over the situation. Thompson (1981) has defined control as the belief that one has at his disposal a response that can influence tolerance to the aversiveness of an event. Three categories of control techniques that have proven effective in the pediatric setting are behavioral, decisional, and cognitive control. One example of *behavioral control* is the self-pacing procedure that many dentists use in which the child is allowed to signal with a buzzer when he wants the aversive stimulation to stop. After an initial short trial period in which the child tests the dentist's veracity, there is a marked increase in his tolerance for duration of ongoing treatment (Neal, 1978).

Decisional control involves giving the child a choice in the pain situation. He is asked which arm for the needle or is offered the choice of regular bone marrow aspiration versus the Mizzy Gun. Decisional control reportedly leads to reduced behavioral upset (see, for example, McClellan, 1984). The essential element is that the choice must be a genuine one in which the child does make the decision and it is upheld. Otherwise, children become resentful and angry on finding that they have been duped (Rogers & Head, 1983). A higher level of decisional control consists of encouraging the child to collaborate with pediatric personnel in mutual problem solving concerning facets of his treatment regimen. Such a procedure could reduce pain perception through several other mechanisms, including distraction and perceptions of self-efficacy (Whalen, 1987).

Cognitive control refers to the child's belief that he is in control of himself. He may believe this on the basis of past experience ("I did it before so I can do it again") or as a result of vicarious learning experiences ("If that little kid can handle this, so can I"). The feeling of control may also stem from the child's ability to use coping strategies effectively. Here the child has a strong feeling of being in control because he is the one who generates the strategy and decides when to use it. He is confident that he can manage environmental threats should they occur. After being taught thought-stopping (Ross, D., 1984), one child, for example, told the nurse, "I'm in charge now."

One interesting feature of control is that it does not have to be exercised in order to be effective; furthermore, in order for it to have effect, it is necessary only that the child perceive himself as being in control, when in fact he might not have any real control at all. Two issues underlie the "effectiveness" idea: one is whether control increases pain tolerance; the other is whether it decreases pain reactivity by raising the pain threshold. Laboratory evidence on the effects of control is mixed. Turk et al. (1983) reported that the subject's perception of himself as in control resulted, in most instances, in higher pain thresholds, higher tolerance, or both. Thompson (1981) concluded that behavioral control does not reduce pain intensity but does increase the ability to tolerate pain. She offered several possible explanations for this phenomenon: Control affects the predictability of the aversive event, thus giving the child time to prepare for it; it can affect the child's sense of competence with the resultant benefit of increased well-being; and it can change the meaning that the aversive stimulation has for the child, from something that is too much for him to bear to something he knows he will be able to stand. Other investigators have not been able to demonstrate these effects. In an analysis of control as a variable, Averill (1973) concluded that the relationship between control and pain reactivity was equivocal and suggested instead that the reduction of uncertainty might be the important variable.

State Anxiety

State anxiety is a transitory emotional state that varies in intensity and fluctuates over time (Spielberger, Gorsuch, & Lushene, 1970). It generally increases in response to physically or psychologically threatening situations or events and results in the heightened activation of attentional mechanisms (Melzack, 1973). Observational evidence of age and sex differences in state anxiety has been reported by Katz, Kellerman, and Siegel (1980). State anxiety was inversely related to age, and there were differences as a function of age in its expression and duration. Younger children exhibited more diffuse verbal and physical expressions of anxiety over a longer duration of time, whereas older children exhibited fewer types. There were also significant sex differences, with girls exhibiting higher anxiety than boys. It should be noted here that many older children, particularly boys, are often reluctant to show their anxiety overtly. Consequently, written self-report measures might have yielded different findings from those reported here.

Clinical experience has shown that acute state anxiety usually heightens the pain experience, whereas reduction of state anxiety attenuates it. On the empirical front, however, attention has been focused on more esoteric aspects. Although the subjects in the following studies were adults, the findings are relevant here. In a study on sensitivity to stimulus change (Uhde et al., 1982), it was found that increased state anxiety was associated with decreased sensitivity in discriminating among randomly administered electric shocks of varying intensities. Extrapolating from this study to children in clinical pain, always a risky procedure, suggests that sequential self-report pain ratings from children who are high on state anxiety may not reflect the changes in pain intensity that have occurred. It would be interesting to study the relationship in nonclinical children between state anxiety induced with a suspenseful video presentation and ratings of the intensity of auditory or visual stimuli. Another study of relevance here is that reported by Weisenberg, Aviram, Wolf, and Raphaeli (1984). State anxiety was found to exacerbate pain reactivity when the source of anxiety was directly relevant to the pain experience, but when the source of anxiety was irrelevant, such as successful performance on a learning task, the anxiety reduced pain reactivity.

Role of Attention

There is substantial clinical support for the role of attention in attenuation of discomfort. The child who focuses intently on ongoing nociceptive input will generally report more severe discomfort and typically show more upset than the one who either is distracted by competing external events or, of his own volition, is able to focus his attention elsewhere. (However, see Kavanagh [1983a, 1983b] for an opposing view.) Examples of distraction by competing events are legion: dentists have often used music (Gardner, Licklider, & Weisz, 1960) or television programs (Lemchen, 1987) as attention-diversion techniques and elements in athletic competitions, such as excitement, may be so attention directing that the participants are impervious to pain perception (Melzack, 1973). Similarly, many children are able to focus their attention elsewhere by means of coping strategies, such as engaging in imagery or taxing cognitive tasks (Ross & Ross, 1984b), and when they do so they appear to be unaware of ongoing aversive stimulation. In a discussion of the small but impressive body of empirical evidence with young adults that attention to pain enhances the aversiveness of the stimulation (Meichenbaum, 1977; Meldman, 1970), Pennebaker (1982, p. 45) offers the following explanation:

> The mere act of attending to a known unpleasant event results in most of the information related to the event being encoded in line with its unpleasantness. . . . The more information you receive, the more extremely you rate [it].

The probability that a child will focus on noxious stimulation is also dependent on the situational context in which the noxious input occurs as well as on the child's interpretation of that input. Being struck in sport, for example, does not elicit as much attention to the noxious stimulation as does corporal punishment in school. An ingenious demonstration of the effects of situational context and interpretation was reported by Dworkin and Chen (1982), who showed that the identical amount of tooth pulp stimulation was rated as less painful in a laboratory setting than in a dentist's office, presumably because the latter setting functions as a provocation ecology for most people in our culture, whereas a laboratory situation does not have this connotation.

Self-Efficacy

Self-efficacy as a situation-specific variable in pain reactivity refers to the child's perception of his capability in specific situations (Bandura, 1981). As such, it overlaps or incorporates some of the situational variables discussed here and also casts further light on the previously described predisposing factors that can intensify or attentuate pain reactivity. It is a construct that is situation specific: As each situation occurs, the child reevaluates his efficacy. It follows that self-efficacy is a contributor to intraindividual differences in pain reactivity in ostensibly similar pain situations as well as across situations. The child's beliefs about his ability to cope with competency pain, for example, may differ sharply from his perceptions of his ability to cope with an apparently equally aversive clinical procedure such as venipuncture.

Judgments of efficacy in pain or other situations are based on four sources of information (Bandura, 1981). The first of these is *previous performance* related to the present situation, a topic discussed earlier in this chapter as a predisposing factor. Successful handling of similar or related pain experiences in the past raises the child's appraisal of his capabilities; failures lower it, particularly in situations in which he has made a maximum effort to cope with the problem. Levels of perceived efficacy can be raised through the mastery of progressively more threatening pain events. The implication is that in the clinical situation pain experiences should be ordered in increasing severity so that the child is likely to cope adequately with them, at least initially. Dentists, for example, should fill the smallest caries first rather than the largest ones. This line of thinking is difficult to reconcile with the widespread preference, especially in children, for "getting the worst over first." It also overlooks the possibility that the child who is confronted with a series of dental sessions would likely become increasingly upset on realizing that with every session the severity or duration of the pain will increase.

Vicarious experiences also exert an influence on the child's assessment of his capabilities. A child who sees his peers cope with equanimity in an aversive situation is more likely to feel optimistic about his own chances than if those ahead of him fail to cope. A further refinement here concerns the effects of coping models, who manage adequately, versus those of mastery models, who behave brilliantly (Thelen et al., 1979). It is possible that the former are of more help to the child because he sees their level of attainment as being within the realm of possibility for himself (Meichenbaum, 1971).

A third source of information is that of *social persuasion,* in the form of others telling the child that he will be able to manage. If this input is credible it will encourage the child to make the maximum effort, which in turn will increase his chance of success. However, if the effect is to encourage unrealistic beliefs, the inevitable discrepancy between the child's expectancies and his subsequent performance will undermine his confidence in his own ability to manage as well as in "support" from others.

The child's assessment of his capabilities is also influenced by his *physiological state.* If, for example, he experiences noticeable increases in cardiac and respiration rates, he is more likely to doubt his ability to cope than he would in the absence of such physiological changes.

The child's judgment of his capabilities will significantly influence how he behaves in the pain situation, particularly in respect to how much effort he will expend and how long he will persist in the face of aversive experiences. A highly intelligent and verbal 6-year-old boy with leukemia, whose friends age 7 and 8 had just died, made a number of comments, when interviewed (Ross & Ross, 1982a), about his determination not to die because "there is too much I have to do yet . . . lots of things I want to do." He had no doubt at all about his capabilities for grappling with the situation and going into remission:

> This is how it's going to be and if God has any other ideas He'll simply have to compromise.

The child did go into remission and has remained there, hanging in doggedly through all the pain and other problems associated with the disease.

Environmental Social Factors

The child's own attributes and experiences are not the sole determinants of his response to a specific pain experience. His pain reactivity may be heightened or minimized by the behavior of others in the situation, mainly his parents and pediatric personnel, as well as other adults and children present but not directly involved with the child. In this section these clusters of potential influence are described along with supporting clinical, empirical, and theoretical evidence and other relevant issues.

Presence of Mother

The effect of mother's presence on children's reactions to aversive medical and dental procedures in clinical settings has been a controversial issue, with equivocal findings reported at the empirical as well as clinical level (Frankl, Shiere, & Fogels, 1962; Lewis & Law, 1958; Murphy, 1982; Peterschmidt, 1984; Shaw & Routh, 1982; Venham, 1979). In the following discussion, *mother* should be interpreted as either or both parents since, realistically, it is usually the mother who is present.

In all instances favoring the mother's presence, the assumption made is that she will behave in ways that are reassuring to the child. The effect then is to diminish the child's fear and anxiety, with a concomitant decrease in pain reactivity and increase in manageability. This effect occurs with medical/dental procedures as well as with spontaneous pain such as earache. Stoddard (1982) reported that with children with burns, the presence of the mother minimized pain. Bradshaw (1985) found that in young children a common reaction concerned the idea that the mother somehow took over the pain:

> It didn't hurt me but it hurt my mom a lot. (Boy, CA 4, needle stick while sitting on mother's knee)

The mother's presence exerts these potent effects for a variety of reasons. Amidst strangers and acquaintances she is a familiar and reassuring link to the safety of home and a consequent source of security. These effects are consistent with attachment theory (Ainsworth, 1964), which implies that the mother's presence helps the child to cope more comfortably with novel or frightening experiences. They are also consistent with affiliation theory (Schachter, 1959) and social ecology theory (Bronfenbrenner, 1979). The mother understands what the child says or means; as an intermediary with the pediatric personnel she is seen as a resource having some control over events. This latter benefit is consistent with the buffering hypothesis (Cohen & Wills, 1985). If the mother is serene and calm, she also functions as a strong, positive model for the child. In one study (Kleck et al., 1976) there was evidence that with undergraduates in an experimental situation outward calm was associated with lower pain ratings. Although extrapolating from experimental to clinical situations, not to mention from undergraduates to children, is a dubious business, still, the calming effect of the model on the child and the consequent effect of the child's calm on his own pain reactivity has some support in the form of clinical reports from experienced pediatric personnel

(Bradshaw, 1985; Peterschmidt, 1984). Consistent with the limited empirical findings are children's ideas on this topic. Almost all the children in the Ross and Ross studies (1984b, 1985) thought that mother's presence was what would have helped most when they were in pain, although they also acknowledged that there was not much the mother could actually do. In other studies, the mother's presence was included in the category of what helped, but it was not ranked first by the children (see, for example, Abu-Saad, 1984c; Gaffney, 1983; Jerrett, 1985; Ross & Ross, 1986; Savedra et al., 1982; Tesler, Savedra, Gibbons, Ward, & Wegner, 1983). The findings from the interview studies are consistent with the social support hypothesis of Cohen and Wills (1985).

An unusual benefit of the mother's presence may occur in children with terminal cancer. These children often muster all their resources to protect their parents from immediate distress as well as grief should they die (Whalen, 1987). Even young children frequently pursue help for their parents with singleminded determination:

> My Mom used to cry a lot, like she'd all of a sudden walk out and then she'd come back and try to smile. So I told my lady that comes [social worker] and they talked to Mom and now she never walks out of the room. I don't have to worry about her now. If I die, the people here'll help my Mom and Dad. (Girl, CA 9, with leukemia, Ross & Ross, 1982a)

Pediatric personnel (Grobstein, 1979) have noted that such intense concern often functions as a distractor, with a consequent attenuation of pain.

If the mother does not behave in a reassuring way, she may heighten the child's pain reactivity, thus turning the situation into a provocation ecology. In any case, the child's anxiety may increase sharply on realizing that the person whom he has seen as a buffer between him and the outside world cannot be counted on to "save" him from the pediatric personnel. Often the parent, previously regarded by the child as omnipotent, suddenly assumes a submissive role, to the dismay of the child:

> And Pop goes like, "yes, doctor, no, doctor," and never says another thing and he never goes like that and right off I knew he can't help me if they're mean. (Boy, CA 7, in emergency room for fracture, Ross & Ross, 1984b)

Anxiety would further escalate, and with a concomitant increase in pain reactivity, should the mother scold the child for not cooperating or, even worse, help the doctor by holding him down.

The mother may initially be reassuring, but in the face of the child's treatment may flinch, cringe, or gasp; she then becomes a model in pain, with a consequent negative effect on the child. Indeed, maternal affective reaction may better define the child's response than the nature of the aversive stimulus itself (Barr, 1982; Crockett, Prkachin, & Craig, 1977). Hahn (1983) has emphasized the need to prepare parents for the sight of noxious procedures: They may need to observe the procedure with another child or be primed on how to respond. This is an essential step that should be routinely included in the child's treatment sequence. An all too common incident in pediatric settings is the child who, having been reassured by pediatric personnel, is reasonably relaxed and ready for the procedure only to have his calm irrevocably disrupted by his mother's response. Slosberg (1977, p. 41) has described a textbook picture of disruptive maternal behavior transforming a carefully constructed rarefaction ecology into a provocation ecology in a matter of seconds. In this episode, a highly skilled male nurse had used information, reassurance, distraction, and peer modeling to prepare a boy for his first dialysis session, had inserted and secured the needles, and had turned on the machine, with the child still reasonably calm:

> Technically, David's first hookup had been perfection. The needles, the tubes, the machine—it was all textbook. Emotionally, it had been worse than a disaster. . . . the tissue-thin little world that Feldman [nurse] had built lovingly, painstakingly for David . . . was smashed . . . when his mother hit the floor . . . the look in his mother's eyes . . . was, I could see, more shattering than her fainting. The look, when she came to, of fear and loathing for the machine. David saw it. And from then on he, too, would fear and loathe the machine.

Absence of Mother

When the child is alone with the pediatric personnel, it is reasonable (Ainsworth, 1964; Bronfenbrenner, 1979) that he might feel abandoned, thus creating the sequence of increased fear → heightened pain reactivity and increased upset. However, Shaw and Routh (1982) contend that having the mother absent should create a positive sequence. Their rationale for this stand is as follows: Increased behavioral distress and heightened pain reactivity would be more likely to occur with the mother present because typically she rewards these behaviors with attention and reassurance. Maternal cues that previously have been present in clear-cut sequences of child hurt → mother present → mother comforts are now present, so the child reacts as he ordinarily would when he is hurt and his mother is nearby. However, with the mother absent, the cues that could be expected to elicit increased upset and pain reactivity are also absent, so consequently there could be less upset. Empirical support for the advantage of mother absent comes from a study (Shaw & Routh, 1982) in which 18-month-old and 5-year-old children who were undergoing routine immunization procedures were randomly assigned to mother-present and mother-absent conditions. Although many infants in the latter condition showed upset at their mothers' departures, when the injections were done the behavior of the mother-present infants was rated as significantly more negative. The older children's behavior in the mother-present conditions was also significantly more negative during and after the injections. Shaw and Routh (1982) concluded that infants and young children may inhibit protest in a minor pain experience if their mothers are absent. The finding of less upset in the mother-absent condition cannot, however, be interpreted as evidence of a reduction in amount of pain experienced, although Kleck et al.'s (1976) results on the effect of outward calm on ratings of pain intensity would support this possibility. It is also possible that the children inhibited distress responses from a fear of strangers or hopelessness, since there was no one to comfort them, or that there was less upset because the pain event was accomplished more quickly in the mother's absence since there was no interference in the form of hugging the child or having him reach for the mother.

Pediatric Personnel

Young children are fairly knowledgeable about the social roles of doctors and patients, in that they often understand the consultation interaction (Haight et al., 1985). However, they frequently do not understand clinical procedures: If they see the doctor's actions as threatening or deliberately unkind, the resultant increase in fear, anxiety, and tension will heighten their pain reactivity. Frankl (1964) believed that suffering could be endured if the "victim" could invest it with some kind of meaning. Certainly, the leukemic children who understood why the painful diagnostic procedures were necessary soon brushed aside the pain of finger sticks and venipuncture as unimportant and often exhibited remarkable tolerance for the more severe bone marrow aspirations and lumbar punctures because they could see the reason for them (Ross & Ross, 1984b). The same effect is apparent in biographical accounts (Bruce, 1983; Schorlemer, 1984).

Lack of trust is another important variable contributing to the fear/anxiety → increased pain reactivity sequence, with children feeling betrayed on being deceived:

> Right off [when venipuncture hurt after doctor said it would not] I could tell he was a liar and now everytime I go, I'm scared 'cos whatever he says, I know it could be a big lie. (Boy, CA 7, blood test, Ross & Ross, 1984b)

> I was lying on the X-ray table getting a blood test. I think the doctor must be crazy because he said he couldn't find my vein. The other two doctors from before could. And then he *lied* to me a lot. He promised that he would stop when it started hurting me. He didn't stop at all. (Girl, CA 12, Lewis, 1978, p. 18)

Statements about the temporal duration of pain should be made with great caution, particularly comments about the treatment not taking long. The child's view of "long" usually differs from the doctor's and this discrepancy is heightened by the fact that pain appears to increase estimates of time (Bilting, Carlsson, Menge, Pellettieri, & Peterson, 1983; Ross & Ross, 1983). Instead, length of time should be defined in terms of some routine action known to be familiar to the child:

> So I always know exactly how bad and how long, like he says it will take one riddle and it does, so even though it hurts it's not so bad because I know, he *always* tells me. (Girl, CA 9, wound dressings, Ross & Ross, 1984b)

It is also important to avoid claims that are not completely foolproof: If the child is told that it will just be one little jab and the doctor does not enter the vein the first time, his credibility suffers, to the child's detriment. The trust variable operates in a reciprocal fashion: The pediatric personnel must also appear to believe the child. If the child responds affirmatively to questions about whether he is in pain, and then is told that he "shouldn't be having any pain," this will anger and frighten him. Everything the child says should be taken seriously and sympathetically; if it is necessary to correct him, this should be done without implying disapproval.

It is reassuring to the child if the pediatric personnel show warmth and involvement and treat him as an individual rather than as an inanimate thing ("the fracture"). Calling the child by name also helps to alleviate his all too common television-mediated fear that the doctor does not know which child is which, with the consequent possibility of error in treatment. This approach should begin with the child's first contact in the setting. The following complaint is an example of how an apparently minor incident can contribute to a provocation ecology:

> The reception lady . . . *always* said "the leukemia child." She never once said my name even though it was right there in front of her. (Boy, CA 11, with leukemia, Ross & Ross, 1982a)

Warmth and involvement should be the keynote of the consultation. In setting the rarefaction ecology as a goal in the pediatric environment, it is important to be aware that the genesis of the rarefaction ecology is often the outcome of a series of relatively minor interactions and events, none of which is either difficult to implement or time consuming. In the following accounts of two physicians doing physical examinations, note that initially neither had an advantage over the other. The two patients, five-year-old boys, were scheduled for physical examinations prior to possible treatment interventions; both were new patients, very nervous and uneasy; and both pediatricians knew that observations were being made. In the first case, summarized from Beuf (1979, pp. 45–50), an observer was in the same room; in the second (University of California, 1975) a video recorder was known to be turned on. Despite knowing she was being observed, the first doctor's behavior and demeanor almost immediately served to move the situation toward a provocation ecology, and this process accelerated as the examination proceeded. In contrast, the second doctor started in methodically to create and maintain a rarefaction ecology.

> *Case 1.*   Patient (R.M.) has chronic heart problem, is visibly frightened, and is on bed in hospital examination room with both parents present. Doctor enters, sits down with her back to the child, gets history from mother, and refers to child in the third person as though he were absent [Beuf interprets this as *objectification,* a lack of any real interest in the child]. Midway through the history she turns to child and says, "So you're the baby!" [Beuf sees this as demeaning.] Child shakes his head. After further discussion with parents, the doctor is ready to examine the child, and asks, "What holiday is coming up?" Child covers his eyes. "What do you want for Christmas?" No reply. Doctor then asks in a slightly strained voice, "R.M., why do you cover your

eyes?" No response. She begins to examine him. He is very nervous. She starts to take off his blue jeans; he kicks and cries, but she makes no effort to reassure him and gets them off. Doctor discusses affect-laden matters and his shortcomings in these areas [urination and defecation] with no attempt to temper the effects [child cries when she does this]. Her manner becomes cooler toward the child as she proceeds with the examination, still getting no reply to direct questions. Doctor removes the rubber reflex hammer from the instrument case and says, "Now I think I'll hit you with my hammer for a while." No response. At end of reflex testing series, child starts to cry and says, "I'm scared." Doctor replies, "Oh, come on, there's nothing to be scared of." Child cries when he hears he must return in a month.

Case 2. Patient (J.) has a neurological problem, looks terrified, clings to mother. Doctor enters, asks mother to sit on bed with child and takes history. Doctor sits on a low chair so that he is at eye level with child. Alternates discussion with mother with nonthreatening comments to child, making no attempt to elicit responses. Then gradually asks questions that can be answered with a nod, for example, "Soon it'll be Hallowe'en, do you go trick-and-treating?" and makes demands such as "Stick out your tongue and go *ahhhh* and see if you can sound really scary." Child complies, almost laughs. Doctor takes out reflex hammer, asks child if he'd like to see a trick. Child nods. Doctor produces wooden soldier and says, "See my soldier, his name is Bob and he's standing up straight ready to kick this ball. Now see this [hands hammer to child], feel it, it's soft." Doctor waits while child examines hammer. "Now watch, I just tap his knee like this [soldier is positioned in front of a small ball] and he *kicks* the ball. Do you want to try?" Child tries it several times, laughs in delight, and addresses doctor for first time of his own accord, asking, "What makes him kick?" Doctor briefly explains that there is a special little motor called a reflex, and if you tap it you kick. Doctor asks mother if the child can test her motor. He shows child how to tap gently. Mother kicks. Doctor says to child, "OK if I roll up your pants so we can see how good your motor is?" Child agrees, watches reflex testing with interest, laughs when his leg kicks. Doctor tells child he will have to come back in a week and when he does he can see some other tricks. Child smiles, waves goodbye to doctor when he leaves.

The behavior of the physician in Case 1 was unquestionably inept. However, it is important to keep in mind that the interpersonal skills exhibited by the physician in Case 2 are not emphasized in most medical school curricula and so, presumably, are not valued. This is one of a diversity of curricular shortcomings that has prompted Bok (1984) to call for a massive rehumanization of medical education.

In the pediatric hospital setting, the child life workers constitute a particularly valuable resource for the child. Although they are a part of the pediatric team, they are also in the unique position of having no direct association with disagreeable demands or painful procedures. Consequently, they are often regarded by the children as their only real friends in the hospital setting. In terms of "closest to people in the child's life outside the hospital," they would be ranked first over the rest of the pediatric team. Because they function as powerful sources of reassurance for the child, child life workers should be regarded as an absolute essential for every hospital pediatric department (Rothenberg, 1982; Thompson & Stanford, 1981).

Other Adults and Children

Some pediatric hospitals have two sets of elevators, one for surgery and other serious cases and the other for outpatients, new patients, and the general public (Ack, 1976). Some also have dual access to all departments that have in- and outpatients, in order to avoid having children see fear-arousing sights. Seeing adults crying and looking distraught or hearing them make fear-arousing or ambiguous remarks can cause great anxiety. Similarly, the behavior of other children will have an exaggerated effect when seen through the haze of misconceptions on which many children base their interpretations of events in the medical setting. Seeing a same-age, same-sex peer coping or exhibiting mastery (Thelen et al., 1979) can exert a strong positive influence on the child's behavior (although the mastery model may seem to the child to be beyond his capabilities). Conversely, hearing other children screaming but not knowing why, or seeing them forcibly taken into a room, will almost certainly have a strong negative effect.

The behavior of pediatric personnel toward other children should always elicit an explanation to child onlookers. It is particularly important that adult support be provided (if at all possible) in the high-anxiety areas of the hospital. For the child, the pediatric intensive care unit (PICU) is by far the most traumatic area and one that is open to gross misinterpretation on his part. One 10-year-old boy summed up the PICU experience with the terse comment, "I thought I'd gone to Hell." Its unfamiliar, science-fiction-like surroundings with flashing lights, cardiac monitors, oscilloscope screens, and the monotonous sound of the ventilator (Atkinson, Hamblin, & Wright, 1981); the difficulty the child has in sleeping, with the lights always on, constant activity, and noise; and the fact that the child may be in pain and may be connected to several monitoring devices whose tubes are often seen as ropes so that he feels "captured, a prisoner, tied down," all add up to a terrifying experience (Barnes, 1974; Cataldo, Jacobs, & Rogers, 1982) that makes the child unusually vulnerable and susceptible to distortions of the ongoing activities. Consider the following description of a sequence that is a common occurrence in the PICU, as well as in the emergency room. It is one that could function as a provocation ecology for the child observer, with adults beating up a sick child, or as a rarefaction ecology, in which a reassuring adult explains that pediatric personnel are striving to save a sick child's life:

> An alarm rings, voices call over the PA system, a heterogeneously-garbed group of people rush into the room and gather around the bed of another child. Some of them appear to start hitting the child on the chest, others may restrain him, others start hooking him up to equipment. A veritable stream of people run in and out of the room. Terse orders are given. There is a lot of noise and confusion. The observer is terrified. (Carty, 1982)

Cataldo et al. (1982) have noted the similarity of the psychologically and physiologically noxious events that occur in the PICU to experimentally produced aversive stimuli and have warned that PICU events may result in the same conditioned response suppression and learned helplessness that occur in the experimental situation. The fact that certain events, such as powerful positive stimuli and warning signals that predict the onset of aversive stimulation, can mitigate the effects of aversive stimulation in the experimental setting mandates procedural changes in the PICU. Positive stimulation in the form of attractive toys and attending nonthreatening adults should be introduced into the situation along with scheduled "safe" periods of time during which no aversive procedures occur. Green (1983), in a brief and valuable paper, has emphasized the need for normalization of the PICU across developmental stages.

Environmental Nonsocial Factors

If the pediatric environment is to function as a rarefaction ecology for the child who may experience a pain event, certain of his needs in that environment must be met. Olds (1978) considers these to be the needs to feel comfortable, to feel in control of one's self, and to be purposefully active. Of course, in the pain equation the environment is only one of the factors that can cause the child's pain to escalate or attenuate, so that even under optimal conditions, the other factors will also influence the nonsocial environment effects. Of all the factors, however, the nonsocial environment, being inanimate, is usually the simplest one in which to effect changes: The requirements are an administration that understands the need for apparently superficial changes and is willing to allocate funds for them and creative department personnel with the ability to see the facilities from the child's point of view.

The Need to Feel Comfortable

Physical and psychological comfort can function as major sources of reassurance to the child and, as such, constitute an important contribution to the goal of a rarefaction ecology. Physical comfort is heightened by having furniture and other equipment on an appropriate scale so that the child can safely perform a number of actions independently of outside help. This means that the child should easily reach books and toys on shelves, get drinks from the fountain, and use the toilets and sinks. The scale of the rooms and other spaces should also be appropriate: Large spaces can be broken up with bookcases or shelves serving as partitions or with carpet areas that center play spaces or clustered chairs. Crowded areas are often intimidating to children, so where space is a problem, steps could be taken to minimize a crowded effect: Chairs could be placed in L-shaped groups to provide some privacy rather than in rows where the child is seated among strangers. Outside windows with a reasonably attractive or interesting view are a strong feature. Ulrich (1984) reported that adult postoperative patients with a natural view of trees recuperated faster and required less potent pain killers than did patients with a brick wall view. Cavernous ceilings can be lowered with suspended lattice-type structures; and proper lighting can eliminate much of the institutional look, at least in waiting rooms. Structural changes to reduce noise and monitoring of room temperature are also important.

Closely aligned with the requirements for physical comfort, and in many instances overlapping them, are the requirements for psychological comfort. When there may be some reason for anxiety, children are psychologically most comfortable with the familiar. The more the environment resembles a home, the more at ease the child will feel. The entrance area should be clearly differentiated from its surroundings and have high appeal for children; the waiting room colors, furnishings, and points of visual interest should be carefully thought out. Plants, pictures, toys, and a special play area all help in creating a positive ambience. One hospital that has effectively melded the child's needs for physical and psychological comfort with functional building design is the Children's Health Center of Minneapolis (Lobsenz, 1982). Instead of the usual admissions desk, for example, *Sesame Street's* Big Bird greets the entering child. Windows stretch from floor to ceiling so that even very young children can look outside. Walls are painted in bright colors and covered with attractive, child-appropriate pictures, and play areas are readily accessible with ample space and play materials.

It is essential that these efforts be carried over to other areas, wherever feasible. The contrast between the waiting room and the examination room or cubicle or hospital bed should not be jarring. Potentially frightening equipment should be out of sight or in pleasing containers because there is some evidence that children with the least understanding of instruments report the most anxiety in medically related situations (Siaw, Stephens, & Holmes, 1986). The goal here should be to have the rooms look like a toy store (Jolly, 1981). Semi-gloss, attractive paint colors, pictures, and murals, as well as cushioned chairs and patterned cubicle curtains, all counteract to some extent the essential institutional features. When the transition from one area to the next is marked by a sharp drop in the comfort component, the effect is to create some of the attributes of a provocation ecology. The consequent unease that such a contrast induces is reflected in the following comment by an eight-year-old boy:

> It was real fun in there [waiting room], then I go through this door and I thought, "This is it. This is where it starts." It was terrible and scary. (Ross & Ross, 1985)

Once the child has moved out of the waiting room, particular effort should be directed toward ensuring that he has maximum possible privacy. Proper gowns that preferably he can manage without help, a curtained area where he can undress, and some way for him to let others know that he is ready (a sign that he can hang out or a button that turns on a light) should be a routine part of the procedure. It should be implicitly clear to the child that no one will barge in when he is naked, an unnecessary event that is upsetting for a child used to privacy and embarrassing for most school-age children and adolescents.

Although empirical data on the pediatric environmental variables discussed here are scarce or nonexistent, it is clear from children's comments that they are highly responsive to the setting and atmosphere:

> Sometimes [at Children's Hospital at Stanford] it's almost like I'm on an overnight at a friend's house. Like at night I can see lights in those houses [across the creek] and three boys come and play over there. And see this tree, the same two birds come every day and my nurse puts bread out for them and they look in. It's real peaceful here, they don't have bells ringing all the time and kids screaming and people being crabby. (Boy, CA 9, with asthma, Ross & Ross, 1982a)

> If you have to be in a hospital, this [Children's Hospital at Stanford] is the best one ever. When we first came Daddy looked at this room and said, "*This* can't be right, *this* looks like the Stanford Hilton." Well, this is lots better than a hotel, it's like a friendly house in the country and there's a real nice feeling here. (Girl, CA 7, with rheumatoid arthritis, Ross & Ross, 1982a)

The Need to Feel in Control

The negative impact of even the most dismal setting can be counteracted to a considerable extent if there are features of it that allow the child to feel that in some respects he is in control. The sense of being in control depends in part on feeling competent (Bandura, 1981): Wherever possible, the child should be encouraged to do as many as possible of those things that he ordinarily would do for himself. The physical setting is particularly important here: Easy access to toys and other activities, fountain height, and bathroom facilities have a direct effect on the child's sense of competency. He should also be able to move from one part of the office or hospital without feeling lost or needing help. Many pediatric areas have colored lines on the floor so that he can be told to "follow the yellow arrows back to the play area in the waiting room while your mother talks to the doctor" or "follow the rabbits along the wall." Making one's own decisions is another aspect of being in control. Even the immobilized child should not have to depend on routine checks by the nursing staff but should have some way of signaling when he wants help. Whenever possible he should be given choices such as what to eat, when to get up, how to have parts of the room space arranged. Feelings of control are also enhanced by having him feel that his space (the bed and curtains around it) is truly his. He might put up his drawings; adjust the lighting, blanket, or television set; or personalize the space with posters and messages (Wallace & Cama, 1983). It is not uncommon for a child to become very possessive about his bed: One 5-year-old boy tied ribbon from presents to make a long rope that he then tied around the four corners of his bed and announced that all this land was his. The child also needs the support of personal belongings to form a link with home. He should be allowed to wear his own pajamas rather than the standard gown. As Evans and Evans (1982, p. 596) have pointed out,

> Most children have some form of special object which is vitally important to them. It may be a piece of blanket, silk scarf, sheet, teddy-bear or other doll, etc. Winnicott

(1965) has emphasized the importance of these "transitional objects" in the normal development of a child and described them as intermediate between the self and the outside world. They are used particularly when the child goes to sleep, is sad, lonely or anxious and enables the child to withstand upset of whatever cause. Children should therefore have such articles with them in hospital.

The Need to Be Purposefully Active

Assuming that the child is reasonably well behaved, the setting should allow him some freedom to explore without endangering his safety. This can be done with color ("You can go anywhere in the blue area"), pictures ("Stay in the rabbit rooms"), or lines on the floor ("You can walk all around this floor by following this line and it will bring you back to your room").

In the anxiety-type situation typified by the medical setting, the need for play is strong (Crocker, 1978; Piaget & Inhelder, 1969), particularly at all the waiting points in the treatment sequence, for example, where the child is waiting to be admitted, to get to bed, to be examined, to hear test results. The play materials at these points should be displayed on open shelves; they should be developmentally appropriate and also include other play materials and activities for the less active children. Wallace and Cama (1983) set up an art gallery for pictures by the children. The less active ones might draw pictures for this space. The use of autobiographical scrapbooks (Romero, 1986) should also be considered. Most pediatric departments have playrooms where waiting patients and siblings who have been brought along can go to play. Some of these are particularly appealing with a park-like atmosphere and slides and sandboxes.

Commentary

The pediatric setting frequently functions as a provocation rather than a rarefaction ecology. To reverse this state of affairs, it must first be recognized that the crux of the problem is an imbalance of power, with most of the power being vested in the pediatrician or attendant pediatric personnel. Our thesis here is that a shift to a more equitable power structure would increase the probability that a rarefaction ecology would occur. That such a shift cannot be accomplished by superficial means was epitomized in the patients' rights movement. Advocates of the American Hospital Association Patient's Bill of Rights (1972) naïvely equated the reassignment of rights with the patient's ability to use those rights in the absence of any change in the participants themselves.

If a shift to a more equitable balance of power is to occur, all members of the triad must change their behavior in the pediatric setting (VanderMeulen, 1985). Some of the changes would be common to all; for example, if all three members of the pediatric triad are to share an understanding of the situation, it is essential that they all have the ability to communicate at an appropriate level. Other changes would be directed specifically at one participant. The pediatrician, for example, must acknowledge the distinction between being in charge of the situation and being omnipotent in it. He must make it clear that questions are welcomed and initiate checks to confirm that his explanations and instructions are clearly understood. Probably the most crucial attribute for the rarefaction ecology is a sympathetic imagination, that is, the ability to see and care about how the situation is for the child. The mother, or other adult, must sustain an assertive rather than a passive role. This means pursuing explanations and options as well as assuming the role of child's advocate by putting his welfare above all other considerations, including the convenience of the doctor and hospital regulations. Note how one mother's insistence (Murphy, 1982, p. R8) transformed an incipient provocation ecology into a rarefaction one:

> Recently, our five-year-old son fell and split his forehead open. . . . My husband and I rushed him to the emergency room . . . where we were able to keep Danny fairly calm by reading . . . to him while waiting for the doctor. After examining our son, the doctor told us he would need 10 stitches and asked us to leave the room as he prepared to strap Danny down on the table. Amid Danny's shrieks, I asked the doctor if he would please speak with us outside the room. I told him that Danny was a very sensitive child and that if the procedure were explained to him, and if we were permitted to remain with him, the whole experience would be less traumatic for Danny and easier for him as a doctor. Finally, he agreed, although he said it was against hospital rules. He told Danny he would receive a long shot of Novocain directly into the wound and that this would hurt, but after that, he would feel nothing. Danny held our hands and remained calm throughout the whole operation. Not once did he flinch or move.

The child, too, must learn new responses. By approximately age 6, he must begin to be aware of his rights in the pediatric situation so that he knows when a question or complaint is justified. He must have some control over himself, for example, some skills in managing anticipatory fear and anxiety, and must be equipped and sufficiently informed that he can assume some responsibility in the pain situation.

The kinds of changes that we are advocating are well within the realm of possibility. They could be effected through direct training supplemented by observational learning experiences. It is essential that innovations be introduced in medical school and public school curricula that will equip the pediatrician, parent, and child for coping effectively with the demands of the pediatric consultation and related situations. There is some evidence that the forces that can effect such changes are in progress. There is a readiness for change in the medical establishment, with doctors and medical students becoming increasingly critical of the medical school curriculum (Jonas, 1978; Millman, 1977). One set of complaints centers around the dehumanization of medicine (Folkman, 1981), and there are newly revised curricula designed to remedy this problem (Bok, 1984). A discussion by Lindell (1982) on the humanization of the hospital should be mandatory reading for those genuinely concerned with the improvement of the social and nonsocial facets of the pediatric setting. Similarly, there is active and vocal concern in the lay community as well as in sociopolitical spheres (Jonas, 1978) about the spiraling costs and diminishing quality of health care. One related change in the educational domain has been the introduction of health programs of a most practical nature in the schools (see, for example, Kristein, Arnold, & Wynder, 1977; Lewis, Lewis, Lorimer, & Palmer, 1977; Ross & Ross, 1985). Furthermore, in the last decade there has been an increasing number of powerful and often prestigious models (see, for example, Brody, 1982, on defiance of hospital regulations; Ross, M., & Ross, A. P., 1980, on noncompliance with a painful treatment regimen) who have demonstrated unequivocally that in the intimidating situations of the medical world, the parent has the right to insist on optimum care for his child, rather than passively accepting what is offered (Brazelton, 1986; Rogers & Head, 1983; Stinson & Stinson, 1983).

4
Assessment and Measurement

At a time when impressive advances have been made in techniques for the measurement of a diverse group of pediatric disorders, it is sobering that there is no instrument or test that can be used to directly and objectively measure a child's clinical pain in the way that a thermometer measures body temperature. In the last two decades, rapid and dramatic progress has occurred in the refinement of existing methodology and the development of increasingly sophisticated measurement procedures for a variety of pediatric conditions. For example, the assessment potential of computed axial tomography (CAT scans) had such an extraordinary impact on pediatric neurosurgery that in certain respects current pediatric neurosurgery bears little resemblance to procedures as recent as even the early 1970s (Milhorat, 1978). By comparison, progress in the technology of clinical pain measurement has lagged far behind (Eland, 1983; Jeans, 1983b; Sanders, 1979).

A fundamental and formidable deterrent to progress in developing clinical pain measurement procedures continues to be the divisive issue of whether it is possible to measure pain at all. Some clinicians and measurement theorists have stated unequivocally that clinical pain can never be measured. Hendler (1981, p. 2) comments on "how absurd it is to try to measure pain," and Linton et al. (1984, p. 2) argue that "pain is a *set* of complex behaviors and therefore there is no 'measure of pain'." Savage (1970) contends that the severity of pain is an unmeasurable phenomenon. He believes that since subjective reports of pain are dependent measures of an uncontrollable and generally unobservable event and since there is no independent measure of the nociceptive stimulus (as there is in experimentally induced pain), it follows that the arbitrary assignment of numbers to such reports of pain does not constitute measurement. For the reader who is interested in pursuing different facets of the measurement controversy, there are two papers that should be regarded as mandatory reading. The first, by Chapman (1976), is an outstanding statement on problems and issues in the measurement of pain. The second is an impressive examination by Michell (1986) of the complexity of the problem of choosing appropriate statistics for the analysis of measurement scale data and of the theories of measurement that underlie the continuing "permissible statistics" controversy.

What is needed is a measurable body function that is present or increased when pain is perceived and absent or decreased when pain is not present (Brena, 1978), but no such meaningful and objective physiological indicator has been identified. In commenting on the status of the theory and technology of pain measurement in man, Bonica (1984) states that "only minimal advances" have occurred. This lack of progress ties in with the previously discussed general difficulties inherent in pursuing research on clinical pain, particularly the problem of definition. In this connection, Wolff (1980, p. 174) believes that

> the lack of a generally accepted scientific definition of pain still hampers us . . . measurement is always made difficult if one is not quite sure what one is actually measuring.

In addition, characteristics specific to children further compound the assessment difficulties. Different developmental stages have their own unique problems and issues (Jeans, 1983b): For example, developmental changes occur in the perception of pain, in verbal and nonverbal behaviors, and in the children's cognitions about pain. Regarding methodology, additional design precautions are required when young children are involved. It is essential, for instance, to establish unequivocally that each child understands the measurement instructions; merely asking the child if he does is not sufficient. Other checks such as short practice "tests" must be built into the procedures.

Although there is at present no way to measure pediatric pain directly, the fact remains that pain assessment constitutes a fundamental basis for progress in the clinical as well as the theoretical pediatric arena. It is of crucial importance to refined diagnosis, decisions about treatment regimens, and evaluations of their effectiveness. It is the first step in investigating pediatric pain; it makes feasible the investigation of the correlates of a pain episode and the variables that may modify it. It would also permit the documentation of secondary levels of influence, such as the qualitative transformations in pain experience and expression that occur as a function of developmental, socialization, and cultural factors.

In view of the vital role that the assessment of pain plays in potential clinical and theoretical advances, it is fortunate that other investigators have been undeterred by the current failure to develop a direct measure of clinical pediatric pain. They have chosen instead to approach the problem indirectly by studying subjective reports from patients, observing their pain-related behaviors, and defining physiological correlates of pain. Within their assessment framework, clinical pain can be conceptualized as a complex, multifaceted experience with each of three components, the subjective, the behavioral, and the physiological, lending itself to specific assessment and measurement procedures. In using measures specific to these response systems, it is likely that comparisons either within or between response systems may yield different findings. The apparently discrepant findings should not be interpreted as evidence that the respective measures lack validity (Syrjala & Chapman, 1984). Instead, they should be seen as representing different facets of the complex problem of pain. For this reason, these indices generally cannot stand on their own, but in combination they can serve as a useful basis for coming to some conclusion about the degree and quality of pain the child is experiencing.

The *subjective component* requires verbal or nonverbal input from the child. It has been assessed with a diversity of techniques, including direct questions, self-rating scales and scale derivatives designed specifically for children, graphic procedures such as pain drawings, and projective tests. A reluctance to rely solely on the child's subjective estimate of his pain has led to the development of *behavioral measures* incorporating parameters that are thought to be related to pain severity and that are measurable objectively. Included here are observation scales of a global nature to determine the presence or absence of pain as well as schedules that focus on specific pain-related behaviors such as linguistic (complaints) and paralinguistic (crying, screaming) vocalizations. *Physiological measures* are completely objective indices of pain-related parameters but are not measures of pain per se. The physiological correlates of pediatric pain that have proved useful include thermogram data and cardiac rate.

This chapter describes and evaluates the assessment and measurement procedures for each of these components and suggests directions for future research in these areas. The focus is on pediatric pain; measurement procedures for adult pain are referred to only when they have implications for some facet of pain in children. Basic to the evaluation is an understanding of psychometric criteria, that is, of standardization, reliability, and validity.

Psychometric Criteria

Standardization

Standardization means uniformity of procedures for administering and scoring an instrument; it is prerequisite to the task of obtaining satisfactory reliability and validity. Uniformity of procedure requires that detailed instructions be provided. These describe the target population, specify the materials to be used, provide the explanation to be given to the child, outline the practice sessions, describe how to handle the child's questions, discuss the use of specified probes as well as when and how to give other help, and conclude with instructions on scoring the responses and interpreting the results (American Psychological Association, 1974). Some pediatric pain assessment procedures have been carefully standardized (see, for example, Lollar et al., 1982), but the majority are characterized either by a lack of concern for this step (Beyer & Knapp, 1986) or, even worse, apparent ignorance of the need for it.

Reliability

Reliability means consistency. It is a general term that includes several specific types of reliability, the ones of interest here being test-retest and interrater reliability.

Test-retest reliability, expressed numerically as a reliability coefficient, describes the extent of agreement between the scores or other information provided by the same individual on two separate occasions. The assumption is made that the phenomenon of interest is a relatively stable one, such as IQ. When the variable under consideration is subject to fluctuation over time, establishing test-retest reliability is difficult because the resultant coefficient indicates only that instability is present but provides no information as to its source. In the case of pain, with its random temporal fluctuations as well as diurnal variations (Lloyd, 1977), the use of test-retest reliability is most appropriate with measures of moderate postoperative and tissue injury pains. It is not appropriate for use with severe to excruciating pain such as the pain associated with the removal of the innermost layer of bandage in burn dressing changes (BDC). In the latter case, the acknowledged severity of this pain (Szyfelbein, Osgood, & Carr, 1985) would likely result in the child's consistently selecting the extreme point on any pain intensity rating scale. The resultant high test-retest reliability coefficient is more accurately regarded as a ceiling effect than as evidence of reliability. Guidelines such as these should be viewed with caution. For example, moderate postoperative pain measures lend themselves to the establishment of reliability coefficients because this pain usually follows a diminishing path and is transient. However, in some chronic pain conditions such as juvenile arthritis there is a similar decrease in the magnitude of the child's responses or pain ratings even though all clinical signs point to the intensity of the pain being unchanged. In this case, habituation to the pain has occurred rather than a decrease in the pain itself, and the reliability coefficient does not reflect this basic distinction.

Interrater reliability describes the extent of agreement between independent observations of behavior, categorizations of verbal data such as recorded interviews, or scoring of test forms. It concerns stability on the observers' rather than the subject's part. It should be reported whenever some evaluative judgment is made of observable events: Observers would simultaneously but independently rate behavioral aspects of an ongoing pain experience, such as the presence or absence of specific verbal and motoric responses in a child, or would look at a child's drawing of his pain and rate it in terms of specified characteristics. The level of agreement between the resultant sets of observations/categorizations/codes is expressed as a reliability coefficient. It is customary to require an r in the .90s, with zero or blank responses excluded from the computation. This high a level of agreement is not difficult to achieve with well-trained raters if the rating categories are discrete, clearly defined, and accompanied by explicit examples. However, artificially high rs may occur on rating scales having just three or four points, because these scales require only gross discriminations on the rater's part.

Validity

Validity refers to the extent to which an instrument measures what it purports to measure (Wiggins, 1973). The necessity for establishing the validity of an assessment tool influences the decisions and choices that are made at each stage in its development. Four types are relevant to the evaluation of pediatric pain.

An instrument has *face validity* when what it measures coincides with the respondent's view of what it measures. Although some researchers view face validity as a relatively inconsequential requirement (MacRae, 1977), it is, in fact, an essential one, because what the child perceives as the real purpose of the evaluation may determine his response. When asked to rate the intensity of his pain, a child who believes his response will determine whether or not he will be given an unwanted shot (Eland & Anderson, 1977; Ross & Ross, 1984b) will likely respond differently than if he sees it as helping the doctor understand how he feels at that moment.

The evaluation instrument has *content validity* if it contains a selection of behaviors that are representative of the domain of interest. One of the best examples of a tool having content validity is the McGill Pain Questionnaire (Melzack, 1975). Among other things, it requires the patient to assess qualitative and quantitative aspects of his ongoing pain, specify location and describe temporal aspects of it, and provide a global assessment of the pain's overall intensity.

Concurrent validity is determined by correlating pain scores with one or more external variables considered to be a more direct, objective index of pain. In a study by Scott et al. (1977), pain intensity ratings of children with juvenile chronic polyarthritis were correlated with independent assessments on four-point scales of the activity of the disease (swelling of joints and a blood test) and its severity (number of joints involved and their functional status). Abu-Saad and Holzemer (1981) had nurse-observers record the frequency of body movement, facial expressions, and vocalizations (considered by experienced pediatric nursing professionals such as Meinhart and McCaffrey [1983] to be indices of pain) and correlated these ratings with several physiological measures, including temperature, pulse, respiration, and blood pressure, that often become elevated when the child is in pain. One difficulty in using concurrent validity with clinical pain is that pain is not simply and directly related to quality and intensity of noxious stimulation and behavioral and physiological changes do not always correlate in pain experience.

The extent to which pain assessment scores conform to what would be expected on a theoretical or empirical basis is referred to as *construct validity*. In establishing that a rating scale has construct validity, one would select a behavior or other response having a known pattern of reaction and correlate the rating scale scores with points within the known pattern. It can be expected, for example, that as the wound resulting from an appendectomy heals, the intensity of pain should decrease; a rating scale of pain intensity completed at intervals during the recovery period should reflect this pattern of decreasing pain intensity. Szyfelbein et al. (1985) used a thermometer-like numerical rating scale to obtain pain intensity ratings of BDC every minute from severely burned children. They then demonstrated a significant relationship between these ratings and the well-documented and rapidly changing pain levels of the BDC procedure.

Subjective Assessment Procedures

The assessment of the subjective component of pediatric pain entails having the child provide an estimate of his pain. As Bond (1979, p. 26) has stated,

> There are methods which, though they cannot tell us what is experienced when pain is felt, do give us information representing the subject's interpretation of the experience modified by what he or she wishes us to know about it. . . . [These methods] enable us to use the patient's own estimate of pain as a basis for treatment.

Although it is almost impossible with the available methodology to establish that the child's estimate of his pain experience is reliable and valid, this failure does not negate the clinical utility of the data collected. Instead, it makes essential strict adherence to certain conditions when collecting subjective data: Estimates should not be viewed as measurements, nor should they constitute the sole basis for making a judgment about the degree of pain. The estimate procedures must be sensitive enough to detect reasonably small variations in the pain experience, but at the same time, they should be characterized by brevity, clarity, ease of administration, practicality in the clinical setting, and versatility in respect to clinical and experimental use. Finally, to the maximum extent possible, they should conform to the criteria of measurement methodology discussed above. Investigating the subjective component of the child's pain experience has unavoidable weaknesses, but these can be at least partially mitigated by combining the data with those collected through behavioral observation and physiological measures. The subjective procedures to be described here include verbal, pencil-and-paper, graphic, rating scale, and projective test procedures.

Verbal Self-Report

Although verbal self-reports are the most frequently used pain estimation procedure (Agnew & Merskey, 1976), their value is a subject of controversy among clinicians and investigators working with adults. One group has given them strong endorsement:

> Verbal self-report is one of the most important means by which the practicing physician may routinely assess the quality and quantity of pain experienced by his patients. (Bailey & Davidson, 1976, p. 319)

> The single most reliable indicator of how much pain a person is experiencing is the subject's verbal report. (Jacox, 1980, p. 86)

A second group of clinicians and investigators has sounded a cautionary note. Representative of this position is the statement of Liebeskind and Paul (1977, p. 42) that in measuring human pain, verbal report is naturally relied upon heavily to provide the most direct access to subjective experience; yet it is occasionally forgotten that even verbal report is only behavior from which we infer the internal state, sometimes incorrectly.

In commenting on this issue with respect to children, P. A. McGrath (1987c) has stated that

> the triangular validation model has demonstrated that verbal reports of clinical pain are acceptable provided the patient's frame of reference has been established either through experimental pain matching or some brief standardized inventory.

Certainly, with many children at the preschool and school-age levels, verbal reports are a valuable source of information about the pain experience. They are generally sensitive to variations in ongoing pain states as well as to the effects of treatment. It is often possible to use them to establish facts that are inaccessible with other measurement procedures and that otherwise might be overlooked. Furthermore, they convey more information about the intensity, quality, and nuances that comprise pain than is usually the case with behavioral observational data or physiological measures. Consider the following description of a stomachache by a 9-year-old girl:

> It feels like a cramp that hurts, like somebody just punched you. It's not a dull pain, it's more like sharp and your stomach gets tight like you were holding your breath.

There is no question that verbal reports have their limitations. The verbal self-report procedure is an obtrusive one and may sensitize the child to the demands of the situation. The resultant distortion may be in either direction: The child may exaggerate the intensity of his pain or he may mitigate it. Scott et al. (1977) reported instances of arthritic children exaggerating the intensity of their pain because it was under the discriminative control of their parents, who wanted them to have increased dosages of analgesic medication.

Reasons for mitigating pain are particularly interesting. The child may have learned in the process of socialization to inhibit or attenuate complaints of pain, a response pattern that is particularly characteristic of victims of child abuse. If he has difficulty using language to convey his thoughts, he may find it easier to say "no pain" than to struggle with verbalizing. Fear, particularly in the pediatric hospital setting (Eland & Anderson, 1977), may also act as a response inhibitor. Children are often convinced that an admission of pain will result in a loss of privileges, such as eating lunch in the pediatric playroom, or painful treatment, such as shots (Ross & Ross, 1982a). Sometimes the child believes that an emphatic denial of pain will speed his release from hospital:

> *Pain? Me?* No, no, no, *I'm* not in pain, Nurse. In fact, I was just wondering why I'm here at all. I *should* be at home. It's *bad* to take a bed when . . . some other kid . . . *really* needs it. (Boy, CA 9, less than 24 hours after emergency appendectomy, McCarthy, 1972)

Minimizing Error and Maximizing Quality in Verbal Reports

Despite their limitations, verbal reports *can* be of value in obtaining a picture of the topography of the child's pain—its degree, duration, location, and intensity pattern over time. The goal is to maximize the probability of accuracy in the child's response by minimizing the known sources of error as well as to upgrade the quantity and quality of information obtained. Because the child may be afraid to admit that he is in pain, it is essential to preface a question with an accurate, but nonthreatening, explanation for asking the question, accompanied by the maximum reassurance possible that the child's admission of pain will not result in noxious or unwelcome consequences. Note, however, that we are not advocating lying to the child. Whenever possible, use open-end questions that require the child to generate answers (Ross & Ross, 1984a), such as, "What does your stomachache feel like?". Maximum information is obtained when the wording of the question provides a structure that facilitates the child's response (Ross & Ross, 1984a). For example, the aforementioned question should be set in the following context:

> Suppose your best friend came to the door right now and wanted you to go for a bike ride. You wouldn't feel like going with this stomachache, would you? Let's pretend that your friend has never had a stomachache. What could you tell him/her about how this stomachache feels so he/she would know just what it feels like?

The alternative is the supplied format question, which spells out the direction that the child's answer must take (for example, "Is your stomachache a stabbing pain?" and "Did you have trouble sleeping?") and requires only a yes or no answer. The direction indicated in the question may be one that might not otherwise have occurred to the child, thus creating a biasing effect that would raise doubts about the validity of the information obtained. In addition, this format tends to elicit minimal information with little elaboration. The generate format is clearly more time consuming, but it avoids the bias problem and usually yields relevant information of considerable value. It is essential to create a set that what the child has to say is important, and that in certain respects he is even something of an expert since only he can supply the information about his pain. The generate format lends itself well to this requirement:

> I have a young man working with me today who is just learning how to be a doctor. He has never had arthritis. What could you tell him about the pain you have so that next time he sees a girl like you with arthritis he'll know a lot about how it feels?

Equivalence of meaning of commonly used pain words should not be assumed. In the assessment of pediatric pain, the words *pain, ache, hurt,* and *owie* are often used interchangeably on the assumption that they convey equal intensity of pain. However, these words have different meanings for children (Ross & Ross, 1982a) as well as for adults (Gaston-Johansson, 1984), so the meanings the words have for the child should be determined before verbal report questions are initiated. The fact that these familiar words do differ in meaning for different children supports Wilkinson's (1984, p. 353) contention that

> even when the child has acquired speech, he may express his pain in his own special language which has to be learnt if his communication is to be understood.

Sometimes it is easier for the child to provide information about his pain if he is asked to compare it with a previous episode of the same pain or a different one. Children often spontaneously use a specific pain experience as a basis for the description of another pain (Ross & Ross, 1982a):

> It [broken elbow] felt like scraping your knee, only harder. (Boy, CA 7)

> Probably it [worst tension headache] was equal to my sprained wrist when it first happened. (Girl, CA 9)

> An earache is equal in pain to a strep throat. (Boy, CA 10)

Sensory pain matching has the advantage of minimizing communication difficulties. The child who gropes unsuccessfully for pain descriptors may have less difficulty retrieving the names of previously experienced pain conditions. It also represents a move toward an objective way of handling a subjective experience: If the pediatric professional knows the child well, it provides the professional with a basis of comparison for the immediate pain event.

The issue of the accuracy of the child's long-term memory is relevant to the sensory pain matching procedure, because should the memory of pain events deteriorate over time, the validity of asking a child to compare an ongoing pain with the faded memory of a prior pain is questionable. As we noted in Chapter 2, the available clinical (Hahn & McLone, 1984; Hawley, 1984; Peterschmidt, 1984; Travis, 1969) and empirical evidence (Ross & Ross, 1982a) shows that preschool and older children can recall noxious events accurately and sometimes in surprising detail. Further, the mood-state-dependent memory phenomenon (Bower, 1981) posits that recall will be facilitated if the child's emotional state at the time of recall is similar to his state at the time of the previous event (Bartlett, Burleson, & Santrock, 1982). Since pain events of childhood are frequently associated with negative affect, it is likely that the child's emotional states during the previous and current pain events would be affectively congruent. This increases the probability of the accuracy of sensory pain matching by the child.

Apart from the memory issue in sensory pain matching, it is not known how the recalled severity of a prior pain experience may influence the subjective estimate of an ongoing pain (Wallenstein, 1982). Women in labor who previously had had severe pain unrelated to the pregnancy cycle rated their labor pain on the McGill Pain Questionnaire (Melzack, 1975) as low to moderate; those with no prior severe pain experience rated it as severe (Niven & Gijsbers, 1984). Children who have previously undergone bone marrow aspirations (BMAs) often rate another severe pain as milder than would a child with no prior severe pain experience (McGrath, P. A., 1987c). When pain matching is used with children, the implications of this finding should be kept in mind.

Duration of Pain Of relevance to diagnosis and treatment decisions is the duration of the child's pain. Response accuracy on this dimension depends, in part, on the child's developmental level and concept of time. The young child is generally unable to report the duration of events of any kind. In the case of pain, this difficulty can partly be overcome with prompts using temporal anchors: "Was the pain there at breakfast? Was it still there at lunch?" Even children in kindergarten can pinpoint the time of onset of pain when this approach is used (Ross & Ross, 1986). As one might expect, older children generally have little difficulty on this point:

> Not more than a minute for the whole thing [penicillin shot] because he [pediatrician] always asks me riddles when I get shots and he only asked two. (Girl CA 8, Ross & Ross, 1985)

In a study with adults, Bilting et al. (1983) reported that the subjective estimate of time showed an increase with pain, with the amount of increase correlating with the clinical estimate of pain severity in different diagnostic groups. As Weeks (1983) has pointed out, one shortcoming in the Bilting et al. study was the failure to report the reliability of the time estimates. However, it is an interesting hypothesis in that it raises the possibility that time estimation might prove useful in children in assessing the intensity of clinical pain that follows a predictable course (for example, postoperative pain). Some evidence that children's estimates of the time required for iatrogenic procedures may be indicative of how painful they perceive the procedure to be comes from a study (Ross & Ross, 1985) in which children who described the pain of shots as "torture" and "terrible" estimated the duration of time needed to administer a shot as significantly longer than did those who were more matter of fact about the pain. It would be interesting to identify a group of iatrogenic procedures that all take about the same actual time and then have children estimate the time for each one and rate the severity of pain associated with each procedure. The data should throw some light on the question of whether the apparent duration of time serves as an index of the child's perception of the magnitude of the pain.

Temporal Pattern Another kind of relevant information concerns the temporal pattern, that is, the continuous, intermittent, or pulsating characteristics of pain as well as rhythmic or arrhythmic pounding. A highly verbal child may be able to provide information about this aspect of his pain. For most children, however, a better way to obtain it is to demonstrate the temporal options with simple musical instruments, such as a whistle and drum, and ask the child, "Does your earache go on and on like this and never stop [long unbroken whistle note], or does it stop and start like this [rhythmic beat on drum]?" An alternative would be to use a crayon and paper. In any case, the child would enjoy using the materials since these activities have the distracting quality of a game. As one five-year-old boy said (Sunderland, 1984),

> I can't hear what my earache is like when I crayon, I have to stop and listen and then I'll show you.

In an investigation of children's perception of intermittent versus continuous pain experiences, Scott (1978) used a sheet of paper with two rows of light bulbs. Each bulb in the "on," or continuous pain, row was yellow, with radiating yellow lines to emphasize that the lights were all on; the intermittent pain row contained alternating lighted and unlighted bulbs.

Use of Tangible Objects to Supplement Verbal Report   For the child whose verbal difficulties markedly reduce the content value of his responses, there is a need for objects to supplement his verbal report. In the pain interviews reported by Ross and Ross (1984b), some of the younger children who had difficulty generating pain descriptors used gestures and demonstrations. One 5-year-old boy, reporting a stomachache that "feels like this," first pressed his hands together, then made a squeezing motion. A 6-year-old girl first described an earache as "poking," then shook her head emphatically and said, "No way. Poking's not hard enough" and jabbed at the table with a pencil until the point broke, saying, "*That's* how hard it hurt." A cluster of such incidents suggested that children who experience difficulty in using language as a medium for pain description might communicate better if they were given an assortment of objects such as a same-sex rubber doll, colored Band-Aids, and a safe tool-kit. The result could be information about the location and intensity of the pain and its sensory and temporal characteristics. This proposed procedure is a variation on the well-documented use of doll-play as a medium of communication for the preschool child. It also has affinity to Jolly's (1981) recommendation that the pediatric medical setting should look more like a toy shop than a tribute to modern technology.

Pencil-and-Paper Self-Report

Questionnaires

The Varni/Thompson Pediatric Pain Questionnaire (PPQ) (Varni & Thompson, 1985) is a comprehensive, multidimensional instrument designed for the assessment of pediatric pain. There are three forms: Parent (P), Child (C), and Adolescent (A). Form P is designed to elicit two clusters of information: One set of questions covers general information about the child and family; a history of the current pain problem, including the medication and other management procedures being used; the efficacy of these procedures; a list of pain descriptors for the kind of pain the child is experiencing; visual analogue scale (VAS) ratings of the child's ongoing and average intensity of pain; and a pain map to show the locus of the pain. The other set of questions concerns etiological factors of a psychological nature and is designed to provide a comprehensive evaluation of the child or adolescent's life situation. Topics included here are familial models of acute and chronic pain, the presence of stressors in the home environment, the possibility that the mother's reaction to pain episodes serves to maintain them or that they result in tertiary gains for her, the effect of the child's pain on the family, and the mother's perception of the importance of the pain to the child.

Form C requires the child to generate descriptors of his pain, supplies a checklist of pain descriptors as well as VAS for rating ongoing and worst pain, and a pain map that uses the child's color choices for different intensities of pain. Form A's questions, VAS, and checklists (see Figure 4-1) elicit a detailed report of the topography of the pain: diurnal and seasonal variation, location, current and worst recent intensity, duration of pain episodes, and pain descriptors. In addition, Form A produces information on the effect of the pain on the life of the adolescent and his family, the adolescent's view of what effect it would have on his life and that of his family if the pain were to disappear, possible tertiary gains in the situation, what he calls the pain, and what actions the adolescent could take if the pain continued.

This excellent pain questionnaire has several important features. The forms do not take long to complete, which makes it useful for clinical settings. The verbal descriptors are ones that would be familiar to most respondents. The questions tap factors that may precipitate, exacerbate, or maintain the pain, and this information is of value in planning the therapeutic program. Pain is not viewed as an isolated event. Information is elicited from both the parent and the child or adolescent concerning the place of the pain condition in the life space of the patient and family. The questions are ordered with some care: Respondents are required to generate descriptors before they select words from the checklists, and the order is such that inconsistencies in responses can be identified. Methodologically, this is the optimum combination for eliciting pain descriptors. If only a checklist is used, a follow-up interview should be conducted to determine the basis for the respondents' choices. This additional procedure is essential in the light of findings by Ross and Ross (1984a): In developing their pain interview protocols, they had two experimenters administer checklists to 20 hospitalized and nonhospitalized children ages 5 to 12. A third experimenter then talked informally with the children, the goal being to identify the rationale for their pain descriptor selections. Although there was often a valid basis for the word selected, the responses of some children raised doubts about the checklist format:

> Try to figure out which words are shot words and don't check any of them or you'll get the needle.

> Check all the words, then they'll know your pain is awful and do something about it.

> They always put in some words that aren't real words. Find them, because if you check them they know you're not good at telling what your pain is like. (This child said that someone had taken *easy* and added *qu* to it to make *queasy*.)

There is preliminary evidence of satisfactory reliability and validity of the PPQ from a study of JRA children (Varni, Thompson, & Hanson, 1987). Further evaluation of reliability and validity will be forthcoming from the test developers as well as other investigators who currently are using this valuable instrument (Varni, 1987).

The Children's Comprehensive Pain Questionnaire (CCPQ) was designed by P. A. McGrath (1986) to provide a comprehensive and multifaceted assessment of the child's view of his current pain problem. The topics covered include the to-

---

When did your present pain problem begin? Please also explain the symptoms.

What was your reaction to the pain at that time? Please explain.

Were any major changes in your life occurring then? Please explain.

If your pain were suddenly to disappear, how would it change your life?

How would it change your family relationships?

Assuming that the pain continues, what kinds of things do you think you should do now, which will help later on?

What words do you use to describe your pain?

What day of the week do you have the most pain?

Have you ever noticed something that tells you that you are about to experience a pain episode? (e.g., stiffness, particular thoughts or statements, physical sensations or irritability)

What do you call your pains? (e.g., "headache," "joint pain," "stomachache," "backache," etc.) Please list them in order of severity, #1 being the most severe pain.

On a scale of 0–10, (0 = no pain, 10 = severe pain), how severe is your pain at the following times of the day?
6 A.M.   9 A.M.   12 noon   3 P.M.   6 P.M.   9 P.M.   12 A.M.   3 A.M.

What do you currently do, besides taking medication, to relieve your pain?

Does your pain seem worse when you are (Yes/No to each):
tired, anxious, bored, happy, unhappy, angry, busy, lonely, arguing, upset.

Are there any other situations in which your pain is worse? If yes, what are they?

Please rate how much pain you are having at the present time by placing a mark somewhere on the line.

Not Hurting	Hurting a Whole Lot
No Discomfort ⎯⎯⎯⎯⎯⎯⎯⎯⎯⎯⎯⎯⎯⎯⎯⎯⎯⎯⎯⎯	Very Uncomfortable
No Pain	Severe Pain

Figure 4-1 Sample items from Form A (Adolescent) of the Varni/Thompson Pediatric Pain Questionnaire. Reprinted, by permission, from Varni, J. W., & Thompson, K. L. The Varni/Thompson Pediatric Pain Questionnaire, 1985.

pography of the pain, that is, duration, frequency, location, and whether it is diffused as opposed to localized; temporal aspects and diurnal variation; and causality. The child is asked to estimate on a VAS the efficacy of the ongoing treatment and parent action when he is in pain, as well as the long-term prognosis for his pain. It is not clear whether there is some provision for a practice session prior to the first VAS task. At one point in the questionnaire a checklist of pain descriptors is supplied, and later the child is asked to generate his own descriptors. Facial scales and VAS positioned at different points in the questionnaire are used to assess both pain intensity and the range of intensity. The VAS format is also used for gathering information on the range and level of pain-associated affect and the child's feelings, if any, of sadness, fear, and anger concerning his pain. There are opportunities for the child to report the use of coping strategies as well as secondary gains that are pain related. In connection with the latter line of thought, the possibility is explored that the pain is specific to certain days (for example, school versus weekends) or activities (school versus play). It would be helpful as a last question to ask if there is anything else that the child can tell about his pain, a suggestion that also applies to the Varni/Thompson PPQ.

The CCPQ is suitably brief for the clinical setting but at the same time provides a comprehensive picture of the child's view of his pain. It is an excellent pain questionnaire. The questions that tap coping strategies, pain-related secondary gains, and the child's view of his family's actions and reactions to his pain have particular potential. Different forms of some of the most important questions are used so that a child who finds one question format difficult may subsequently be able to provide the information with another format. The use of VAS at intervals in the questionnaire means that verbal and nonverbal responses are alternated, thus providing a welcome change of pace, particularly for the child who finds verbalizing difficult. We would recommend having the mother independently complete the questionnaire as she thinks the child would as a way of adding another level of information about the child's pain.

The McGill Pain Questionnaire (MPQ), developed by Melzack (1975), was designed for adults, but it is included here (see Figure 4-2) because verbally competent children age 12 and up are able to use it (Jeans, 1983b; Monk, 1980) and it is considered one of the best multidimensional instruments presently available for assessing clinical pain. It is a comprehensive pain assessment instrument that enables the patient to tell the clinician how he perceives his pain on both physiological and psychological dimensions. It can usually be completed in less than 10 minutes if it is read to the person and the person's responses recorded. Self-administration takes somewhat longer. From research with adults, there is some evidence (Klepac, Dowling, Rokke, Dodge, & Schafer, 1981) that the two modes of administration yield different scores.

The MPQ has four major sections. The first contains 20 sets of words that describe the sensory, affective, and evaluative qualities of pain and an additional

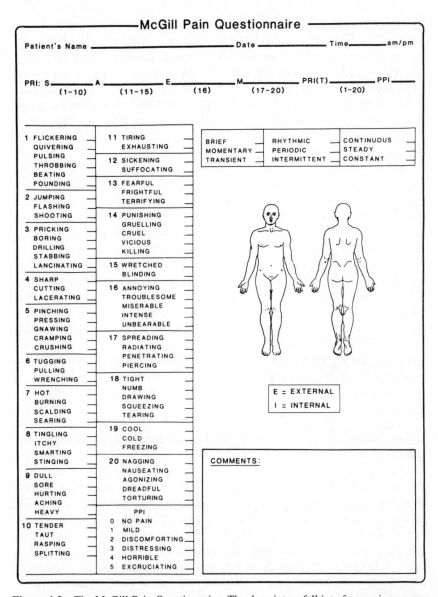

Figure 4-2 The McGill Pain Questionnaire. The descriptors fall into four major groups: sensory, numbers 1 through 10; affective, numbers 11 through 15; evaluative, number 16; and miscellaneous, numbers 17 through 20. The rank value for each descriptor is based on its position in the word set. The sum of the rank values is the pain rating index (PRI). The present pain intensity (PPI) is based on a scale of 0 to 5. Reprinted, by permission, from Melzack, R. The McGill Pain Questionnaire. In R. Melzack (Ed.), *Pain measurement and assessment.* © 1983, Raven Press, New York.

category containing miscellaneous pain descriptors. Within each set, the descriptors are valued from 1 ("least pain") to 4 ("most pain"). In the sensory category, for example, the set of thermal words are "hot" (1), "burning" (2), "scalding" (3), and "searing" (4). The rank values of the descriptors selected by the patient yield a score for each of the categories (sensory, affective, evaluative, and miscellaneous); the total score is called the Pain Rating Index (PRI). Although the subscale score for each category can be used in isolation, research by Turk, Rudy, and Salovey (1985) suggests that the total PRI score is preferable. This section also yields another major pain score, Number of Words Chosen.

The second section contains descriptors that assess the pattern of pain, for example, a brief, rhythmic pattern or a steady nonfluctuating pattern. The next section consists of anterior and posterior line drawings of the human figure on which the patient marks the location of his pain and indicates whether it is external, internal, or both. The fourth section requires the patient to evaluate the intensity of his pain on a 0–5 scale with corresponding verbal descriptors that correlate more highly with the evaluative category in the first section than with either the sensory or affective categories (Melzack, 1975). This section yields the third and final score, Present Pain Intensity, which is the number-word combination selected on the 0–5 scale to represent overall pain intensity at the time the questionnaire is completed. The MPQ also includes questions about factors that exacerbate or minimize pain. The patient is asked to rate the range of his pain, that is, the points at which it is worst and least, and to compare his pain with other types of pain. There is unequivocal evidence of the reliability and validity of the MPQ (Reading, 1983).

Diaries

In the diary approach to self-report, the child is provided with a diary with sections for different entries. The child's task varies depending on the purpose of the data collection. If the goal of the diary activity is to identify the etiology of recurring pain, then the child is asked to (a) record the time of occurrence of each pain episode for a fixed period of time, such as 2 weeks; (b) rate the severity of his pain episodes; (c) provide a record of temporally associated events that occurred prior to the point of onset; and (d) describe what was different, noticeable, or salient about that particular day. If the goal is to evaluate the efficacy of therapy in relation to the time-course of persistent pain, then the child is asked to rate the intensity of pain at fixed intervals throughout the day. He may also be asked to summarize the data and participate in the evaluation of his diary entries.

Richardson, McGrath, Cunningham, and Humphreys (1983) used the pain diary format in a study of the validity of two self-report pain intensity scales. Sixteen children, ages 9 to 17 and suffering from recurring migraine headaches, recorded the intensity of their headaches at fixed time intervals daily for 4 weeks. Their headache diaries contained one of two behavioral pain rating scales along with columns to enter symptoms experienced with each headache, medication logs for amount and type of medication taken, and possible causes of the headaches. In an ongoing study, P. A. McGrath (1987c) is using pain diaries to collect normative data on the pain experiences of nonclinical, school-age children, each of whom is recording and rating the intensity of all the pain experiences that occur over a 4-week period. To evaluate the accuracy of diary accounts, Barr et al. (1987) had parents use diaries to record observations of the frequency and duration of infant crying and fussing and then compared the entries with data obtained from a voice-activated recording system. Parental diaries were found to be accurate measures of these vocal phenomena.

Pain diaries are subject to the same weaknesses that characterize other self-report procedures: It cannot be assumed either that they are free from contaminating biases or that the child will comply with the instructions. There is very little evidence of reliability and validity in their use with children, but it is known that the validity of any self-observation task decreases as the complexity of it increases (Keefe, Kopel, & Gordon, 1978). On the other hand, pain diaries have several strong features. They provide a basis for the study of children's pain experiences from a developmental viewpoint. They are one of the least expensive pain assessment procedures since they can be used as easily in the child's natural environment as in the hospital setting. They heighten the child's awareness of events that might precipitate and exacerbate his pain episodes, thus suggesting, at least in part, a logical explanation for the pain in lieu of a more frightening, mystical, random reason for it. By permitting the child to be a valued and active contributor to the management of his pain problem, his sense of mastery is fostered along with an increase in his self-esteem (Bandura, 1982). In addition, pain diaries involving daily entries are likely to be less subject to distortion of memory and consequently are more valid than are retrospective questionnaires or interviews (Andrasik & Holroyd, 1980b).

Graphic Procedures

Pain Drawings

Children sometimes are able to communicate more effectively through their drawings than they are able to do verbally (DiLeo, 1977), a fact that has encouraged clinicians to use this approach for obtaining information about a child's pain. The child is usually given paper and pencil, crayons, or paint, and is asked to make a picture of his pain. Typically, he requires little encouragement; when he has completed the drawing he is interviewed about his picture (see Figure 4-3). Since there is no standard procedure for this technique, in the interests of replication those collecting data in this way could be expected to provide a description of their method. In fact, such descriptions are rare in the pain literature. Unruh, McGrath, Cunningham, and Humphreys (1983, p. 387) are one of the few groups to describe the approach they used in a study of migraine tension headaches:

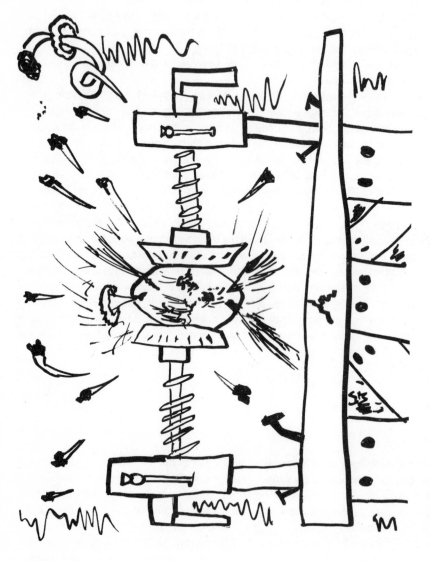

Figure 4-3a Pain drawing of a headache (Boy, CA 10), (Ross & Ross, 1987).

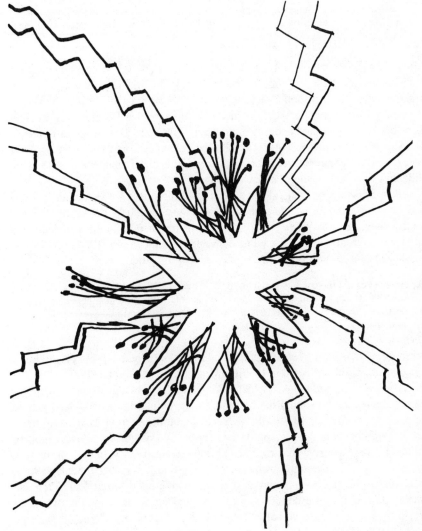

Figure 4-3b Pain drawing of a crashing fall (Boy, CA 12), (Ross & Ross, 1987).

[The] children . . . were given 2 sheets of blank white paper and 8 colored markers (black, brown, blue, purple, orange, red, yellow and green). Each child was asked to draw 2 pictures. The instructions for the first picture were "Please draw a picture of your pain. If we could actually see your pain, what would it look like?" The instructions for the second picture were "Please draw a picture of you when you are in pain." Each child was left alone to complete the drawings and all were able to do so. Drawings were then sorted in categories on the basis of content and definitions for these categories were developed.

Although no evidence of the reliability of the pain drawings was presented, there is some interesting support for construct validity. The drawings differentiated between children with migraine headaches and those with tension headaches and could be reliably categorized by content and dominant color. Despite the age range, there were no age-related patterns in the data; there were also no sex differences. In a subsequent study, Kurylyszyn, McGrath, Cappelli, and Humphreys (1987) have reported that raters were unable to discriminate different intensities of pain in children's drawings of their headaches.

Pain drawings have also been shown to differentiate between children who have been prepared for needle procedures and those who have not (Sturner, Rothbaum, Visintainer, & Wolfer, 1980), as well as between children with acute and those with chronic orthopedic pain. Villamira and Occhiuto (1984, p. 285) reported substantial differences in the drawings of the latter group:

In most cases, the patients with chronic pain emphasize, in their drawings, the bodily district affected by the pain: whereas the patients with acute pain generally emphasize . . . the bodily districts that, in each developmental period, have a particular importance.

Other facets that have been studied include developmental aspects of children's concepts of pain as reflected in their drawings (Jeans & Gordon, 1981).

There are two situations in which asking for pain drawings would be inappropriate: The technique should not be used for the child who is convinced that he cannot draw or for one whose illness has depleted his energy. Apart from these restrictions, the technique is appropriate for a wide range of age and cognitive ability and is responsive to the child's developmental level. Children at the preoperational level, for example, who see pain as a thing (Piaget & Inhelder, 1969), find it reasonable to draw a picture of it. Those with limited verbal skills often find graphic procedures an excellent way to communicate information that would be very difficult for them to verbalize (Ventafridda, Rogers, & Valera, 1984). Even the child who is otherwise quite verbal is sometimes at a loss to describe his pain; for this child pain drawings provide a framework for his answer. Hahn and McLone (1984) reported the case of an 8-year-old girl with a spinal cord tumor who told her doctors (when she was older) that the tumor-related pain had radiated from her back to her stomach area but that, at the time, she could not figure out how to describe the pain. Graphic procedures could have been a useful adjunct in this type of situation.

Pain drawings usually convey considerably more information about the pain than just location and intensity, particularly if color is used. The child tends to project affective and cognitive information about his pain experience into his artwork and subsequently into his commentary about it (Vair, 1981). Often the drawings are rich in details that help the clinician to understand the child's perception of his pain and fantasies about it.

Pain Maps

The pain map procedure was introduced by Keele (1948) to obtain graphic reports from adults of areas of bodily pain involvement. In this procedure, the child is given an anterior and posterior outline of the human body similar to the back and front line drawings of whole figures depicted in Figure 4-4b, but without the horizontal and vertical lines. For the locus of pain, he is asked to mark the specific pain site with an X or, in the case of a diffused pain, to shade in the areas of pain. For the intensity of pain, he is asked to shade in the areas of bodily pain involvement, using the colors of his choice. No quantitative scoring system is used to assess the child's graphic report of painful areas and their intensity. Instead, the pain map is examined visually to determine the accuracy of the locus of pain as well as to decide if the colors used coincide with observed behavioral indicators and the child's self-report of the intensity of pain. See Figure 4-4a for a template, with the figure divided into 45 anatomical areas, which was used by Margolis, Tait, and Krause (1986) to score the pain map after the locus of pain had been marked by the adult subjects.

The pain map has been used in several studies of hospitalized children, with results lending credence to its efficacy as well as its concurrent validity. In the first of these, Eland reported in an unpublished study (see Eland & Anderson, 1977) that all but four of 172 hospitalized children ages 4 to 10 were able to mark accurately and on the correct side of their body the area that coincided with the pathology, surgical procedure, or other painful events that had occurred during the hospitalization period. Similar findings were reported in a second study by Eland (1983) and one by Vair (1981) of postoperative pain. Further support for the concurrent validity as well as test-retest reliability comes from a case history of a 4-year-old boy hospitalized with an immune deficiency (Eland & Anderson, 1977, p. 461):

> The child had been hospitalized for eight weeks for infection that involved his left leg, had gone home for two weeks, and returned with what apparently was a thrombus in the saphenous vein behind his right knee. At the time of his first interview, he placed numerous x's along his left leg and told the investigator that he only hurt at night when his leg was placed in a plaster splint which was being used to prevent a flexion contracture in his left knee. The following day he placed x's along the left leg in the same area

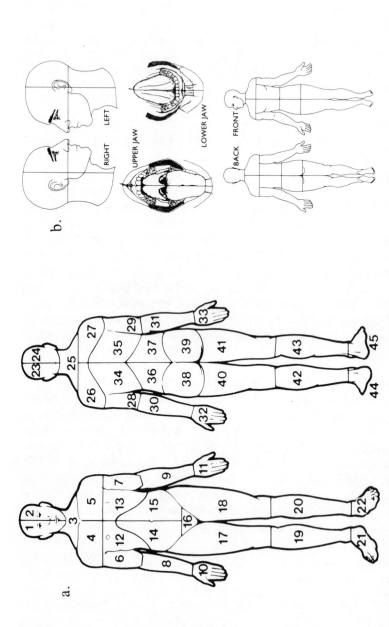

Figure 4-4 Pain maps: a) Scoring template for pain drawing. Reprinted, by permission, from Margolis, R. B., Tait, R. C., & Krause, S. J. A rating system for use with patient pain drawings. *Pain*, 1986, *24*, 57–65. © 1986, Elsevier Science Publishers. b) Distribution of pain sites across body regions. Reprinted, by permission, from Toomey, T. C., Gover, V. F., & Jones, B. N. Spatial distribution of pain: A descriptive characteristic of chronic pain. *Pain*, 1983, *17*, 289–300. © 1983, Elsevier Science Publishers.

as the previous day, and in addition, placed several x's in the region of the lower abdomen. On the third day the patient was diagnosed as having a partial bowel obstruction. He again placed x's on the left leg and abdomen, and then colored brown the whole lower portion of his right leg between his knee and ankle. Two days after the child had colored his right leg brown, a purulent yellow-brown material began to drain from his leg in the area of his right ankle. In reality, the child did not have a thrombus in the saphenous vein but a severe infection caused by seven specific bacteria. It was necessary to incise and drain the area and the child endured an extended hospital stay. Ironically, the child had graphically depicted his pain and pathological condition several days prior to clinically measurable signs and symptoms or the physician's discovery of it.

Another opportunity for demonstrating concurrent validity could lie in a comparison of pain map information with thermography data.

In addition to the advantages characteristic of graphic procedures in general, the pain map procedure offers several advantages specific to it. Logistically, it is sufficiently practical in terms of brevity, appeal for the child, and ease of administration and evaluation for use in the pediatric setting. It is particularly useful where repeated measures are needed, as in the case of children with chronic pain. A potentially useful scoring procedure for these children's pain maps was developed by Toomey, Gover, and Jones (1983) for adults with chronic pain (see Figure 4-4b). In developing their quantified system for scoring the distribution of pain on pain maps, Toomey et al. used enumeration of total sites of pain as the measure of pain distribution. Pain maps are also useful for confirming expected changes in the spatial distribution of pain that occur over time as a result of treatment, and for identifying unexpected pain developments.

Self-Report Rating Scales and Derivatives

Although the multidimensional nature of pain has been widely accepted, the most common approach to pain estimation continues to be unidimensional, in the form of self-report scales on which the patient is asked to rate some facet of his pain, usually its intensity. Depending on the type and number of anchor points supplied, these scales fall into three main categories. The *visual analogue scale* (VAS) consists of a line, without markers other than endpoints, of least to greatest value for the dimension of pain being assessed. The *graphic rating scale* (GRS) consists of a series of words along a continuum of increasing value, for example, "no pain," "mild pain," "moderate pain," "severe pain." The *numerical rating scale* (NRS) uses numbers, for example, 1 to 10 or 1 to 100, reflecting increasing degrees of pain. (Figure 4-5 contains a sample of these three types of scale.) There are derivatives of these scales that are used almost exclusively with children. These derivatives include pictorial representations of faces, animals, and thermometers and frequently use tangible objects such as blocks and poker chips to help children describe their pain. The self-report rating scales have in common certain strengths

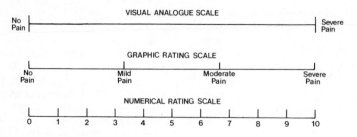

Figure 4-5 Visual analogue, graphic rating, and numerical rating scales.

and limitations. Others that are specific to an individual scale will be described under that scale.

Strengths

All of the scales are notable for their clarity and simplicity. Children usually grasp the idea with little difficulty: There is evidence that children as young as 5 can use the scales or their derivatives providing that the instructions are clear and simple and practice sessions precede participation (McGrath, de Veber, & Hearn, 1985; Ross & Ross, 1982a; Szyfelbein et al., 1985). It is unrealistic to expect a child in pain to use a rating scale with no prior experience. Brevity is another advantage of these scales: They make minimal demands on sick children. The scales are also versatile: They can be adapted to different cognitive levels and are practical for use in a variety of clinical settings. Finally, administration and scoring are both straightforward.

Limitations

The deceptive simplicity and apparently straightforward approach characteristic of self-report rating scales mask several important assumptions underlying their use. One such assumption is that although rating scales are obtrusive procedures that sensitize the patient to situational demands (Syrjala & Chapman, 1984), these scale characteristics do not influence the patient's self-ratings. Another assumption is that what is being measured is a single attribute, such as intensity of pain. In fact, the child's rating is likely to be influenced by his affective state, perhaps misery or loneliness, and these other factors could confound the assessment of intensity. As Chapman (1976) pointed out, the question of whether the child's rating represents only intensity or is influenced by all the components of his discomfort is rarely considered. The oversimplification of the pain experience that occurs when one mark on a scale represents the patient's pain has been strongly criticized.

In commenting on the tendency to rely on single scales, Gracely (1980, pp. 113–114) has stated that

> Simple scales can no more assess the diverse qualities of pain experience than they can assess the nuances of political attitudes or specify the intricacies of personality.

The use of several scales, each relating to a different aspect of pain, partially compensates for this limitation. Johnson, Kirchhoff, and Endress (1975) used this procedure, with one scale measuring the intensity of pain and the other measuring the degree of distress in children undergoing cast removal. The children were asked first to think of pain as a sensation, defined for them as "the physical feel of the pain," and then to judge how much distress the pain was causing them. Distress was defined as "how much these feelings bother you."

The efficacy of using either one or more scales, each targeting a different dimension of pain, is largely dependent on careful standardization procedures. The instructions must specify what is to be rated and the salient terms defined. For example, *intensity* might be defined as "how much the pain hurts," with categories ranging from "just-noticeable" to "excruciating"; *sensory* might be "what the pain feels like, for example, tingling or stabbing"; and *reactivity* might be "how unpleasant the pain is, miserable, horrible."

Even when the scale used is designed to measure only one facet of the pain experience, Gracely (1980) believes that this causes a further problem, namely, the compression of the broad range of the pain experience into an artificially small continuum. As a result, patients tend to spread their responses over the entire scale, regardless of the magnitude of the actual sensation. Huskisson (1974) demonstrated a uniform distribution of results with an unselected population. His finding that there were equal numbers of measurements at all points in the line would appear to support Gracely. However, Huskisson interprets it as confirming the sensitivity of the VAS.

Another difficulty concerns the fact that self-report rating scales are cross-modal; that is, they require the patient to translate some aspect of his feeling of discomfort, usually the intensity, into a mark, word, or object along a linear path, none of which expresses exactly the discomfort he is experiencing (Huskisson, 1983). In addition, pain may not be represented cognitively as a linear experience. In connection with this, Syrjala and Chapman (1984, p. 78) have noted that

> pain intensity (or some other dimension) may not represent itself in private experience in a linear fashion, and the forcing of judgments onto a length scale may be quite distorting.

A final difficulty in using self-report rating scales concerns the choice of the appropriate statistics for analyzing the data. Although the verbal descriptors/numbers/pictures are invariably presented as occurring at equal intervals, there is no evidence that they correspond in a one-to-one fashion with intensity or any other dimension of pain. The scores obtained, however, are often treated as interval or ratio level scaling in the absence of any evidence that respondents have interpreted the numbers in this way. Although many investigators (see, for example, Beaver, 1983) believe that the use of parametric statistics for scale data is acceptable, this is true *only* when two conditions are met: There must be empirical evidence, first, that the patients are in fact using the verbal descriptors/numbers/pictures as though the points at which they occur on the line are equally spaced along it, and second, that the scale ratings are drawn from a normally distributed population (Syrjala & Chapman, 1984).

With these ideas about self-report rating scales in general as background, we now move on to a discussion of the VAS.

Visual Analogue Scale

The VAS consists of a 10-cm line that can be used by a child to provide an estimate of the intensity, or some other dimension, of the pain. There are small stops at each end of the line and at right angles to it to set the limits to the rating area. The end-point descriptors are beyond the stops. Although the end points are defined as the extreme limits (for example, "no pain," "pain as bad as it can be"), they should function as possible choices rather than being so extreme that they are virtually never chosen by the child. The child's task is to put a mark on the line to indicate the severity of his pain. The score, with a range of 1 to 10, is obtained by measuring the number of centimeters from "no pain" to the point where the child puts his mark.

A practice session is essential to ensure feelings of confidence on the part of the child, to emphasize the particular aspect of the pain experience that the child is to scale, and to define the end points. In this session, the child should first be given four objects differing markedly only in size, and then asked which is the smallest, the next smallest and so on. As he responds, the adult puts each choice in a line on the table directly in front of the child, with the smallest piece to the child's left and the largest to his right. This choice/line procedure is repeated with a different set of similar objects, again differing only in size. Next, the child is shown an enlarged VAS scale and it is explained to him that the smallest to the biggest objects could be placed on this scale. The same procedure is repeated first with the remaining objects, then with experiences that the child identifies as differing in fun. If he is able to do these tasks, then he is ready to begin the pain ratings; if not, further practice should be provided.

Research with adults has shown that 10 cm is the optimum length for the line (Revill, Robinson, Rosen, & Hogg, 1976) and that a horizontal line is easier to use than a vertical one (Scott & Huskisson, 1976). The latter variable has been subjected to limited empirical study with children, with conflicting results: Children in the Ross and Ross (1982a) study were unanimous in preferring a horizontal NRS, whereas in the other studies preschool children preferred a vertical facial scale (Beyer, 1985) and older children preferred a vertical pain thermometer (Szyfelbein et al., 1985).

The VAS has proved satisfactory for use with children age 5 and older, some of whom were healthy and others were oncology patients or had arthritis, recurring headaches, and other chronic pains associated with disease or injury (McGrath et al., 1985) or juvenile chronic polyarthritis (Scott et al., 1977). It has also proved satisfactory for use with children age 8 and older having cancer-associated pain (Rogers, 1981) and with 9- to 15-year-old postoperative patients (Abu-Saad & Holzemer, 1981; Vair, 1981). In a series of studies notable for sound experimental methodology, McGrath et al., (1985) first established that children older than age 5 could use two cross-modality matching responses, brightness matching and VAS, to rate the heaviness of metric stimuli in a reliable manner with validation of responses. Next, they showed that children could use the same two cross-modality matching responses to rate with consistency the magnitude of positive or negative affect depicted by nine faces on an interval scale. Finally, in a study of children with cancer, McGrath (1987d) reported that these children's ratings of their cancer-related iatrogenic pain were both reliable and valid.

Strengths The VAS is useful for children with limited language skills because the choice points are not labeled. It offers an unlimited number of choice points between the end points. Although it has been suggested that more structure, in the form of verbal or numerical anchor points, would be less confusing to the child than having an infinite number of choice points, the unsegmented response continuum allows the child to rate his pain within the context of the maximum number of points that he can discriminate. The VAS has proven reliable and valid in studies of children in the postoperative period. Vair (1981) and Abu-Saad and Holzemer (1981) reported that the expected decline in VAS scores occurred in the postoperative pain period. The latter investigators also found the VAS to be sensitive to medication effects over time and to behavioral indicators of pain. Statistically, the VAS is reported to be superior to the GRS (Sriwatanakul et al., 1983; Syrjala & Chapman, 1984).

Limitations In a sense, the VAS represents a pure continuum with a quality of abstractness that could be a handicap for the patient unable to conceptualize his pain intensity linearly and with only end point terms (Kremer, Block, & Gaylor, 1981). There are recurring complaints about adults being unable to complete the VAS, but in each instance no mention is made of whether there were practice sessions. Walsh (1984), for example, reported that of 98 consecutive patients, 26 were unable to complete the scale. It would be a simple task to have the patient rate other experiences prior to completing the VAS. If abstract thinking limitations are a factor, then children who are unable to complete the VAS after a practice trial should have no difficulty with either the GRS or the NRS, and this has yet to be established empirically.

Graphic Rating Scales

Dissatisfaction with certain aspects of the VAS led to the development of the GRS, which is a straight line continuum with from four to seven verbal descriptors placed in ascending order of severity at equal intervals along the line. Usually the scale is intended for assessing the intensity of pain, so descriptors such as "none," "mild," "moderate," "severe," and "unbearable" are used. Sriwatanakul, Kelvie, and Lasagna (1982) have reported that the descriptors "some" and "terrible" are probably the least useful terms for assessing pain in adults. No empirical data are available on the most useful terms for children to use. This scale can also be used to assess aversiveness or any other aspect of pain that lends itself to description by a series of adjectives that can be ranked in ascending order of magnitude. The GRS has been more widely used with children than the VAS, possibly because the anchor points provide more structure than the VAS end points do. McGrath et al. (1985) and Scott et al. (1977) have reported that children age 5 and older have used it effectively.

It is important to note that the GRS *classifies* the child's pain experience according to the category descriptors provided. It provides no basis whatsoever for assigning numerical values to the categories and using parametric statistics in analyzing the data. Using analysis of variance to analyze rank ordered data is acceptable when the assumption can be met that differences between successive steps on the ordinal scale are perceived by the respondent as being equal. With adults, at least, there is evidence (Heft & Parker, 1984; Sriwatankul et al., 1982) that the word categories do not represent identical steps in pain intensity. Attaching numerical values, for example, severe = 4 and some = 1, means at best that the numerical scores are ordinal or rank-ordered scores, with nonparametric statistics then being the appropriate tool.

Neither the descriptors used nor their placement at equal distances along the line necessarily reflects the child's interpretation. The same descriptor, such as "moderate," may not have the same meaning for each child; that is, the descriptors do not have universal anchorage, as is the case with "yes" and "no." As far as placement is concerned, the child should show where on a line he would locate the words; then he should rate his pain according to *his* placement of the words (Heft & Parker, 1984; Sriwatanakul et al., 1982). This methodological change would result in individualized scales that reflect interindividual differences in interpretation of pain descriptors. A further complication has been raised by Shapiro (1975), who has pointed out that in addition to interindividual differences in interpretation of the scale points, some of the points may not even be regarded as lying on the same dimension.

Because the format of the GRS restricts the child to the descriptors provided, the scale has limited sensitivity in that the descriptors may not express exactly what the child is experiencing. Increasing the number of pain descriptors is not the answer, because it is generally difficult for children to conceptualize more than five descriptors, a difficulty that is due to semantic rather than scaling limitations. Unlike the VAS, the GRS does not cover all contingencies: A child with mild pain that improves slightly but is still present has only one category of improvement, "no pain"; the child is then forced to continue using the descriptor "mild" when in fact his pain has actually improved.

Face Interval Scales   Using cartoon faces, several investigators (Kuttner & LePage, 1983; McGrath et al., 1985; Pothmann & Goepel, 1984b; Rogers, 1981) have developed derivatives of the GRS for use with children. These face interval scales measuring pain affect operate on the same principles as the GRS: The child is shown a set of cartoon faces that usually vary in expression from tears or total misery through neutral to smiles and laughter and is asked which picture tells how he feels right then. The cartoon association is a positive one, the facial expressions are familiar, the child need only point to his choice, and the task is interesting. Furthermore, it represents a global index of how the child perceives his pain. Using this procedure in two studies of iatrogenic pain in children with cancer, McGrath et al. (1985) obtained evidence of its reliability and validity with children age 5 and older. Their work is particularly important because the actual value of affect depicted by each face was determined from the perspective of healthy children and child oncology patients. The children used two cross-modality matching responses, brightness matching and VAS, to rate the magnitude of negative or positive affect depicted by each face. Each of the nine faces was presented four times in random order, and the children's responses were then averaged to obtain a mean affective value for each. The results provided empirical evidence that the intervals on this nonmetric scale were indeed unequal (see Figure 4-6). McGrath (1987c) is currently using the facial scale with the VAS to assess differences in intensity and affect as a function of intervention; she is also using this combination

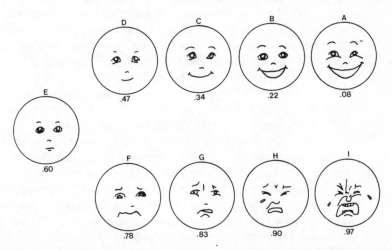

Figure 4-6   Facial scale with mean affective magnitude for each face determined from children's direct scaling using brightness matching and visual analogue scales. Each value represents the geometric mean of 132 responses (four trials per child) averaged over 33 children. The mean values were then transformed to a 0–1 scale on which the maximum negative affective value equals 1 and the maximum positive affective value equals 0. Reprinted, by permission, from McGrath, P. A., de Veber, L. L., & Hearn, M. T. Multidimensional pain assessment in children. In H. L. Fields, R. Dubner, & F. Cervero (Eds.), *Advances in pain research and therapy, Vol. 9.* © 1985, Raven Press, New York.

of scales to study the ratio of affect to intensity, a very interesting and potentially valuable line of inquiry.

Photographic Scale   A second derivative of the GRS is the Oucher (Beyer, 1984), which is designed to elicit self-reports of pain intensity. The assumption is that the Oucher should allow pediatric personnel to quantify the intensity of children's pain more accurately than is the case with children's verbal descriptions alone. This instrument consists of two scales. In the one for younger children, a series of six color photographs of the face of a young preschool child is arranged vertically from "no hurt" to the "biggest hurt you can have." For the older children, a numerical rating scale from 0 to 100 is arranged vertically. The pictorial part of the Oucher has good instructions, particularly in respect to the practice trials. In these, the child is asked to rate pains he has had, such as falls or needle procedures. If the scores vary appropriately, the child is asked, "How much hurt do you have right now?" Like all the pictorial scales, the Oucher is useful for children with language difficulties. Initial evaluation of the Oucher is promising. There is some evidence of content and construct validity and test-retest reliability with children in the 4- to 12-year-old range (Aradine, Beyer, & Tompkins, 1987; Beyer, 1984, 1985; Beyer & Aradine, 1986, 1987a, 1987b). Beyer and her associates have shown commendable diligence in the pursuit of satisfactory reliability and validity.

The Oucher has some shortcomings. There is no firm empirical basis for the placement of faces at equal intervals adjacent to the numerical scale. Such placement could bias ratings based on either scale. The fact that most children ordered faces correctly does not then justify either equal intervals or specific numerical values. There is also one procedural change that should be considered. Although the manual describes the photograph child as a boy, there are no clues to identify the child's sex. It would be preferable to treat the photograph child as the same sex as the patient. The issue of photographs versus cartoon faces deserves some research attention. Cartoon faces would appear to be more clear-cut in terms of expressions, but children might see the photographs as "more like me."

Poker Chip Tool   The Poker Chip Tool, developed by Hester (1979), consists of four white poker chips that are equated to degrees of hurt. The child is asked, "Did it [immunization shot] hurt?" A response of "no" is scored zero; if the response is "yes," the child is given the four poker chips and told, "These are pieces of hurt—one chip is a little bit of hurt, and four chips are the most hurt you could ever have. Did you have one, two, three, or four pieces of hurt?" The number selected by the child is then recorded. In a modification of the Poker Chip Tool, Molsberry (1979) made several improvements. Red chips were used for pain, with a white chip for no pain; the instructions were improved; and a practice session was introduced. Reliability and validity data are limited for either form: Hester (1979) conducted a study of 24 children's perception of pain during immunization injections. The children were ages 4 to 8. The Poker Chip Tool scores were highly correlated with the children's verbal and behavioral responses to the injection, indicating some evidence of concurrent validity. Molsberry (1979) used the tool to measure postoperative pain in children ages 4 to 7. The decreasing scores reflected the diminishing pain, thus providing some evidence of construct validity.

Although the Poker Chip Tool has the advantage of appealing, easy-to-use materials whose use does not depend on verbal facility, the scale makes some questionable assumptions. The word *hurt* was used in the instructions on the assumption that most 4- to 8-year-old children do not know the meaning of *pain* but do understand the word *hurt*. Several studies have shown this assumption to be false (Bibace & Walsh, 1980; Gaffney, 1983; Ross & Ross, 1984b). Children using this scale are assumed to have mastered the number concepts of 1 to 4. This is a debatable point, particularly for the preschool child. One possible change here would be to have four poker chips differing greatly in size from very small to very large, since size concepts are grasped at an earlier age than are number concepts (Piaget & Inhelder, 1969). There is also the problem that preschool children might not see their hurt as "bits of hurt" but rather as one big thing. A 4-year-old boy (Ross & Ross, 1982a) described pain as

> a big thing [gestures a half circle, like a tent] that gets all over you [repeats gesture]. Not an *animal* thing, no [shakes head decisively] or a *people* thing, it's just [pauses] like a *big* thing . . . [On the source of pain] When the pain comes, the thing is there . . . [On how mother's presence helps] She gets in with me [makes another tent-like gesture].

The cross-modality matching involved in expressing pain in terms of poker chips may also be difficult for the youngest children (McGrath et al., 1985). In fact, in Molsberry's (1979) study, children under the age of 6 years, 2 months had some difficulty with the task. Just because the child is able to do a task, such as picking up poker chips or putting a mark on a line, does not mean that he understands the task. When assumptions of the kind made by Hester underlie an assessment scale, it becomes crucial that the instructions incorporate checks at each stage of the practice session task to determine whether the child's responses are in fact based on understanding. See McGrath, Cunningham, Goodman, and Unruh (1985) for a brief review of this and some of the other procedures in this section.

Numerical Rating Scales

The general format of the NRS consists of a straight-line continuum numbered 0 to 10 or 0 to 100. The verbal instructions to rate the severity of the pain usually use the anchor points from the VAS, that is, "no pain" and "worst pain." The NRS is generally viewed as an attempt to approximate the VAS but in a form that allows the patient to respond orally (Syrjala & Chapman, 1984). However, any child using the NRS must know his number concepts. Numbers do have the advantage in that they permit more definable choices than does the GRS and so are useful for patients who have poor abstract abilities. They also increase the sensitivity of the instrument, but whether this increase with the 0 to 10 or 0 to 100 choices as com-

pared with the four to seven choices of the GRS is bought at the expense of reliability has not been determined. The investigator who is interested in the numerical approach to the assessment of pediatric pain should consider two variations of
the NRS, the 101-point NRS and the 11-point Box Scale, developed for use with
adults by Jensen, Karoly, and Braver (1986).

In the clinical use of this scale, some investigators believe incorrectly that
certain anchor words are essential if the child is to conceptualize the intensity of
his pain in terms of numbers. If the instructions establish the relationship between
the numbers and the child's pain experience, no anchor words are needed. In the
interview study of Ross and Ross (1982a), each child was shown a 0 to 10 scale and
asked if he knew what a Richter Scale was. Almost all the children were familiar
with the meaning of points on the Richter. After this was established, the child was
asked if he had had a cluster of common pains (blister, scraped knee, finger stick)
and where he would rate them, then was asked where he would put his worst pain
(identified through prior questions). There was no evidence of any difficulty in
using an NRS. However, the scale was used only as a warm-up item because test–
retest reliability checks made one week apart showed that the only reliable item
was the "worst pain" placement.

There is limited sensitivity in the NRS using the 0 to 10 format rather than the
0 to 100 format. Some investigators have pointed out that there are preferred digits
(0, 5, 7) that may appear too frequently to satisfy statistical needs for probability
and homogeneous distribution (Murrin & Rosen, 1985). Statistically, the intervals
cannot be assumed to be equal: The pain change between zero and three divisions
on the rating scale cannot be assumed to be equal to the pain change that has
occurred between the sixth and ninth intervals. Although rank statistics can be
used, the use of parametric statistics cannot be justified.

Pain Thermometer   Pain thermometers are simply graphic representations
of a thermometer graded on a numerical scale (0 to 10 or 0 to 100) with zero indicating "no hurt" and the highest number indicating "the most possible hurt" (see
Figure 4-7). The pain thermometer is the only important derivative of the NRS.
The child is instructed to point to the place on the thermometer to show the intensity of his pain. Szyfelbein et al. (1985) established empirically that of seven different pain scales used by children to assess the rapidly changing pain levels of
BDC a thermometer-like vertical rating scale was the almost unanimous choice as
the best way of expressing degrees of pain. Pain scores on the thermometer correlated well with those obtained with a conventional 5-point GRS. Another version
of a thermometer (called a "hurt thermometer") was used by Molsberry (1979),
but limited reliability and validity data were reported and the instructions contained words that one could not assume the child would know.

Pain Color Matching

The first formal use of pain color matching was reported by Stewart (1977), who
developed the Stewart Pain Color Scale in 1974 for use with adults. Stewart had

found that when asked to choose from an array of colors the ones that best represent pain, nearly everyone picked red for intense pain, oranges or orange-reds for milder pain, and yellows for little or no pain. Subsequent studies with children and adolescents (Abu-Saad, 1984a, 1984c; Eland, 1981; Jeans & Gordon, 1981; Loebach, 1979; Savedra et al., 1982, 1985; Schroeder, 1979; Scott, 1978; Vair, 1981) using a variety of color choice tasks confirmed Stewart's finding, with one exception. Abu-Saad (1984b) reported that a group of Arab-American children chose black and blue before red.

The pain color matching procedures are reported with no accompanying evidence of reliability or validity. With the exception of Vair (1981), no one has asked the children what their choices represent, so it is only an assumption on the investigator's part that the colors represent intensity of pain. Furthermore, the procedure appears to be unappealing to some older children and adolescents: Savedra et al. (1982, 1985) found that many hospitalized children in the 9- to 12-year-old range reported that pain had no color or that they did not know what color it was, and many adolescents showed disinterest in the question.

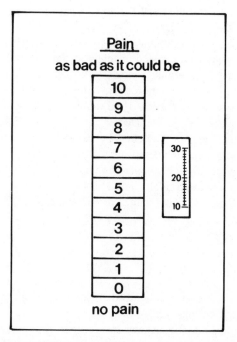

Figure 4-7 A thermometer-like numerical rating scale used to assess pain in acutely burned children during dressing changes. The figures are white on a crimson background. Reprinted, by permission, from Szyfelbein, S. K., Osgood, P. F., & Carr, D. B. The assessment of pain and plasma β-endorphin in immunoactivity in burned children. *Pain*, 1985, *22*, 173–182. © 1985, Elsevier Science Publishers.

It is difficult to see that any theoretical advances or applied benefits will accrue from further investigations in which the child's task is simply to choose a color that describes his pain. In the absence of some purposeful relationship to the pain experience of children, the continued use of this approach represents an exercise in futility. However, two methodological innovations in pain–color matching suggest that some researchers are pursuing more productive directions. Eland (1981), for example, has developed a procedure that permits the child to construct his own vertical color scale which he then uses to rate his pain during immunization injections. The procedure takes into account interindividual variations in color choice, an approach subsequently advocated by Sriwatanakul et al. (1982) for the measurement of pain using a GRS. Although reliability and validity data on Eland's scale are limited, as yet, the approach is methodologically sound and a promising development in color scale design. In the second innovation, Nayman (1979) has developed a color scale variant designed for continuous subjective pain recording. Although intended for adults, it is included here because a combination of its best features and Eland's (1981) procedure would result in a pain assessment procedure of great practicality and high appeal for children.

The Nayman scale consists of five colored lights set vertically in a wooden box similar to the vertical set of traffic lights. The lights are in a fixed ascending order of white, yellow, orange, red, and purple. The light box is placed close to the patient's bed with a small light-control hand set. Pressing a button changes the light reading. The buttons are coded tactually so that the patient can change the light reading by touch. An audible click alerts the patient to report his present pain intensity and the light readings are recorded on a moving paper. This device has great potential for use with children. If all the lights were white, the child's own scale of pain colors could be assembled very quickly using Eland's procedure and colored gels for insertion over the lights. The audible click could be replaced by a more interesting sound and the device presented as a variant of traffic lights. On the one hand it would have great appeal for children. It would have appealed, for example, to the children in Szyfelbein et al.'s (1985) study who were undergoing burn dressing changes and were required to record the intensity of their pain every minute. On the other hand, as a diverting and distracting activity it could affect what it was measuring.

Comment

The self-report rating scales have considerable potential as useful tools for children's assessment of various dimensions of their pain. As a group they represent one avenue of approach to the difficult and complex problem of pain assessment. In terms of refinement, however, they are at a primitive level: Attempts at standardization are sketchy, reliability and validity data are in most instances weak or nonexistent, and there are no large clusters of studies supporting or extending their use. If the self-report scales are to achieve a reputable place in the pediatric pain assessment field, the specifications delineating one from the other must be respected. The VAS is only a VAS if it involves a straight line without markers other than end points of least to greatest value for whatever dimension of pain is being assessed, the basic idea being to offer the patient an infinite number of choices. An increasing number of researchers are violating the specifications of the VAS by adding numbers or vertical divisions, which means that what they are calling a VAS in fact is no longer one. The same trend is apparent in GRS to which numbers and extra divisions have been added, and in numerical rating scales with word descriptors added. This procedure makes it impossible to evaluate a particular scale, such as the NRS, or to make comparisons with other scales. For example, on a GRS to which numbers have been added, it is not known whether the children are using the words, numbers, or both, so support for the superiority of the GRS over the VAS cannot be claimed. Similarly, reliability and validity data on these "modifications" have little value for making interscale comparisons because the underlying specifications for the scales have been violated. We are saying, in effect, that if the use of the VAS, GRS, or NRS is reported in a study, the reader should be able to assume with confidence that the scale's specifications have been adhered to. If this assumption cannot be met, then the scale should be identified with some descriptor other than VAS, GRS, or NRS.

Projective Tests

During the 1970s sporadic attempts were made to use projective test methodology in assessing children's perceptions of pain. Scott (1978), for example, used two cartoon sequences that showed a child experiencing self-inflicted pain in the form of an accidental hammer blow and experiencing other-inflicted pain in the form of being given a shot. The purpose of the test was to assess color, shape, texture, pattern, and time sequences in the child's perception of pain. It was administered to young children in outpatient clinics and school settings. Scott reported some evidence of developmental trends in the children's perceptions of pain, but in the absence of test-retest reliability data the results do not stand up under scrutiny.

During this period, projective tests were also thought to have potential as a means of facilitating communication concerning ongoing pain. Eland (1974) developed a series of instruments designed to help the preschool and young school-age child convey his feelings about the intensity of ongoing pain. One of these is the Eland Projective Tool, which consists of five pictures of a dog cartoon character in five situations. Four of these depict the animal in a series of painful situations familiar to children (such as hit in head by swing, paw caught in car door). The fifth picture depicts the animal in the same painful situation that the child is encountering, that is, an injection. The child is instructed to rank the four pictures in order from the picture of the event that hurts least to the picture of the one that hurts most. The fifth picture, replicating the child's situation, is then inserted by the child in the ranked series. There was no consistency in the children's ordering of the pictures, and Eland did not pursue further work with this instrument. Noteworthy, however, is the methodological procedure of supplying a scale with a series of choices and requiring the child to order his choices in terms of his own perception of the intensity of pain for each choice.

A much more refined instrument is the Pediatric Pain Inventory (PPI), a structured projective test developed by Lollar et al. (1982) to assess how children perceive pain experienced by themselves and by their parents. It is a model of careful development. The PPI consists of 24 pictures in clusters of six, with each cluster relevant to one of four potentially pain-evoking situations: medical, recreational, psychosocial, and common daily activities (see Figure 4-8). The child is first asked questions concerning responsibility in the picture situation, whether the picture child needed help, who would help, and what would be done. Then the child's task is to rate the pictures for intensity and duration of the perceived pain. The child's parents are asked to complete the PPI as they perceive the situations in relation to him.

Preliminary findings based on the test's administration to 240 children and adolescents between the ages of 4 and 19 indicate that the test has potential for the assessment of pediatric pain. The reliability and validity data are sufficiently high to warrant its continued development. Correlation data for the intensity and duration constructs were low ($r = .08$), indicating their independence from one another. Medical pain was perceived as lasting longer than pains in the other three situations. Of particular interest was the finding that psychosocial pain was perceived as the least intense of the four situations. This assessment was in marked contrast to findings in a number of the interview studies mentioned previously in which many of the same psychosocial pains on the PPI were cited by the 11- to 12-year-olds and up as their worst pain experiences. A significant difference was found between how the children perceived their own pain intensity and how adults perceived the children's pain intensity, with the adults erring in the direction of underestimation. This finding is consistent with that of Eland and Anderson (1977) that adults tend to underestimate children's pain experiences and with Ross and Ross's finding (1982a) that mothers' choices of their children's worst pain differed from the children's choices. Those children who described their own pain experiences as relatively intense perceived medical pain as lasting significantly longer than did children who described their own pain as less intense. This finding ties in with that of Bilting et al. (1983), who reported that the subjective estimate of time by adults is shown to increase with pain with the amount of increase correlating with the clinical estimate of the pain severity. When the 24 PPI pictures were rank ordered for intensity of pain, the highest rank was assigned to the picture of the child sitting on a doctor's table with a bandaged leg. Being given a shot ranked 17th in intensity and 23rd in duration, which would appear to support the idea that as distance from the medical setting increases, children's fear of shots decreases.

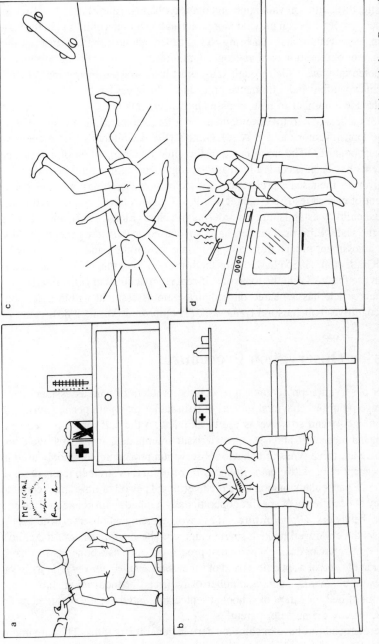

Figure 4-8 Pain-evoking situations from the Pediatric Pain Inventory: Medical (a) getting a shot and (b) receiving stitches; Recreation (c) falling off a skateboard; and Activities of Daily Living (d) burning hand on a stove. Reprinted, by permission, from Lollar, D. J., Smits, S. J., & Patterson, D. L. Atlanta Pediatric Psychology Associates, Tucker, Georgia, 1981.

Comment

Despite the difficulties in validation and other problems, careful use of self-report assessment procedures can provide more information about a child's pain than any other single procedure and can bring to light facts about it that are inaccessible with behavior observation or physiological monitoring. The wealth of information that is potentially available through self-report has attracted increasing research interest in expanding and refining the procedures. Progress has been encouraging. In this decade a number of new assessment instruments have appeared, some of which are models of careful development (see, for example, Lollar et al.'s [1982] Pediatric Pain Inventory and P. A. McGrath's [1986] Children's Comprehensive Pain Questionnaire). The importance of the children's perception of assessment instruments has been accorded increased recognition, with careful consideration being given to their scale preferences (Szyfelbein et al., 1985) and their value placement of categories (McGrath et al., 1985). Scales have been tailored to the individual child by establishing his ordering of colors (Eland, 1981) before having him use the scale. Empirical interest has also focused on the more general question of what assessment procedures are appropriate for children and at how early an age: McGrath et al. (1985) have established, for example, that children age 5 and older can use the VAS. On the topic of self-report procedures in general, an excellent review article has appeared on pediatric pain assessment within a developmental cognitive-biobehavioral framework (Thompson & Varni, 1986).

Behavior Observation Procedures

Behavior observation procedures approach the problem of pain assessment from the vantage point of behavioral indices of pain rather than pain per se (Syrjala & Chapman, 1984) and so serve as useful adjuncts to the self-report procedures, physiological measures, and documented tissue trauma data available to the clinician. There are three types of behavior observation procedure commonly used in the assessment of pediatric pain. In *behavior rating scales,* trained raters observe the child in a particular situation for a predetermined period of time and record the frequency of occurrence of specific, operationally defined, pain-related verbal and nonverbal behaviors. *Global rating scales* involve having an observer who generally knows the child well make a single judgment about some facet of the child's pain-relevant behavior during a particular procedure, such as a bone marrow aspiration, or at the end of a specific period of time. *Indirect measures of pain* focus on pain-relevant behaviors, such as number of requests for medication, time spent playing out of bed, or extent of school absenteeism, and these are recorded by an observer, usually the nurse or parent.

These procedures have in common certain general strengths. They are unobtrusive and so avoid the biasing effects likely when a child knows he is being observed. They extend the boundaries covered by self-report methods and offer refinements not available through them. Neonates and infants can be rated, verbal level is irrelevant, the problem of having procedures intelligible to the child does not exist, and data on nonverbal expressive behavior can be obtained. Fluctuations in the child's behavior that occur as a result of changes in the social and nonsocial environment, such as mother present/mother absent (Shaw & Routh, 1982), can be detected. In addition, these procedures are considered to be more objective and reliable than self-report procedures and are not subject to the cognitive- or affective-mediated distortion by the child that may occur with self-report (Syrjala & Chapman, 1984).

The behavioral observation procedures also share some limitations, a major and basic one being the issue of the validity of the behaviors selected for rating. This serious problem arises because of the paucity of pain-related behaviors that are uniquely or invariably associated with pediatric pain (Craig & Prkachin, 1983). Children in pain may engage in a diversity of verbalizations marked by negative affect: Even very young infants may emit paralinguistic vocalizations such as cries and screams, exhibit facial contortions and expressions suggestive of discomfort, show increased or decreased activity, and make postural adjustments such as stiffening or hunching the trunk. But with the possible exception of pain-specific variants of facial expression and pain cries in infants, none of these responses is solely or invariably associated with the experience of pain (Craig & Prkachin, 1983). Consider the following report (University of California, 1975) from a mother who was doing a jigsaw puzzle with her 6-year-old hospitalized son:

> Ben was feeling great, he was in *really* good form. . . . He was trying to get the whole corner finished and he was sighing and groaning, scowling and rocking to and fro—he always acts like that when he does puzzles. A nurse going by stopped and looked at him and looked kind of startled. About two minutes later she was back with pain medication for Ben. I had the hardest time convincing her that this wasn't pain—it's just how Ben acts when he does jigsaw puzzles—he looks like a child in a trance and in a state of misery all at the same time and he's loving the whole thing.

With these general points in mind, we shall now move on to a more detailed description of the available procedures and related research, beginning with the behavior rating scales.

Behavior Rating Scales

The format of these scales, with many categories for each behavior being rated, lends itself to a fine-grained analysis of pain-related behaviors. The data are very objective: The precise operational definitions for each category effectively eliminate the need for subjective inferences on the part of the raters. By definition, these scales are time limited. When a brief, but complete, treatment procedure is rated, this is not a problem; however, in other instances it is a limitation that needs to be considered in the total assessment plan.

Infant Pain Behavior Rating Scale

The Infant Pain Behavior Rating Scale (IPBRS) was developed by Craig et al. (1984) for assessing the pain behaviors of infants and young children (CA 2 to 24 months) who were undergoing routine immunization in a clinic setting. With this time-sampling scale, ratings were made once every 5 seconds of behaviors that included vocalizations (crying, screaming, use of language expressing stress), expressive body responses (rigidity, kicking), and facial expression. Concomitant behavior ratings were made of the mothers and pediatric personnel involved in the procedures. The behavioral categories used were precisely defined (see Table 4-1) and clearly have the potential to elicit information about the social contingencies that could influence pain reactivity early in life. The context in which the ratings were obtained was described precisely, making it possible for other investigators to replicate the study or extend its parameters.

Table 4-1 Sample of Definitions of Behavioral Categories from the Infant Pain Behavior Rating Scale

Subcategory	Brief definition
Infant Vocal Actions	
Crying	Vocal expression characterized by high-pitched, prolonged rhythmic and perhaps broken manner. Excludes meaningful utterances.
Pain vocal	Nonverbal expression distinct from crying, i.e., screaming (single high-pitched sound), groaning (deep sounds without wailing or sobbing), whining, moaning, gasping, choking, whimpering, and sniffling.
Pain/Fear verbal	Use of language to express physical stress or fear. May include attempts to delay action or expression of physical discomfort indicative of autonomic activity.
Other	Any verbal/vocal expression that cannot be classified otherwise—defined by exclusion.
Mother/Nurse Verbal Actions to the Child	
Praise	Statement positively evaluating or approving of prior, ongoing, or future actions of the child.
Criticism	Statements negatively evaluating or disapproving of child's actions.
Distraction	Statement endeavouring to distract from medical procedure or its sequelae.
Soothing	Attempt to calm child or alleviate pain.
Procedural statement	Statements informing about current immunization procedure.
Other verbalizations	Those not encompassed by the above.

Note. Reprinted with permission from *Social Science and Medicine,* Vol. 19, No. 12. Craig, K. D., McMahon, R. J., Morrison, J. D., & Zaskow, C. Developmental changes in infant pain expression during immunization injections. © 1984, Pergamon Journals Ltd.

Craig et al. reported interrater reliabilities of .70 or greater for responses that occurred with some frequency in all members of the triad (infant, mother, nurse). There is indirect support for the scale's content validity in that pain-specific variants of two of the scale's behavior categories have been reported. Izard, Huebner, Resser, McGinness, and Dougherty (1980) have identified a *facial expression* specific to the pain response in young infants: Eyebrows are lowered and together, nasal root broadens and bulges, eyes are closed tightly, and the mouth is angular and squarish. Johnston and Strada (1986) have used the Maximally Discriminative Facial Movement Coding System (Max) (Izard, 1979) to demonstrate this pain expression in 2- to 4-month-old infants. They consider facial expression to be the most consistent across-infant indicator of pain available. There is also evidence of a *pain cry* (Grunau & Craig, 1987a; Johnston & Strada, 1986; Wasz-Höeckert, Lind, Vuorenkoski, Partanen, & Valanné, 1968; Wolff, 1969), a high-pitched cry followed by a relatively long period of apnea, then a period of dysphonia, and finally a gradual return to the basic rhythmic rising and falling cry. Although the pain cry can be differentiated electronically from other cries (Wasz-Höeckert et al., 1968), it cannot be identified by experienced caregivers without the assistance of other measures of distress and knowledge of contextual variables (Hollien, 1980; Owens, 1984).

The IPBRS has great potential and practicality for use in the clinical situation. It would be excellent for documenting developmental changes in pain expression in infants and very young children as well as for improving pain management procedures. A strong feature of the IPBRS is its inclusion of data from the social environment in recognition of the marked influence that this environment may exert on the child's pain behaviors. A mother who gasps, becomes tense, and looks horrified when the needle is inserted is almost certain to have a negative influence on her child's reaction, whereas one who radiates serenity will communicate this feeling with positive effect (Craig, 1978). Furthermore, Craig et al. (1984) are to be commended for the restraint shown in interpreting the significance of their findings with this scale, while at the same time making it clear that the preliminary data are most encouraging.

Facial Movement Coding Systems

Another important methodological contribution to the assessment of pain reactivity in infants has been the development by Izard and his associates (Izard, 1979; Izard, Dougherty, & Hembree, 1983) of the anatomically based facial movement coding systems, Affex and Max. Affex, described by Izard, Hembree, and Huebner (1987) as the more efficient of the two, is a system for affect expression identification by holistic judgments of videotape records. It allows coders to watch the entire face in slow motion and assign emotion labels to facial expressions as they are identified. Max is seen as more objective and more microanalytic. It requires a separate, slow-motion (frame-by-frame) run of the videotape for each of three facial regions (brow, eye, and mouth), with coders judging only the presence or absence of facial movements, each of which is designated by a code number. Rater reliability for both coding systems was satisfactory in a recent longitudinal study of infants' emotion expressions to the acute pain of diphtheria-pertussis-tetanus (DPT) inoculations. Of particular interest during this evaluation was the evidence of stability of individual emotion-expression patterns over the first $1\frac{1}{2}$ years of life. The type and duration of emotion expressions of 2- to 7-month-old infants ($n = 25$) in response to DPT inoculations predicted their emotion expressions to the same event at 19 months of age. This study also replicated two previous findings (Izard, Hembree, Dougherty, & Spizzirri, 1983), namely, that particular expressions to aversive stimulation occur consistently in infants and that the duration of these expressions changes differentially with age.

Children's Hospital of Eastern Ontario Pain Scale

Developed by McGrath et al. (1985) for use with young children, the Children's Hospital of Eastern Ontario Pain Scale (CHEOPS) assesses six categories of behavior: crying, facial expression, pain-related and non-pain-related verbalizations, torso activity, tactual responses, and lower limb responses. Behaviors in each category are assigned a score value according to the following criteria: 0 = behavior that is the antithesis of pain (smiling, positive comment), 1 = behavior neither indicative of pain nor of its antithesis (child is not crying, child complains but not about pain), 2 = behavior indicating mild or moderate pain (moaning or complaints about pain), 3 = behavior indicating severe pain (full-lunged cry). The observation schedule calls for 5 seconds of observation time followed by 25 seconds of recording time, a very sound practice that contributes directly to higher reliability coefficients. CHEOPS, in fact, does have excellent interrater reliability, with agreement for all categories exceeding 80%. However, the reported coefficients may be spuriously high in view of the gross nature of the rating discrimination required, given the wide disparity between categories. Another positive feature is its scoring procedure, which allows the nominal descriptive information provided by the raw data to be transformed into ordinal data, thus permitting the use of a more refined statistical analysis.

Preliminary evidence (McGrath et al., 1985) of the validity of CHEOPS is encouraging. Postoperative assessments of young children's CHEOPS scores have proved comparable to blind VAS ratings by recovery room nurses, and changes have occurred in CHEOPS scores as a function of intravenous narcotic administration. In a social validation test, teachers rated video clips of children in the recovery room on a VAS and a trained rater rated each video clip on CHEOPS. A significant correlation was obtained between the VAS and CHEOPS scores. Although McGrath et al. report lower correlations for each of the six behavior categories, this drop is to be expected. Subscores on any scale or test seldom achieve a correlation as high as that of the full-scale score because of the restricted range of possible scores. Further research is being done to determine which children and pain conditions could be assessed with this scale.

Several teams of investigators have developed behavior rating scales to measure *behavioral distress,* the term used to describe the combination of anxiety and pain that typically characterizes the pediatric oncology patient who is undergoing a discrete painful iatrogenic procedure.

Procedural Behavior Rating Scale

Katz et al. (1980) developed and subsequently revised the Procedural Behavior Rating Scale (PBRS). It consists of 13 behaviors that young oncology patients exhibit prior to, during, and after BMAs. The PBRS has an interrater reliability of .85, but there is little data on its validity. One problem specific to this scale is that it does not discriminate intensity of upset but, instead, merely documents the occurrence or nonoccurrence of the 13 behaviors during the aversive procedures. This means that a few tears and violent sobbing are given identical ratings and a child who exhibits a variety of behaviors will be scored higher than one who exhibits only a few. The simplicity of this form of scoring generally yields high interrater reliability but at the expense of the quality of information obtained.

Procedure Behavior Check List

On the basis of behavior observations and extensive interviews with leukemic children regarding their pain experiences, LeBaron and Zeltzer (1984) selected eight behaviors that were identical or similar to those of Katz et al.'s (1980) PBRS to form the Procedure Behavior Check List (PBCL). In this adaptation, operationally defined behaviors are rated for intensity on a Likert 1 to 5 scale, with 1 = "very mild" and 5 = "extremely intense." A major problem with the PBCL is overlapping of categories: "Physical resistance" often includes "muscle tension," for example, and "screaming" sometimes includes "crying." Since these behaviors can occur together or independently, rater reliability can become a problem. However, in this study interrater reliability was satisfactory. There was also evidence of concurrent validity: Significant positive correlations were obtained between independent observers' ratings of the children's pain and anxiety made at three points during the BMA procedure and their total scores on the PBCL.

Observational Scale of Behavioral Distress

The Observational Scale of Behavioral Distress (OSBD) (Jay & Elliott, 1986) is a model of careful scale development. It is an eight-item modification (see Table 4-2) of the PBRS that introduces two important refinements in the PBRS procedure. Behaviors are recorded in continuous 15-second intervals within each of the four phases of the medical procedure (first 3 minutes in treatment room, first

Table 4-2   The Observational Scale of Behavioral Distress

Information Seeking (IS)

Definition:	Any questions regarding medical procedures.
Examples:	"When will you stop?"; "Is the needle in?"; "Is the drip coming?"
Nonexamples:	"Will I get a toy?"

Cry (C)

Definition:	Crying sounds and/or onset of tears—usually nonintelligible but can be double coded with verbal categories.
Examples:	Sobbing; screnching up face—obvious onset of tears; booohooohoo; crying sounds; tears (code as long as still <u>flowing</u> and/or sounds).
Nonexamples:	Sniffling; heavy breathing.

Scream (S)

Definition:	Loud vocal expression at <u>high pitch</u>/intensity, usually nonintelligible, but can be double coded with verbal categories. High pitch distinguishes this category from <u>Cry</u>.
Examples:	Sharp, shrill, harsh, high tones; shrieks.
Nonexamples:	Loud yelling but at low pitch.

Restraint (R)

Definition:	Child must be physically held down by staff member or parent with noticeable pressure and/or child must be exerting force, resistance in response to restraint attempts by staff. Sometimes it is not clear if the child is exercising pressure back due to tightness of restraint (i.e., child *cannot* move). In such cases where restraint is obvious and child's resistance is not clear, code Restraint.

Verbal Resistance (VR)

Definition:	Any verbal expression of delay, termination or resistance.
Rule:	Must be intelligible.
Examples:	"I want to go"; "I want to go to the bathroom"; "No, no, no"; "I don't like this"; "Let me loose"; "Take me home"; "Don't hurt me"; "Stop"; "No more"; "Don't"; "Let me rest"; "Take needle out"; "I don't want it."

Emotional Support (ES)

Definition:	Verbal or nonverbal *solicitation* of hugs, hand holding, physical or verbal comfort by child.
Rule:	Code *initiation* only for physical behaviors.
Examples:	"Hold me"; "I love you"; "Momma"; "Daddy"; "Momma please"; "Help me"; grabbing at others; reaching out to be held. (Do not code *Mommy* if part of the statement is appropriate for another code, e.g., "Mommy, get me out of here" = Verbal Resistance, not Emotional Support.)

Verbal Pain (P)

Definition:	Any words, phrases, or statements which refer to pain, damage or being hurt, or discomfort.
Rule:	Must be intelligible. May be in <u>any tense</u>. Can be anticipatory as well as actual. Has to be a statement, <u>not a question</u>. This category is distinguished from <u>Cry</u> by coding discrete intelligible <u>words</u> as pain ("Owh, " "ouch") and nonword crying sounds as <u>Cry</u>. Only exception is that groans without crying are coded as Verbal Pain ("Ahhh").
Examples:	"That hurt"; "It stings"; "Owwwh"; "Owwhee"; "Will it hurt?"; "You are killing me"; "You are pinching me"; "Oh!"

continued

Table 4-2–*Continued*

Flail (F)

Definition:	Random gross movements of arms and legs or whole body. Flail often occurs in response to restraint (out-of-control behavior).
Rule:	Must be random.
Examples:	Pounding fists; kicking legs repeatedly and randomly; flapping arms on self or otherwise; child's back moving back and forth repeatedly during procedure.

Note. Reproduced, by permission, from Jay, S. M., & Elliott, C. Observational Scale of Behavioral Distress—Revised. Unpublished paper, 1986.

cleansing of site and Mizzy Gun, second cleansing and aspiration, removal of needle and postprocedure recovery) rather than recorded once for occurrence or nonoccurrence over an entire phase. Each of the eight behavioral categories is weighted according to intensity: For example, "nervous behavior" is 1.0, "verbal resistance," 2.5; and "Scream," 4.0. The reliability and validity of the OSBD are satisfactory (Jay, 1987; Jay, Ozolins, Elliott, & Caldwell, 1983). The OSBD is more complex than the PBRS and PBCL and the information it provides is more precise (Katz, Varni, & Jay, 1984).

For children in the diagnostic category for which these scales were developed, a painful test such as a BMA has an overlay of desperation that is absent in the case of children who are undergoing a painful test with no particular life-threatening implications. The developers of all three scales believe that anxiety and pain cannot be separated out in the oncology children's behavior: No distinction can be made between behavior that is primarily anxiety based and behavior that represents pain. This position comes in for considerable criticism because it does not distinguish between the anticipatory crying of a child in the waiting room that almost certainly reflects anxiety and the crying during the needle procedure from pain. In a discussion of this issue, subsequently replied to by Katz, Kellerman, and Siegel (1981), Shacham and Daut (1981, pp. 468–469) point out the importance of recognizing pain and anxiety as two different constructs:

> Although anxiety can be part of or can amplify the pain experience . . . and pain can cause anxiety . . . the distinction between these constructs . . . is important from both a theoretical and a clinical point of view. For example, methods used to reduce distress related to pain are often quite different from those used to reduce anxiety.

These three scales illustrate the value of building on others' work in seeking to develop a sound instrument. Although their suitability only for pediatric oncology patients is often seen as a limitation, this restriction of target is the optimal way to build up an information base on pediatric pain. The focus *should* be on groups of children who are homogeneous in some respect such as diagnosis (as is the case here), developmental stage and procedure (as in Craig et al., 1984), or simply type of pain (as in McGrath et al.'s [1985] study of postoperative pain).

Expressive Pain Interaction Coding System

A very promising recent development in the behavior observation field has been the Expressive Pain Interaction Coding System (EPICS) developed by Russell and his colleagues (Russell, 1984; Russell, Strassberg, & Speltz, 1986) to provide an objective base for the social learning analysis of children's pain experiences. This 29-category, sequential, 6-second time-sampling behavioral scoring system is designed to provide moment-by-moment recording of children's pain and nonpain behaviors along with concomitant facilitating and inhibiting responses from the immediate social environment. Thus the EPICS provides an empirical basis for analyzing potential controlling social stimuli. At the same time, a variety of discrete behaviors can be sampled. Russell (1984) has presented preliminary evidence of satisfactory rater reliability and content, construct, and concurrent validity. Although the EPICS is one of the most objective and sophisticated observation instruments developed for use in pediatric settings, it is also a very complex, expensive procedure. It requires extended observer training, uses costly videotape equipment, and requires time-consuming data analysis. However, it can yield important information concerning the behavioral contingencies that influence children's pain reactivity and parent responses. Although it is more suitable for empirical investigations than for clinical use, it is described here because the rigor and attention to coding detail that underlie its development could serve as a model for other developers of behavioral observation procedures.

Global Ratings

Global ratings are gross measures based on the observer's conclusion about some aspect of the child's behavior during a specific treatment procedure or over a certain period of time, such as 1 day. The rating instruments used include VAS, GRS, and NRS, as well as Likert scales. In the last case, the scales usually consist of a 1 to 5 continuum, with "1" indicating "no evidence" of whatever pain-related parameter is being assessed and "5" indicating "extreme" evidence of it. Global ratings are widely used in research and clinical settings. They are simple, quick, and, as far as scoring procedures are concerned, require little training. Those using the scales are usually personnel indigenous to the setting, such as the nurse or mother, who know a lot about the child and can place his immediate behavior in its broader context. Although significant correlations have occasionally been reported between nurses' global ratings on Likert scales of children's anxiety and behavior rating scales (LeBaron & Zeltzer, 1984), such results are more often an indication of observer skill than of rating scale strength. In the main, global ratings do not stand up to empirical scrutiny because of rater variability. Contributing to this variability is the fact that observer characteristics, such as attitude and experience, can have a major effect on the ratings. New nurses, for example, assessed pain as more severe than experienced nurses did (Jacox, 1980; Lenburg, Burnside, &

Davitz, 1970), and in the Lenburg et al. study nurses from different cultural settings also varied markedly in their global assessment of severity of pain. In a standardized hypothetical situation, nurses with less time on burn units rated pediatric and adult patients' pain during debridement as more severe than did those with more time on those units (Perry & Heidrich, 1982).

Indirect Measures of Pain-Related Behavior

Indirect measures consist of procedures in which pain-related behaviors are counted, timed, or otherwise recorded. Mechanical devices and instrument systems that automatically record the behavior have been used with adult chronic pain patients (Sanders, 1980), but manual recording by observers is the most common procedure with children. Usually the target behaviors are simple and gross, such as time spent playing or number of times the child leaves his bed. Often a cluster of behaviors is counted for one child (Varni, Gilbert, & Dietrich, 1981) throughout the baseline and treatment conditions, the purpose being to demonstrate the comparative efficacy of operant conditioning programs.

The major weakness in the use of these indirect measures is one that is common to all the behavior observation procedures but assumes even greater importance here: There are at this time no behaviors that are indicators solely of pediatric pain (Craig & Prkachin, 1983). Consider, for example, requests for medication. As an index of the presence of pain, this behavior is generally appropriate for use with adults. However, in the case of children, it becomes problematic because the children's misconceptions concerning the request effectively invalidate it. The child in pain may refrain from asking for medication because his fear of needles and shots is stronger than the pain itself (Eland & Anderson, 1977; Ross & Ross, 1982a); he may see the need for medication as evidence that he is not getting better, so he rejects help in order to avoid being confronted by this cognition; or he may associate oral medications with an unpleasant taste and vomiting.

Restlessness is another behavior frequently associated with pain. The assumption of validity of this behavior as an indicator of pain stems from biochemical evidence for increased restlessness with the onset of sudden, swiftly rising pain (Cannon, 1929) and from the fact that voluntary body movements may sharply increase during acute pain episodes (Abu-Saad, 1981; Johnston & Strada, 1986; Meinhart & McCaffrey, 1983). However, restlessness can also be a strategy for coping with pain, a point that is well documented in the clinical pediatric literature (Eland & Anderson, 1977; McCaffery, 1969) as well as in children's advice to peers who are scheduled for hospitalization (Ross & Ross, 1982a):

> Move round a lot if it hurts and just think about the moving parts. (Boy, CA 7)

> I'd tell him [peer] to start as soon as it hurts to move to a different part of the bed. If it hurts there, move again. Keep moving faster and faster. (Boy, CA 9)

Restlessness may also represent boredom or an attempt to elicit nurse attention for some reason other than pain, or may stem from the conviction that a show of activity will result in playroom meal privileges or earlier release from hospital. Decreased activity, often misinterpreted as "resting quietly," may also be a coping response for avoiding treatment and handling ongoing pain (Ross & Ross, 1982a):

> Keep very, very still, it's the only way to be sure not to get a shot. (Boy, CA 8)

> If it starts to hurt, stay *real* quiet, be still like you're dead and the hurt won't get any badder. (Boy, CA 9)

Comment

The behavior observation field is notable for a methodologically sound approach to the development of assessment instruments. Under rigorous conditions the nonobtrusive procedures can be regarded as objective: The behavioral data are quantifiable, and reliability is higher than is the case with self-report. Even the major problem concerning the validity of the behaviors selected as indicators of pain can be somewhat circumvented by selecting a cluster of different behaviors rather than a single one and by including subjective report and physiological measures in the data set. In other words, the behavior observation procedure cannot stand alone but when used in conjunction with other data sources, it becomes a most useful tool for collecting information about the child's pain experience.

Particularly noteworthy has been the development of instruments for use with infants: General indices of pain (Craig et al., 1984) as well as specific indices such as crying (Grunau & Craig, 1987a; Levine & Gordon, 1982; Wasz-Höeckert et al., 1968) and facial expression (Izard et al., 1980) have been investigated in a systematic way. However, the major advance has been the increasing acceptance of the importance of social context in identifying pain behavior. Russell's (1984) work on the EPICS sets the analysis of children's pain in a social learning framework, and Craig et al. (1984) include adult-infant interactions in their IPBRS.

Physiological Measures

The search for a reliable, pain-specific, physiological reaction to clinical pain has drawn a limited amount of investigative energy. The potential value of such a pain parameter would be inestimable in determining the validity of other pain measures as well as in assessing pain in infants, young children, and others whose relative lack of communication skills precludes the use of most, if not all, self-report procedures. In pursuit of this goal, two clusters of physiological events have been studied. One cluster, which includes muscle tension, occurs concomitantly with pain and plays an active part in a variety of pain states such as recurrent headaches

(Andrasik, Blanchard, Arena, Saunders, & Barron, 1982; Sanders, 1979) and back pain (Chapman, Casey, Dubner, Foley, Gracely, & Reading, 1985). Of particular interest, however, is the second cluster, which includes physiological events such as cardiac rate and palmar sweating. These responses occur concomitantly with pain and in proportion to it, but there is no evidence of a causal link between the two. Within this group there is a wide range in complexity of measures, with respiration, cardiac rate, and blood pressure being procedurally simple and palmar sweating, galvanic skin response, and endorphin levels being more complex.

Although all of these physiological events have demonstrated fluctuations with the onset of pain, particularly acute pain (Chapman, 1978), none has been shown to covary with pain report. Instead, attempts to establish that any autonomic indices or other physiological measures are correlates of pain have generally yielded equivocal or contradictory results (Gracely, 1980; Owens, 1984), the only exception being the thermography investigations. Most pain states are characterized by a global pattern of physiological arousal that includes increases in blood pressure, cardiac rate, and respiratory depth, as well as pupil dilation, rather than by precise changes in specific autonomic signs. The problem is that while this nonspecific arousal pattern often does indicate a pain state, it also is indicative of physiological conditions and psychological states that are unrelated to pain (Wallenstein, 1982). Consequently, the use of these parameters as indices of pain is subject to potential error. This problem with the validity of physiological measures parallels that of the behavioral measures: In both cases "pain" responses occur that also have other causes. In addition, autonomic responses are far less reliable and stable than are voluntary responses. When pain persists for several hours or days, autonomic responses such as the galvanic skin response are modified by a process of adaptation so that measures return to near normal (Wolff, 1980). As a result, nurses or other observers whose method of pain assessment depends largely on such signs (Jacox, 1980) may conclude that the long-term acute or chronic pain patient is not in pain when in fact he may just not be exhibiting any of the physiological signs of it. There is also clinical (Eland & Anderson, 1977; Wallenstein, 1982) and empirical evidence (Chapman et al., 1985; Melamed, Yurcheson, Fleece, Hutcherson, & Hawes, 1978; Shapiro, 1975) that although physiological signs are not as subject to voluntary control as subjective reports are, they may be attenuated or amplified by psychological factors, such as fear, expectancy, and social reinforcement factors. For example, in stoical individuals physiological signs that may be indicative of ongoing pain are minimized or absent. Outward demeanor can have a similar inhibitory effect, at least in the laboratory setting. In a study with college students (Kleck et al., 1976) those who were instructed to inhibit their facial responses or did so because they believed they were being observed also attenuated their autonomic and self-report pain responses in response to noxious stimuli. When these subjects were told to exaggerate facial displays in response to pain, their autonomic and subjective responses to the noxious stimuli increased. These results justify further exploration with children to determine if inhibiting expressive displays of pain has a positive influence on physiological responses and self-report pain assessment and whether this influence extends to the pain experience itself. In the following sections, a selected group of measures of physiological arousal are described.

Cardiac Rate

In the study of pediatric pain, cardiac rate is a potentially important dependent variable if used in conjunction with other indices of pediatric pain. Changes in cardiac rate are bidirectional, with general increases in rate to strong stimuli and decreases to moderate and mild stimuli. The measurement technique for it is relatively unobtrusive, producing neither pain nor discomfort, and it has the immense advantage of having been extensively studied in a diversity of pediatric populations and settings so that the norms for infants and children are well established and the procedures carefully standardized.

Owens's (1984) discussion of the complexities of cardiac rate receives indirect support from the ambiguous and often contradictory research findings about it, particularly those involving infants undergoing routine medical procedures. Although sharp increases in cardiac rate in response to noxious stimulation were demonstrated in studies of heel lance (Owens & Todt, 1984) and routine immunization (Johnston & Strada, 1986), the results in other studies have been ambiguous. Williamson and Williamson (1983) reported a marked increase in cardiac rate in infants undergoing unanesthetized circumcision, but the findings were muddied because the rate for infants in the penile block conditions decreased significantly below the baseline to a relative bradycardia during parts of the cutting and clamping procedure. Dale (1986) reported increases and decreases in cardiac rate in infants receiving routine immunizations; Field and Goldson (1984) were able to demonstrate increases in cardiac rate in only one of three groups of neonates undergoing heel lance procedures.

Studies with older children have focused on cardiac rate as an index of anxiety in children undergoing painful treatment procedures, and here too the results are not clear-cut. Cardiac rate increases and self-reported needle avoidance were positively correlated in children having routine immunizations (Shapiro, 1975). For those who were about to undergo a BMA, cardiac rate and blood pressure both proved to be reliable and valid indices of their anxiety (Jay, Elliott, Katz, & Siegel, 1984). However, in a study of pre- and postoperative anxiety, cardiac rate neither correlated with other measures of anxiety nor discriminated between treatment groups (Peterson & Shigetomi, 1981).

Palmar Sweat Index

Emotional sweating as opposed to exertional sweating provides another potential physiological index of pain or stress. The procedure involves attaching tape bands to the left index finger for 3 minutes and then having raters judge the darkness of the finger print on a 10-point scale. (For a detailed description of the procedure, see McNair, Droppleman, and Kussman, 1967). It is simple, inexpensive, and painless. Rater reliability poses no problems, but test-retest reliability and validity are problematic because the procedure is highly sensitive to nonrelevant sources of sweat production, such as room temperature. In the previously noted study by Shapiro (1975), for example, palmar sweat was completely masked by room temperature. This finding underscores one of the hazards of conducting pain research in naturalistic settings, namely, the contribution of extraneous variables to score data. In a study of infants undergoing heel lances, Harpin and Rutter (1982) reported a significant increase in palmar sweat during the procedure, with a return to baseline as the infants settled after it. In the case of older children, results from studies by Melamed and her colleagues (Melamed & Siegel, 1975; Melamed et al., 1978) supported the efficacy of the palmar sweat index in measuring anxiety related to surgery and dental procedures, but their findings were not supported by those of Jay et al. (1984).

Biochemical Assessment

The discovery of endogenous opioid peptides has generated considerable research activity concerning pain modulation (Terenius, 1981; Terenius & Wahlstrom, 1979). The release of these substances from various body sites into the blood can result in an analgesic effect that may persist for 2 or 3 hours. Studying these effects requires the use of invasive procedures that involve some pain, as well as costly equipment. However, biochemical assessment of this kind does have the potential to cast some light on the issue of individual differences in pain reactivity, which in turn could facilitate a more precise selection of pain interventions. It also must be seen as having potential as an objective index of pain.

Olness, Wain, and Ng (1980) reported a pilot study in which plasma endorphin levels were measured in five children before and after they used self-hypnosis for pain control related to treatment-induced and clinical pain. Results of the radioimmunoassay showed no detectable levels of β-endorphin immunoactivity in the pre- or postpain plasma samples. Possible explanations for this finding are that these children tolerated the procedures better than most children or that hypnotic analgesia is not mediated through opiate receptor sites. An alternative explanation suggested by Goldstein and Hilgard (1975) is that hypnosis-related relaxation may diminish endorphin levels rather than increase them.

The possibility that the plasma level of the endogenous opioid peptide β-endorphin might serve as an index of the level of perceived pain was investigated in a study of acutely burned children ($n = 15$, CA 8–17) by Szyfelbein et al. (1985). Pain levels were assessed during 33 BDCs, an extremely painful procedure that the acutely burned child must endure at least twice a day. Pain scores were obtained on a 0 to 10 pain thermometer once every minute during the pro-

cedure. The children were asked to volunteer any changes in pain level that occurred during the 1-minute intervals. To determine β-endorphin immunoactivity
at multiple intervals before and after the BDC, Szyfelbein et al. used highly sensitive radioimmunoassay procedures. The results showed that over the entire sampling period, self-reports of pain experienced during the BDC related inversely to
plasma β-endorphin immunoactivity and body weight, and varied directly with
the extent of the burn injury. In an earlier study, of children (CA 4–18) undergoing
lumbar puncture, Katz et al. (1982) used a thermometer scale to obtain one overall
assessment of pain experienced after the lumbar puncture procedure. They reported a positive but not significant relationship between self-report of pain and
β-endorphin immunoactivity level in cerebrospinal fluid (CSF).

Although Szyfelbein et al. offer possible explanations for the discrepant results, major differences in design would appear to make comparisons between the
two studies meaningless. The disparity in β-endorphin immunoactivity measures
(plasma versus CSF) is one possible explanation offered by Szyfelbein et al., since
changes in one fluid compartment are not always reflected in the other. Also important, however, is the procedural difference in timing: There is no way in which
a single score obtained after the event can be treated as similar to multiple scores
obtained throughout it. If comparisons are intended, investigators should ensure
that the studies will be comparable in all essential respects. If major improvements
over the original study are incorporated into the design of a later one, then this
becomes a different matter. In a field as recent as the study of the endogenous
opioid peptides and pain, it would be better to pursue the latter course in an attempt to establish a base of information than to force the comparison of noncom-
parable data.

Thermography

Thermography is an electro-optical means of translating variations in skin surface
temperature into visual images (Nerlinger, 1976). The human skin emits infrared
radiation primarily as a function of its temperature: The warmer the skin, the more
intense the energy emitted by it. The temperature of the skin is not uniform, but
instead is like a weather map rippled with many lines called *thermolars,* each of
which has a different temperature. Normally, a thermolar is symmetrical in that its
temperature is constant throughout. A video machine called a thermograph scans
the patient with a high-speed mini-camera that detects even the slightest variation
in temperature within each thermolar. It then converts the results by computer into
either black-and-white pictures, with white patches representing the hottest areas,
or colored pictures in which red represents heat. These heat pictures are called
thermograms.

The simple principle underlying thermography, that irregularities in the
body's temperature pattern are an indication that something is wrong, is neither a
new nor a recent idea (Barnes, 1976, p. 1):

The detection of disorders and pain by thermography has a historical precedent. Almost 2,400 years ago, Hippocrates painted his patients' bodies with a slurry of wet clay. The clay dried faster on warmer parts of the body, producing a pattern that reflected variations in skin temperature. Hippocrates did not understand the cause of these variations, but he concluded that if one side of the body, or one arm or buttock, was warmer or colder than the other, something had to be wrong. That reasoning is the basis for almost all thermographic interpretation today.

It is the irregularities in the temperature pattern relative to the pattern for anatomically identical areas on opposite parts of the body that is the criterion in thermography, rather than the absolute temperature of any part (Helwick, 1982). An inflamed appendix, for example, often shows up as an area of elevated temperature on the skin on one side of the abdomen, whereas the temperature in the identical area on the opposite side of the body is lower (Barnard, 1981).

A thermograph can be set to register temperature variations of less than 0.2°F at a range of several feet. Even changes in the temperature of a patient's lips and nostrils as he exhales and inhales can be detected (Barnard, 1981). Because it is so highly heat sensitive, thermograms must be made in a draft-free room at a temperature between 68°F and 72°F. Patients rest for approximately 20 minutes at room temperature in a special room, wearing only a hospital gown so that the temperature of the body, particularly that portion affected by the pain, can adjust to room air temperature. The procedure is completely safe: It involves no radiation, drugs, or discomfort, and it may be repeated as often as is necessary (Uematsu, 1983). It is a fast, noninvasive procedure capable of simultaneously measuring large surfaces of the body without skin-to-instrument contact (Freedman, Lynn, & Ianni, 1982), and it does not require that other pathways be intact.

Thermography has a high reliability and validity (Helwick, 1982). Whereas in the past, pain had always been an invisible sensation that the patient could only report, through the medium of thermography pain can now be "seen." When used in conjunction with the patient's history, complaints, and physical examination findings, thermography has solved many diagnostic puzzles. Kavaler (1981) reports the case of a small boy at the Mississippi Rehabilitation Center who kept complaining that his wrist hurt, although standard diagnostic techniques could find no reason for the pain. However, a thermogram showed a small area that was 3.6°F warmer than either the rest of the boy's arm or the identical area on his other arm. A surgeon subsequently found an embedded rose thorn under that warm spot.

Comment

There is a tendency to dismiss physiological indices of pain on the grounds that no physiological response is unique to pain and no uniform pattern of arousal exists in response to it. Although physiological indices do not begin to match self-report, they should still serve as one of the components in the pain assessment triad along with subjective report and behavioral observation. In view of the difficulties inherent in the assessment of pediatric pain, particularly of pain in infants, no source of information having any potential value should be abandoned. There is no question that physiological input should be a part of pain assessment and that the study of these responses should continue. Although the consensus is that these indices have limited value (Syrjala & Chapman, 1984), the fact is that at least one, thermography, has proven value and another, the endorphins, has great potential value.

Potential Applications of Adult Assessment Procedures

The development of effective assessment procedures is of critical importance to the understanding and competent management of childhood pain. The investigator who is interested in the challenge of assessing pediatric pain should familiarize himself with recent developments in adult pain assessment since many of the measures used with this age group have potential applicability to children and adolescents.

Consider, for example, the Analogue Chromatic Continuous Scale (ACCH), a procedure intended for adults but having methodological features that should have high appeal for older children and adolescents. It is a variant of the VAS developed by Grossi, Borghi, Cerchiari, Della Puppa, and Francucci (1983). It is essentially a ruler with a continuous color stripe with seamless gradations in value ranging from pale pink (no pain) to dark red (unbearable pain). Instead of the 100-mm line of the VAS, there is a colored stripe 100 mm long and 2.5 cm wide on one side of a double-sided ruler-like device. On the back is a 100-mm scale on which the points 0 and 100 mm correspond exactly to the ends of the ruler. To indicate his pain position on the scale, the patient sets a transparent double-sided slider containing a narrow line at right angles to the stripe at the point corresponding to the intensity of his pain. The millimeter value of the patient's pain can thus be read by turning over the ruler.

The ACCH is viewed by its developers as an improvement on the standard VAS. They believe that it is easier for the patient to understand, with the color changes providing more guidelines, and that it makes fewer demands in terms of good visual perception and muscular coordination and requires less physical effort by the patient. Grossi, Borghi, and Montanari (1985) have reported that it was used successfully by more patients than the VAS, with no reduction in sensitivity, accuracy, and reproducibility. Whether the ACCH really is superior to the VAS remains to be seen. However, with its apparently more technical, slide-rule affinity it should have high face validity, an attribute that is particularly important for adolescents.

Another of the procedures for assessing adult pain that has considerable potential for use with children and adolescents is the card sort method of pain assessment developed by Shapiro (1961) and adapted by Reading and Newton (1978). In this procedure, the patient is shown a series of cards each containing two words, one above the other and in balanced order to remove the effects of position set. His task is to sort each card according to whether the top or bottom word more closely resembles the pain he is experiencing. It is possible to obtain a refined evaluation by moving from gross differences between word pairs to increasingly fine differences. For example, early cards in the sequence might contain such pairs as "no pain/severe pain" and "mild pain/severe pain," moving on at later points to variations of "moderate pain/severe pain," and finally to combinations such as "severe pain/unbearable pain." Or, the focus might be on pinpointing the quality of the pain being experienced, quite apart from its degree of severity, in which case the word pairs would reflect this focus. For children, the procedure should become a paired-comparison task, rather than a card sort, with an adult holding up each card and pointing to or reading each word pair. Although the procedure's potential value would be greatest for children with good reading skills, it could also be adapted to younger children by using a pictorial format, such as facial expression, for the item pairs. At the adult level, the card sort procedure has proved to be reliable and valid (Reading & Newton, 1978). It is quick and simple to administer and is well suited to individual case study analysis. The only problem in adapting it for clinical use with children and adolescents is that the construction of the word or picture pairs for subgroups of the pediatric population is likely to be time consuming. If researchers working independently on the development of items pooled their efforts, an item bank could be built up and drawn on in subsequent attempts to refine and extend the item targets.

5
Management
Physical Interventions

Prompt and adequate relief of pediatric pain is of vital importance (Bonica, 1985b). Continuing pain rarely serves any useful function once its onset has alerted the child and his caregivers to the presence of a problem. If severe pain is not adequately relieved then abnormal physiological reactions may ensue, frequently causing complications. Unrelieved postoperative pain, for example, is often associated with reflex responses, such as inability to cough, that can cause serious complications (Willis & Cousins, 1985). Negative psychological reactions, such as anxiety heightened by loss of sleep, may also occur, with consequent demoralizing effect on the child that further depletes his psychological reserves. In this chapter general guidelines underlying the effective management of pediatric pain are delineated, followed by descriptions here and in the next chapter of specific procedures that either have an empirical basis for their efficacy or have the potential to be of use in the management of pediatric pain. These interventions can be classified in several ways, for example, whether they are under external control, as in the case of pharmacotherapy, or internal control, when a child is able independently to initiate a coping strategy; and whether they are primarily adult- or child-directed. The classification system that we are using here is based on Fernandez's (1986) trimodel system of pain management, which places the various interventions into three major groups: physical interventions directly involving the body, behavioral manipulations, and cognitive procedures involving thoughts and private events in which the point of entry is the mind.

General Guidelines for Management

Establish a Reassuring Atmosphere

The pediatrician and the pediatric team should convey confidence that alleviation or elimination of pain is possible. In the case of treatment-related pain, be accurate and specific about the probable degree of pain, for example, "It will hurt but we will help you. It will all be over before you can count to 10." Avoid generalities such as, "It won't hurt much" or "It won't take very long." Be scrupulously honest. Dishonesty will never be forgotten by a child; at best, it will cause him to be fearful and apprehensive; at worst, he will be terrified. For impending pain events, tell the child as much or as little as he wants to know. Some children want to know all the details, others do not (Ross, S. A. 1984), and these differences do not appear to be age or sex related (Ross & Ross, 1982a):

> And I go like, "Don't tell me. I don't want to know *nothing* about it, okay?" (Boy, CA 5)

> Because I like to know *when* I'm gonna go there [lab tests] and *what'll* happen so there won't be no surprise. I like to know *everything* and how bad and I think about it a lot and then I'm ready, even if it's real bad, I'm ready. (Girl, CA 9)

> The resident wanted to show me what he was going to do and the needle and all and I felt like screaming because I hate seeing things like that and I shut my eyes tight and said, "Just do it, don't explain anything" and I blocked my ears hard and I just did that till it was over. (Girl, CA 11)

> So the first time I go to a doctor or dentist for *anything* I get them to tell me all about it first. Then I check and find out if they're lying. . . . It's best to know. (Boy, CA 12)

In stressful situations children often regress cognitively, so after first establishing that the child wants information, gear explanations to a slightly younger developmental level than his chronological age would indicate. The child who does not really understand what is going to be done will interpret what he is told in his own framework of understanding, a reaction likely to lead to frightening misconceptions. One child who was given an explanation of dialysis using a washing-machine analogy arrived for his first dialysis session thinking that he was going to be flung into a washing-machine and whirled around. The only way to avoid this kind of situation is to make periodic checks during the conversation: First tell the child what is going to happen and ask if he has any questions. Do *not* ask if he understands. From an early age children learn to respond affirmatively to such questions because this pleases adults and generally terminates the discussion, usually to the child's relief. Instead, if the child has no questions, ask him to tell you what is going to happen. If he is unable to do this, start again and with absolutely no show of disapproval repeat the sequence until it is obvious that he does have a clear picture of the next events. Wherever possible in the discussion, illustrate with concrete objects what is being proposed. Ack (1983, p. 133) reports an example of misinterpretation that would not have happened had the aforementioned procedure been followed:

> A 4-year-old child visits an ophthalmologist who suggests to the mother, in the presence of the child, that an eye muscle is weak but before deciding upon surgery, he wanted to patch the eye. The child became unmanageable, anxiety stricken whenever mother tried to approach her, and the situation became so bad that mother contacted me in an emergency situation. Only then was the child able to suggest that she would not let mother sew up her eye.

For many children, predictability is reassuring in a stressful situation. Whether such a need exists can only be determined by talking to the individual child. For those who seek predictability, there are a number of opportunities in the pediatric setting for meeting this need. The child will feel a sense of comfortable stability if he knows the nurse and other pediatric personnel handling his case. It is a great help if he knows when he goes for an appointment that he will not be continually seeing strangers. As Crocker (1980) has pointed out, the child has a need for consistent contact with significant people in pain-related situations. Once in the situation, it helps if the child can be familiarized with some procedures, such as the blood pressure routine, by showing him the equipment and giving a brief demonstration before the doctor arrives (Siaw et al., 1986). Predictability is of particular importance for the hospitalized child who often feels at the mercy of pediatric personnel:

> Once they've got you in there [hospital] it's you against all of them. (Boy, CA 7)

The child who is constantly confronted by the unexpected pain procedure begins to think that any environmental event means pain. Consequently, many children, especially those in hospital, are in a more or less constant state of anxiety about what will happen next. The fact that often these children are quiet is erroneously interpreted as indicating that they are reasonably content. If the hospitalized child is to have multiple or recurring pain procedures over a period of time, establish whether he would like "signals" (Shorkey & Taylor, 1973) indicating if anything painful will happen before lunch or in the afternoon. The advantage here is that he then knows that some periods are "safe times"; the disadvantage is that he knows far in advance if a pain event is slated. For those having recurring procedures such as burn dressing changes involving considerable pain, it is a help if the procedure is always done in the same place. If at all possible, such procedures should never occur at the child's bed because this should be seen as a safe place. It may also be better to use one staff person as the "bad guy" for the procedure in order to spare the rest of the staff from the role and allow the child to find support among the other nonthreatening staff (Kenny, 1975).

Some behaviors that the pediatrician may think are reassuring instead have a negative or intimidating effect on the child. Children's spontaneous comments and information that they gave in the course of responding to nonspecific interview questions (Ross & Ross, 1982a) indicated that they deeply resented behaviors that they viewed as inappropriate in the pediatric setting. A frequent complaint concerned pediatric personnel who hummed or whistled under their breath while performing a painful treatment procedure. One group perceived such behavior as mindless happiness in the person who was inflicting pain. For many children there was a link between a mad scientist, the Happy Torturer, in a science fiction story who whistled while he worked on his victims and with another fictional character called the Singing Sadist.

The children were also very disapproving of joking, an apparently friendly behavior that is often used to establish preliminary rapport. When asked what advice the child would give to his best friend, one boy (CA 12) stated tersely that he would warn him to "look out for the ones [doctors] who laugh and joke a lot, they're the worst" (Ross & Ross, 1982a). In a similar vein, a girl of age 7 offered the following tactful advice for any young doctor who was just starting out:

> If he's telling a joke or if he's trying to be jokey, he should look around and if he's the only one laughing, it would be better to just stop.

What was particularly interesting was the fine line between the acceptable and the unacceptable. Riddles, for example, were quite acceptable and even welcomed by a number of children.

Involve the Child

The goal here is active involvement rather than passive endurance. Whichever happens depends to a great extent on the verbal and nonverbal messages that the child gets from the pediatric personnel. The child should feel that he is a member of the team:

> Being here is like—well, your whole team is really rooting for you. (Boy, CA 7, with asthma, wearing a baseball cap in bed; Ross & Ross, 1982a)

He should be addressed by name rather than as an object, disease, or condition, and an open pattern of informational communication should be kept up at a consistent, supportive level. Note the bitterness and resentment when the impersonal approach is the norm:

> Being in hospital is sort of like you're a table or chair or something. They do this, they do that, they move you round, they never say what's going on or how you're doing . . . they don't answer if you ask them something but, of course, chairs and tables aren't *supposed* to ask things. (Boy, CA 10, Ross & Ross, 1982a)

Include the child in discussions about his case or delay the discussion until the child is absent. Above all, avoid ambiguous comments or fragments of conversation within the child's hearing that could be misinterpreted or distorted. The pediatrician's frame of reference concerning the harmless comment differs so greatly from the child's that a concerted effort must be made if situations such as the following are to be avoided:

> The pediatrician and a consultant were in the hall discussing whether to remove the dressing from an 8-year-old boy's leg laceration before he was discharged. He was scheduled for discharge the next day but had not yet been told. They entered the room and were now within the child's hearing. This is the child's account of what happened next: . . . my doctor and this other guy came in and they don't look at me or say anything to me, they just stare at my leg. I'm feeling pretty good and I'm thinking

about playing ball . . . and then this other guy goes, "You better take it off," and my doctor starts to look real funny. And all of a sudden I get real cold, you know? . . . and I think, "Holy Jesus, they're going to cut off my leg like that kid on TV and how can I play ball with only one leg?" And then my doctor goes, "We better do it now, he might not be here tomorrow," and then I know I might die like that kid on TV if they don't cut it off now. And I just started to scream. I couldn't stop. (Boy, CA 8, Waechter, 1971)

Capitalize on the child's resources, for example, if he is good at self-distraction or other coping strategies, encourage him to use them. Emphasize that in doing so he is taking action against the pain and that he is the only one of the team who can take that particular action.

Work Within the Child's Conceptual Framework

During ongoing pain it is helpful to consider the child's behavior in terms of an active/passive dichotomy. In a stress situation, active behavior is generally more adaptive because it implies that the child is trying to cope. In young children this behavior may take the form of struggling or manipulation: "I have to go potty" or "I hear a little boy crying—you go and help him." On the surface, this behavior is undesirable, irritating, and a hindrance, but, in fact, it is an appropriate response for the child to make. Passive behavior, on the other hand, while apparently desirable because it does facilitate carrying out the procedures, may represent withdrawal and feelings of helplessness (Seligman, 1975), so that the "good" child reacts in a helpless, passive way. Some of these behaviors may be eliminated if the adult is able to see the child's pain within his conceptual framework (Cowherd, 1977). Finger sticks, for example, may threaten the body integrity of the preschool child because he may think that if his finger is pricked, all his blood will run out and he will die (Sheridan, 1975). For the school-age child, pain threatens his self-control, so that it is not uncommon for this group to say that they can stand anything as long as they do not cry. This is particularly true of the later middle-childhood years and adolescence, and many are able to verbalize their feelings when given an opportunity to do so:

I can stand anything if I just don't start crying—once I start to cry I just fall apart and I'm just like a baby. (Girl, CA 9, Ross & Ross, 1985)

If the older child does break down and cry he is likely to be almost as upset about the loss of self-control as he is about the pain. When this happens, an accepting, matter-of-fact attitude on the part of the pediatrician or nurse can do much to neutralize the ensuing distress and embarrassment. One effective gambit is to pick up a box of tissues, hand it over to the child, and continue talking. It is important to convey, preferably by nonverbal means, that crying is acceptable. Boys often feel worse about crying than girls do and consequently may have a greater need for security objects (Evans & Evans, 1982) such as their own blanket. Because boys are usually more reluctant to express such needs, these objects should be presented as a routine part of the procedure not warranting a choice on the child's part.

Within the whole sequence of painful treatment, the older child may be confident beforehand, fearful and silent during the treatment-induced pain event, and jaunty and somewhat obnoxious after it. See this behavior for what it is: awkwardly expressed relief that the procedure has finished and an attempt to recoup any loss of face occasioned by the child's performance during the procedure. By contrast, the younger child may whimper before, during, and after the painful treatment. Often the young child is unfairly scolded by pediatric personnel for whining when the treatment is over because they do not realize that the child likely does not have the concept of "over," and as he is still in the "bad" place, the treatment must therefore be continuing.

Treatment is facilitated if areas of concern relevant to a specific illness or injury can be identified from the pediatrician's pool of clinical experience so that reassuring comments can be worked into the conversation without the child's asking about them. Pain can be heightened by concern for the future ("Will I be ugly after the burns heal?") and worry about the past ("Did this happen because of something bad that I did?"). Presenting this information as though it were a passing thought lowers the emotional temperature, reassures the child that the pediatrician understands his feelings, and makes it easier for the child to bring up other topics that might be worrying him.

Personal control is of central importance in the child's attempts to cope with stressful or aversive events, and it can attenuate pain (Thompson, 1981). Accepting the child's need for personal control is prerequisite to recognizing the importance of making apparently minor changes in the pediatric situation in order to at least partially meet this need. Although it is a factor across a wide age range, the forms of meeting this need differ with increasing age (see Erlen's [1987] model of the changing rights of the child in the treatment situation as a function of his level of cognitive development and competency). For the younger child, control over the situation can be enhanced by allowing him to retain some degree of autonomy in decisions such as the amount of information that he wants about impending pain procedures as well as about events that do not in any way disrupt treatment, for example, which of two procedures should come first, which hand for a finger stick, or which color gown. Personal control is also enhanced if some normality of routine can be introduced (Crocker, 1980). To the degree possible, the child should be allowed to carry out self-care activities such as undressing himself, putting on a gown, and getting up on the bed. Children in pediatricians' offices are often enraged and humiliated when a nurse insists on helping them unnecessarily. While the pain procedure is underway, assign the child a task with distraction potential, such as holding a tongue depressor tightly in one hand while blood is taken from the other arm. Note the distinction between offering the child opportunities for legitimate control as opposed to rewarding him for using stalling techniques. In the latter instance, the child attempts to postpone aversive stimulation by asking incessant questions or carrying on a disjointed conversation. Such tactics should not be rewarded by permitting a delay in the procedure. However, the need for them can be considerably reduced if the procedure is presented to the child in a way that takes into account his anxiety. The following quote (Hyson, Snyder, & Andujar, 1982, p. 141) is an excellent example of a child's use of avoidance strategies with a pediatrician who either was indifferent to the reasons for the child's behavior and his needs in the situation or was unaware of them:

> The doctor says, "Hello, how's everything?" "Don't put something on my foot," Tim (CA under 5) says. Mother says, "I'll hold your hand." "I'm going to school," Tim tells the doctor. The doctor checks Tim's ears while Tim sits with his mother holding his hand. The doctor gets out the blood pressure apparatus. Tim speaks up, interrupting what the doctor is doing. "Look what I have—money for candy," he says, pulling money out of his pocket and extending it to the doctor. The doctor starts to adjust the blood pressure cuff. "Mommy," Tim says. He starts to cry.

In this episode, Tim first reverses roles by giving an order to the doctor. That failing, he tries delaying tactics, and perhaps bribery before resorting to tears.

With older children and adolescents, personal control is of particular importance because control is central to the developmental task of becoming independent (Erikson, 1963). The hospitalized adolescent is confronted with two pain- or illness-specific problems related to the issue of control. He must adjust to the regression that results from the loss of ego control during pain and also to strangers and frightening procedures. Helplessness and lack of control are heightened during severe restriction of activity (Seligman, 1975). The restrictions are perceived by the adolescent as a threat to his sense of autonomy: He is deprived of control over daily routines, privacy, and peer relationships. For an excellent statement on the developmental needs of the hospitalized adolescent and strategies that can be used to meet these needs, see Denholm and Ferguson (1987). In an attempt to maintain some sense of control, the adolescent may use confrontation and negotiation with pediatric personnel (Hoffman, Becker, & Gabriel, 1976), with the latter strategy often taking the form of a trade-off. Pugh (1985) reports the case of a 16-year-old girl who, because of previous negative experiences, could not accept any of several anesthesia induction techniques when given a choice. She finally sidestepped the issue by telling the anesthesiologist that he could use whichever procedure he wanted, if she could wear her hiking boots to the operating room. This case is an excellent example of accommodating the adolescent's needs without compromising essential procedural requirements although clearly violating customary practices. Before routinely rejecting the adolescent's (or child's) various nonconforming demands, each demand should be evaluated in terms of its actual consequences on the conduct of the treatment procedure. If minor inconvenience and tradition are the only obstacles, the demand should be granted.

Meet the Special Needs of the Chronic Pain Patient

Although children and adolescents with chronic pain are similar to those whose pain is not chronic in respect to the various needs described above, they do present a different management problem. Generally, they know why they are having their pain problems, tolerate painful procedures well, do not regard their pain as punishment, accept that it will be a recurring problem, and are knowledgeable about the prognosis (Beales, 1979; McCollum, 1981; Ross & Ross, 1982a; Travis, 1969). For these children, continuity of nursing care is an absolute essential and is of immense importance to their morale. They usually do not want to have their problems rehashed but instead find solace in the fact that the pediatric personnel, especially their nurses, know all their problems but do not discuss them:

> They all know about me so they don't ask any dumb questions like how am I? They *know* how I am, and they know that I know, and even though it's scary—like this time I might die—it's real comforting to have them know all about me. (Girl, CA 8, with blood disorder)

> Like you can get uptight, you know? Or you can be cool. I like that best. Last time [most recent hospitalization] my very, very favorite nurse was waiting and she said, "Thank goodness you made it in time to see [special entertainment]." Now that's cool. I know she knows things aren't good but we don't make a big thing of it. (Girl, CA 9, with arthritis and kidney problems, Ross & Ross, 1982a)

In managing children with long-term chronic pain, it is essential to be alert to the possibility that difficulties related to their pain conditions may exist that could interfere with the successful accomplishment of developmental tasks, in which case, intervention should be initiated. A model of such intervention is an innovative summer program (Mogtader & Leff, 1986) in which chronically ill adolescents are employed as child life assistants. This program is directed toward areas of stress and concern characteristic of the chronically ill adolescent, such as social isolation and poor body image.

Many of the interventions described in this and the following chapter have resulted, on occasion, in astonishing pain relief. It is important that when such effects occur they not be attributed automatically to specific factors intrinsic to the intervention procedure. Pain is a complex perception. When pain attenuation occurs, the mechanism of effect may reside wholly in the intervention procedure, it may reflect the individual's beliefs and expectancies, or, more commonly, it may be an intervention × cognitive factor interactive effect. It is generally accepted that a considerable proportion of the pain variance in pain reactivity can be accounted for by psychological factors (Melzack & Wall, 1983). One of the most dramatic examples in the pediatric pain literature of the extraordinary effect that cognitive factors can have on pain perception has been reported by Chapman (1984, p. 1265). A 9-year-old boy who had undergone a nephrectomy was given no postoperative medication because he was involved in a clinical trial of the efficacy

Table 5-1 Trimodal Classification System for Pain Interventions

Physical interventions[a]	Behavioral interventions[b]	Cognitive interventions[b]
Pharmacotherapy	Operant conditioning	Hypnotherapy and self-hypnosis
Acupuncture	Modeling	Cognitive coping strategies
Biofeedback	Psychotherapy	Thought-stopping
Physical relaxation	Talking the child through	Self-pacing

Note. This classification is a modification of Fernandez (1986).
[a]This chapter.
[b]Chapter 6.

of transcutaneous electrical stimulation for the relief of postoperative pain. Electrodes had been attached under the bandages, and stimulation was initated before the boy regained consciousness. As the child lay in bed with his hands outside the covers, his surgeon and associates asked him several times if he was experiencing abdominal pain. The boy repeatedly assured them that he was not in any discomfort. Everyone was impressed with the success of the intervention. When the surgical group had gone, the boy talked casually with the others in the room:

> When asked whether there was anything he feared, he began to cry and confessed his terror of the expected operation that would remove his kidney. His surprised nurse tried to reassure him that the surgery had already been done, and that there was nothing to worry about. He refused to believe her. "But don't you remember?" she contended, "That's why they put you to sleep this morning—so they could do the operation." The little boy looked very threatened. "It's not true!" he shouted, "It's not true!" When asked why it couldn't be true, he asserted confidently, "Because I haven't got any bandages." We asked him to feel his belly, since his hands were outside of the bedclothes. When he did, an expression of astonishment came over his face, and he broke into tears, screaming, "It hurts! It hurts!" Thus, the boy's "analgesia" occurred because no one had told him that he had been operated on and not because of our stimulation therapy.

The procedures to be described here follow Fernandez's (1986) trimodal system of categorizing pain management, which is based on differences in the point of entry in treatment. (See Table 5-1 for our modified version of this system.) The major procedures within each of the three categories are ordered from those involving the most external control to those involving the least. Some of these procedures have variations that are described within the same section even though the source of control for the variation differs from that for the procedure itself.

Pharmacotherapy of Pain

Pediatric pain is most commonly treated with the administration of narcotic and nonnarcotic drugs having analgesic properties (Jeans & Johnston, 1985). There is no ideal analgesic. However, Bond (1984) and others (Huskisson, 1984; Levine,

1983) have identified a cluster of properties considered critical for such an agent. It should markedly reduce or completely relieve the pain without interfering with the other senses. It should have the capacity to produce one specific effect in preference to others, because the greater this selectivity, the less the likelihood of undesired effects and the greater the margin of safety. A wide range of age and pain levels and disorders should respond to it, and its mode of administration should not influence its efficacy. It should be inexpensive. Few if any side effects should result, and these should be minor and temporary, disappearing rapidly after the drug is discontinued. By contrast, duration of drug action should be prolonged in order to keep to a minimum the number of doses ingested per day, that is, it should have a long effective half-life ($t_{1/2}$). There should be minimal tendencies to produce *drug tolerance* (decreased analgesic effectiveness of a given dosage after repeated doses) or physical and psychological *drug dependence* (withdrawal and other symptoms on discontinuing the drug). The latter state is a pharmacological effect that should not be confused with *drug addiction,* a voluntary behavior forming a pattern of overwhelming involvement with obtaining and using a drug.

Pharmacotherapy for Infants and Children

Although the analgesics currently available will, for the large majority of patients, adequately control even pain that appears to be intractable (MacLeod & Radde, 1985; Stewart & Stewart, 1984; Vere, 1984), the safe and effective treatment of infants and children with these drugs remains problematic. The infant and young child are undergoing rapid physiological development marked by substantial qualitative and quantitative changes in parameters such as plasma proteins and gastrointestinal motility. Some of the changes that occur are neither gradual nor predictable, and all contribute to the difficulty in determining the effective therapeutic dosage of drugs for these age groups (Hahn, Oestreich, & Barkin, 1986).

We shall briefly describe the pharmacokinetic parameters (absorption, distribution, metabolism, and excretion) that, along with drug dosage, determine the concentration of a drug at its site of action and control the temporal course of the drug effect. Each of these parameters may show marked variability with age (Hahn et al., 1986): Although a drug may undergo the same processes in children as in adults, the distinctive physiology of children changes this age group's response to pharmacotherapy. The rate and completeness of drug absorption in the child vary as a function of the route of administration. Certain physiological differences, such as slower gastrointestinal tract motility, reduce absorption of orally administered drugs. Drugs administered intramuscularly are absorbed erratically in young children, particularly in infants and neonates, in part because of their relatively low muscle mass, but also because of variability in regional blood flow to specific muscles and tissues. The overall distribution of a drug is influenced by plasma protein binding, body mass, and membrane permeability. The degree of drug binding is an important parameter here because it is only the unbound fraction of a drug that is therapeutically active. In children, more unbound drug is available than is the case with adults because children have fewer protein-binding sites and more competition by endogeneous substances for those sites. Children, particularly infants, have a higher percent of body fluid and a lower percent of body fat than do either adolescents or adults, so distribution volumes for water-soluble and lipid-soluble drugs are altered accordingly. The passage of drugs at certain body sites is limited by specialized distribution barriers such as the blood-brain barrier. The immaturity of the child's blood-brain barrier allows certain drugs to penetrate into the central nervous system (CNS) more readily than is the case with adults, thus increasing the risk of CNS toxicity (Evans, Bhat, & Vidyasagar, 1985; Hahn et al., 1986).

Following drug absorption and distribution, the body eliminates some drugs metabolically by biotransformation and then by excretion; others such as penicillin are eliminated unchanged. The most important organ for drug metabolisim is the liver. The destruction of the drug during passage through the liver is called a *first-pass effect*. It explains why the bioavailability of some drugs, particularly narcotics such as propranolol, is so much lower for oral (PO) as opposed to intravenous (IV) administration. Oral administration of some drugs is contraindicated because the first-pass effect renders them virtually useless. The first-pass effect can be eliminated or minimized by using the oral or pharyngeal mucosa as an administration route because the drugs that are absorbed enter the systemic circulation directly without having to pass through the liver (Hahn et al., 1986). Both the size and metabolizing enzyme systems of the liver change with development (Evans et al., 1985). The immaturity of the infant's liver results in decreased metabolism of many drugs and a consequent increased risk of toxicity. Biliary excretion and excretion by the kidneys are the primary routes of drug elimination. An infant's glomerular filtration rate in the first month of life may be only 5% of an adult's, but it reaches the adult level at about 1 year; his tubular secretion rate reaches the adult level at about 6 months. The relationship between biological age and rate of drug elimination is of crucial importance, particularly in the neonate and infant. Failure to adjust dosage and dosage interval to meet age-related fluctuations in rate of elimination can result in either the accumulation of the drug to toxic levels or inadequate therapeutic regimens. It is important to emphasize that children cannot be treated as small adults even when their height and weight equal that of adults. In the case of smaller children, age-related formulas based on recommended adult dosages are to be avoided. Instead, dosage should be calculated on the basis of weight or body surface area.

The child's distinctive physiology is not the only factor markedly differentiating pediatric from adult pharmacotherapy. There are several more specific reasons why the management of pediatric pain with analgesic and adjuvant drugs continues to be problematic. The knowledge base about their use is incomplete: Only

25% of all therapeutic drugs in pediatrics and neonatology have been subjected to adequate pediatric evaluation (Radde & MacLeod, 1985). A contributing factor is undoubtedly the significant ethical restraints that have existed against pharmacological research with children; however, even when pediatric drug research that falls within ethical bounds has been possible in the clinical setting, such research has not been undertaken by the pharmaceutical industry. For a detailed discussion of these and other difficulties inherent in pediatric clinical pharmacological research, see Maxwell (1984, pp. 375–380) and Radde and MacLeod (1985, pp. 435–439).

A further difficulty is that there is no available objective and satisfactory measure of pain relief (Syrjala & Chapman, 1984), so the pediatrician is seriously hampered in making judgments about the efficacy of analgesic intervention. Adding to the difficulties of effective management of pediatric pharmacotherapy are the complexities of the individual child: Marked genetically and environmentally determined individual differences in capacity to absorb, metabolize, and eliminate drugs cause variability in drug response (Vesell, 1982), and physiological and psychological factors cause fluctuations in ongoing pain independent of pharmacological intervention.

Despite these very basic problems, it is possible to set out general guidelines for the use of analgesics in clinical pediatric practice. Table 5-2 contains a summary of these guidelines. In addition, it should be noted that the pharmacotherapy of pain control does not depend on analgesics alone.

The usual treatment approach to a child (or adolescent) in pain begins with a nonnarcotic drug. For patients in whom anxiety is a prominent feature of their pain, the nonnarcotic alone may not suffice. An anxiolytic agent will then be added. If satisfactory pain relief is still not achieved, a combination of a nonnarcotic and a weak narcotic will be given. Since most narcotics combat the reactive component, the anxiolytic agent may be discontinued. If the nonnarcotic-weak narcotic combination proves ineffective, a more potent narcotic will be tried. Should pain relief still not occur, potentiating agents will be added.

Table 5-2 General Guidelines for the Use of Analgesics with Children

The goal is to provide effective pain relief.
The drug should be effective with different ages and different degrees of pain.
The effect should be independent of the route of administration (that is, effective by a variety of routes).
There should be long duration of action—slow absorption, slow elimination (long half-life), with duration of effect exceeding time present in blood (for example, central nervous system half-life should be greater than blood half-life).
Side effects, including interference with other senses, should be few and minor and should disappear rapidly after discontinuation of the drug (that is, effects should be specific, conferring a margin of safety).
There should be minimal tendency to tolerance or dependence.
The drug should be inexpensive.

Pharmacotherapy for Adolescents

The basis for pharmacotherapy for the adolescent has been described by M. I. Cohen (1980, pp. 45–46) as unsound. In a symposium on adolescent medicine he commented,

> The rationale for the pharmacotherapeutic approach to the adolescent patient . . . is often a transcript of information taken from an adult or much younger subjects, lacks precision and specificity, and avoids the concept of a somewhat unique biologic and psychosocial process of maturation during this particular period of human development. Although drug doses have been adjusted to meet special needs of . . . the young child and the very elderly, little attention has been directed at the pharmacologic principles involved in the care of the adolescent.

The reason for this omission is that usually there is only a brief interval during which both the distribution of drugs and the individual's response to them changes from the pattern of childhood to that of adulthood (Radde, 1985). This shift occurs at the development of the physical signs of puberty or just prior to it. During this period, the change in drug handling depends on a cluster of events including changes in the size of various body compartments and in hepatic metabolic capacity as well as on the occurrence of high levels of circulating steroids and the adolescent's excretory capacity (Radde, 1985).

In calculating drug dosage for adolescents, M. I. Cohen (1980) and others (see, for example, Radde, 1985) emphasize the consideration of several biological factors that influence drug metabolism during this period. Included is the substantial change in body mass that characterizes the period of adolescence. In the absence of firm guidelines for drug dosage for this age group, clinicians typically resort to using body weight as the basis for drug dosage in small adolescents and adult dosages for those of near-adult size. Body composition is also of considerable importance in planning drug regimens. Sex differences in body composition that occur during the growth spurt, specifically, the greater gain in lean body mass in males versus the increase in fat in females, must be considered. Pubertal factors, such as the potential for pregnancy in the female and the increased circulating blood volume that is secondary to the increase in lean body mass in the male, plus ongoing organ maturation, must also be taken into account in calculating drug dosage. M. I. Cohen (1980, p. 48) has concluded that "the current approach to clinical drug dosage regimens in adolescent patients remains one of trial and error" despite the knowledge of the foregoing factors. As a start in remedying this state of affairs he has strongly urged the use of therapeutic drug monitoring techniques.

With these general ideas in mind, we can now consider the specific characteristics of the two main categories of analgesics: the peripherally acting analgesics and the centrally acting ones (see Table 5-3). Traditionally, the former have

Table 5-3 Classification of Analgesics

Nonnarcotics	
Nonsteroidal anti-inflammatory drugs	Drugs without anti-inflammatory action
Aspirin Ibuprofen[a] Mefenamic acid[a] Naproxen Tolmetin sodium	Acetaminophen (paracetamol in the United Kingdom)

Narcotics			
Agonists		Agonist-antagonists	
		Nalorphine-type	Morphine-type
Weak	Strong	Weak	Strong
Codeine Meperidine Oxycodone	Morphine Fentanyl Methadone	Pentazocine	Buprenorphine

[a]Not labeled for use with children by the U.S. Food and Drug Administration.

been designated as mild and nonaddicting and the latter have been considered to be strong, with addiction potential. As is the case with so many other attempts to impose order on complex medical events, these two categories are no longer mutually exclusive: there are now peripheral analgesics that can be described as strong (see, for example, Martino, Ventafridda, Parini, & Emanuelli, 1976) and central analgesics that are nonaddicting (Martin, 1979). Nevertheless, the two categories provide a convenient framework as long as one keeps in mind the potential for overlap.

Our intent in this discussion is to provide a general picture of the analgesics that are used in pediatric clinical practice. Unfortunately, the relevant literature is characterized by gross contradictions in recommended dosages and side effects as well as in general information about specific analgesics. The source most helpful on dosage and other specific aspects of pediatric analgesics is Benitz and Tatro's (1981) concise and well organized manual, *The Pediatric Drug Handbook*. Comprehensive information on the analgesics described in this section is available in the major pharmacotherapeutic texts such as the series edited by Goodman, Gilman, and their associates (for example, Gilman, Goodman, Rall, & Murad, 1985).

Nonnarcotic Analgesics

The peripheral analgesics most commonly used in the treatment of mild to moderate pain in children are acetaminophen and a group of drugs known as nonsteroidal anti-inflammatory drugs (NSAIDs), which include such widely used agents as aspirin, naproxen, and, for children age 12 and older, ibuprofen (Korberly, 1985). The locus and mechanism of analgesic action of the peripheral analgesics differ. Salicylate compounds, such as aspirin, act by blocking the synthesis of peripheral pain-producing substances (prostaglandins) in the tissues that trigger the inflammatory response to tissue damage. Para-aminophenol derivatives, such as acetaminophen, are thought to produce analgesia by a central as well as a peripheral effect (Flower, Moncada, & Vane, 1980). The peripheral analgesics have proved to be highly effective for a diversity of problems of an acute nature, such as headache, musculoskeletal pain, dental pain, and minor physical trauma, as well as chronic pain of somatic origin. Although in analgesic doses these drugs are characterized by a selectivity of target, causing no mental disturbance or change in sensory modalities other than pain, they do not meet the criteria for the ideal analgesic because they relieve only mild and moderate pains (Levine, 1983). Typically, one or more of these drugs is given an adequate trial before the pediatrician resorts to the more potent central analgesics.

Acetylsalicylic Acid (Aspirin, ASA)

Aspirin is the prototypic agent of the peripheral analgesics and is the standard against which other such analgesics should be compared. In terms of efficacy none of the peripheral analgesics has proven to be more than marginally better than aspirin (Huskisson, 1984). Because of its efficacy and low cost, it is the most widely used of all analgesics. Although it is a nonprescription drug judged by the U.S. Food and Drug Administration (FDA) to be safe for use without medical supervision, it is erroneously considered by laymen to be completely safe. It does have side effects, some of which are potentially lethal. It is irritating to gastric mucosal cells and may result in nausea and vomiting. It may prolong bleeding time, or cause tinnitus. A very serious side effect is the strong association purported to exist between the use of aspirin and Reye's syndrome in children and adolescents with viral infections, especially influenza and chicken pox (*Morbidity & Mortality Weekly Report*, 1985). Radde (1985), however, has criticized this claim on the grounds that it is based on retrospective studies involving recall of drug intake. In large doses salicylates can accumulate, and chronic salicylism can occur along with increased risk for developing dehydration and seizures in children (Gaudreault, Temple, & Lovejoy, 1982). In infants and young children it is a sometimes fatal intoxicant. Aspirin also possesses anti-inflammatory as well as antipyretic efficacy, that is, the capability of reducing elevated body temperature. It is particularly effective in relieving mild to moderate pain directly related to inflammatory processes. (When the pain is etiologically related to a noninflammatory process, however, salicylate therapy is ineffective.) It is the basic pharmacotherapy for juvenile rheumatoid arthritis (JRA) because its anti-inflammatory and analgesic properties facilitate more effective physiotherapy and its antipyretic action helps control the fever in systemic JRA (Ansell, 1980). It has proved effective in the treatment of dysmenorrhea (Klein, Litt, Rosenberg, & Udall, 1981).

The recommended pediatric dosages by weight for aspirin as well as the other peripheral analgesics are shown in Table 5-4. Aspirin is administered orally and is rapidly absorbed from the gastrointestinal tract. It should not be given to children in an enteric-coated form or by suppository because absorption then becomes highly variable (Maxwell, 1984). Nor should it be given to those with aspirin sensitivity, a condition that occurs in 0.3% of the general population and in approximately 4% of those with asthma (Korberly, 1985).

Acetaminophen (Datril, Tempra, Tylenol)

Acetaminophen has analgesic and antipyretic properties similar to those of the other NSAIDs but differs from them in having little or no anti-inflammatory action. It is expensive. Side effects are infrequent and mild and include skin rashes and drug-related fever. The most serious one, which occurs as a result of overdosage, is the possibility of hepatic failure. Unlike aspirin, acetaminophen does not irritate the gastric mucosa and for this reason is regarded as an important analgesic for use with mild to moderate pain in pediatric practice. It is considered to be the alternative of choice for children who are allergic to aspirin, cannot tolerate it,

Table 5-4 Peripheral Analgesics

| Generic name | Trade name | Dosage | Absorption | | Half-life |
			Oral	Rectal	
Acetaminophen	Tylenol	10 mg/kg/dose q 4 hr to max. 2.6 g/24 hr	Rapid, nearly complete	Adequate	1–3 hr
Aspirin	ASA	10–15 mg/kg/dose q 4 hr to max. 60–80 mg/kg/24 hr	Rapid	Slow and incomplete	15–20 min dose dependent
Ibuprofen[a]	Motrin	30–70 mg/kg/24 hr divided t.i.d.-q.i.d.	Rapid, complete	Not available	2 hr
Mefenamic acid[a,b]	Ponstel	Adolescents 250 mg q.i.d.	Rapid	Not applicable	3–4 hr
Naproxen[a]	Naprosyn	10 mg/kg/24 hr divided b.i.d.	Rapid	Not applicable	12–15 hr
Tolmetin sodium	Tolectin	15 mg/kg/24 hr divided t.i.d.	Rapid, complete	Not applicable	1–3 hr

[a]Not labeled for use with children by the U.S. Food and Drug Administration.
[b]No recommended dosage for children.

or have bleeding disorders (Stewart & Stewart, 1984). Yaffe (1981) believes that dose for dose, acetaminophen has a safety profile superior to that of aspirin and should be regarded as the nonnarcotic analgesic of choice.

Other Nonsteroidal Anti-Inflammatory Drugs

A variety of other NSAIDs are available, and some of these have been shown in clinical trials to have significant analgesic effects. However, many of these are prohibitively expensive, their principal advantage over aspirin being increased patient tolerance as a result of minimal gastrointestinal irritation. Included in this group are ibuprofen, naproxen, and tolmetin.

Ibuprofen (Motrin) Ibuprofen has been the target of extensive investigation (see, for example, Miller, 1981). It is effective for mild to moderate pain but not for postoperative pain. It is generally considered to be more effective than aspirin for relief of pain from dysmenorrhea (Gilman, Goodman, & Gilman, 1980). Side effects are minimal, the most frequent one being gastrointestinal upset but to a degree significantly less severe than that from aspirin. Sold in the United Kingdom without a prescription, it has been approved in the United States for use with children older than age 12 (Korberly, 1985). Although it is one of the least expensive of the NSAIDs, it is 10 times the cost of aspirin.

Naproxen (Naprosyn) Naproxen is similar to ibuprofen except that its long half-life allows twice-daily administration and it is better tolerated (Gilman et al., 1980). However, it is also far more expensive. It has been shown to be effective in the relief of mild to moderate postoperative pain and is well absorbed. Mäkelä (1977) compared naproxen with aspirin in the treatment of JRA in children and reported fewer adverse side effects with daily doses of 10 mg/kg of naproxen in treatment periods ranging from 1 to 26 months than with 65 mg/kg of aspirin for 14 days. Although there were fewer side effects with naproxen, those associated with bleeding were more serious than they were with aspirin: 42% of the naproxen group experienced significantly prolonged bleeding time compared with 16% of the aspirin group, and pathological thromboplastin times were reported in 21% of the naproxen and 11% of the aspirin group. Mäkelä's statement (p. 193) that naproxen "appears to be at least as effective as aspirin in the treatment of JRA" seems at best a dubious conclusion.

Tolmetin (Tolectin) Tolmetin is a NSAID that has been approved in the United States only for use with children with JRA (Korberly, 1985). Although in recommended dosages it is approximately equal in efficacy to aspirin, it is usually better tolerated (Gilman et al., 1980). The most common side effects are gastrointestinal, including epigastric pain, nausea, and vomiting; and prolongation of bleeding time. Less common are CNS side effects such as anxiety, drowsiness, visual disturbances, tinnitus, and vertigo. In comparison with aspirin, the incidence of the latter two is lower and less severe with tolmetin. In an open double-blind trial of tolmetin for JRA, Levinson et al. (1977) reported that with doses of

15–30 mg/kg, tolmetin had anti-inflammatory properties comparable to those of aspirin and showed little evidence of hepatotoxicity. At this dosage tolmetin does not appear to modify the systemic fever of JRA (Ansell, 1980), although there is some evidence for such an effect at higher doses of 35–40 mg/kg (Gewanter & Baum, 1981).

Narcotic Analgesics

Narcotics are natural or synthetic drugs with a morphine-like pharmacologic action. In this discussion the terms *narcotic* and *narcotic analgesic* are used interchangeably with *opioid* to designate these morphine-like drugs.

A narcotic is generally recommended for a child when appropriate therapeutic doses of simple analgesics have not effected adequate pain relief or such relief can be obtained only at a dosage level at which toxicity would increase the child's state of discomfort. Contrary to common belief, the narcotics are often more easily tolerated than are nonnarcotic agents such as the NSAIDs.

The narcotics act centrally to depress activity of the nervous system by binding to specific opiate receptor sites in the CNS, with a resultant activation of an endogenous pain suppression system. Their relative analgesic potencies usually, but not always, parallel their affinities for the opiate receptor sites. An example of an exception is nalaxone hydrochloride (Narcan), which is characterized by high affinity but no potency as an analgesic. *Affinity* is a measure of potency referring to the strength of the narcotic-receptor attachment. Drugs with a high affinity generally displace drugs with less affinity by competing for the receptors (Twycross, 1984). The greater the affinity of a narcotic, the greater its propensity to bind with a given receptor and the smaller the concentration of the drug needed to produce a specific intensity of analgesic response. It would follow that a drug having a lesser affinity for the same receptor would require a greater concentration to match that specific intensity of analgesic response. In fact, this relationship is far more complicated because affinity is not the sole variable in the binding process.

Narcotics can be categorized in terms of potency as strong or weak. However, a more informative method (see Table 5-5) is to group them according to their relationship to morphine with respect to their agonist and antagonist properties. *Agonists* are narcotics, such as codeine and methadone, that have morphine-like effects; *antagonists,* such as naloxone, are narcotics that have the capability to reverse the effects of morphine. Naloxone is the only clinically used pure antagonist; it binds to the receptors for opioids but does not exert analgesic or other central morphine-like effects. Narcotics that have agonistic effects when given alone but are antagonistic when given with or following an agonist are termed *agonist-antagonists.* There are two major classes of agonist–antagonists: *Partial agonists* are morphine-type agonist-antagonists that are not antagonistic at low dosages, whereas the *nalorphine-type* agonist-antagonists are antagonistic at any dosage and also antagonize partial agonists. It is essential to be cognizant of these drug

Table 5-5 Pharmacokinetics and Dosages of Narcotics

Agent (trade name)	Half-life (hr)	Duration of action (hrs)	Relative potency	Bioavailability (%) oral	Dosage	Route of administration
Buprenorphine (Buprenex)	2–3	10	35		Not established. Only available in Europe	IM
Codeine	3–4	4–6	0.08	40–70	0.5 mg/kg/dose to 5 mg/dose q 4 hr	PO
Fentanyl (Sublimaze)	4–6	½–1	80		Under 2 yrs, not recommended; 2–12 yrs, 0.001 mg/kg/dose	IM, IV
Meperidine (Demerol)	3–4	2–4	0.1	50	1–1.5 mg/kg/ dose q 3–4 hr p.r.n.	IM, IV, PO, SC
Methadone (Dolophine)	17–24	6–8	1–1.5	90–100	0.7 mg/kg/24 hr divided q 6 hr	IM, PO, SC
Morphine	2–4	4–5	1	20–30	0.1–0.2 mg/kg/ dose q 2–4 hr to max. 15 mg/ dose	IM, IV, SC; PO is not recommended
Oxycodone (Percodan)	4–5	4–5	1	50	0.05–0.15 mg/ kg/dose to 10 mg/dose q 4–5 hr	PO
Pentazocine (Talwin)	2–3	2–4	0.3–0.5	10–30	Not established for children under 12 yrs	IM, IV, SC

actions because uninformed administration of certain combinations or sequences of narcotics could fail to provide any pain relief for the child and in some circumstances could cause withdrawal symptoms (Twycross, 1984).

The narcotics are alike in a number of respects. Their pharmacologic profiles are essentially similar. They all have the ability to induce and maintain some degree of physical and psychological dependence and to develop tolerance. There is a widespread and long-standing conviction that the narcotics affect the perception and interpretation of aversive stimulation rather than inducing change in the aversive stimulation itself. Support for this belief comes from adult and child reports that the pain is still present but is no longer troubling (Gilman et al., 1980). A recent study by Price and his associates (Price, Harkins, Rafii, & Price, 1986) of the analgesic effects of fentanyl on clinical and experimental pain casts some doubt on this belief. Their results indicated that low to moderate doses of fentanyl reduced both the sensory and affective dimensions of both kinds of pain. Although fentanyl had the most effect on the affective dimension of clinical pain, this effect was by no means the exclusive one that has been commonly reported. Instead, the findings strongly suggest that changes in pain affect are primarily a direct result of reductions in pain sensation intensity. The pain relief that does occur is selective in that it does not impair sensation; that is, there is little alteration in sensory phenomena other than pain. With the exception of morphine, and of fentanyl, which is not available PO, the narcotics are generally absorbed quite well from the gastrointestinal tract, reach peak concentrations in 30 to 60 minutes, and are rapidly distributed throughout the body. However, all of them are associated with frequent and sometimes severe side effects such as nausea and vomiting due to a central stimulation of the vomiting center, constipation, and dose-related respiratory depression. Drowsiness and mood changes are common, the latter sometimes being of a euphoric nature but sometimes also dysphoric, especially in children. The sedating effect is of therapeutic value especially for the child who needs sleep.

The narcotics also differ in several basic ways, including chemical structure and degree of side effects. Marked differences occur in duration of analgesic action (see Table 5-5), which coincides with the rate of metabolism. It is important to distinguish between *efficacy* and *potency*. When one narcotic is described as more potent than another, this means that it can achieve a specific analgesic effect with a lower dosage than the other narcotic. Some are very potent in low doses but also have a relatively low upper limit or analgesic ceiling effect. Consequently, the efficacy of a more potent drug with a low ceiling effect would be lower than the efficacy of a less potent drug with no ceiling effect.

Narcotics may be administered orally, sublingually, subcutaneously, by intramuscular injection, time-contingent intramuscular injection, intermittent intravenous injection, continuous intravenous infusion, patient-regulated intravenous infusion, and by epidural injection. Certain narcotic analgesics such as propranolol are far less effective when given orally than when given parenterally because of a first-pass effect, while others are equally effective with either route of administration. The "on demand" intramuscular (IM) injection is the conventional narcotic regimen. Selecting the IV route over the other two (IM and subcutaneous [SC]) allows the physician to sidestep the fear-of-injection problem that characterizes many children and adolescents (as well as adults). There is considerable anecdotal evidence that fear of injection may outweigh the need for pain relief. In any case, the fear variable makes assessment of pain difficult here. If an IM injection must be given, the ventrogluteal site is reported by Eland (1984) to be less painful than other alternatives, such as the rectus femoris, and the pain that does occur can be further minimized by using a coolant (Eland, 1981).

Patient-regulated IV injection is a procedure often used for the control of severe pain. It involves the use of a machine that gives the patient control of his own pain relief; that is, it is essentially p.r.n. analgesic delivery, the major difference being that the patient administers the drug, rather than the nurse. The machine is an infusion pump, a small unit that delivers a predetermined small dose of narcotic intravenously. Although the pump gives the patient control over when the drug is taken, a limit is placed on the size of the dose by a sophisticated microprocessor that enables the unit to be programmed to release a specific amount of narcotic at a push of the button and then remain inactive for a certain period of time. In this way safeguards are built into the system to avoid overdosage. Although this procedure has proved to be relatively safe, serious overdosing has been reported (Jewell, 1985). The advantages are patient oriented: The patient feels less anxious and consequently feels less pain with the security of knowing that there would be no delay because he controls the drug administration; the procedure allows for individual differences in pain tolerance; and for adolescent patients, the resultant feeling of being in control is a strong plus. The disadvantages are largely technical: Availability is limited by high costs, and use at present is restricted to the hospital setting because the machines are not yet portable. However, some patients are uneasy about using the system or do not understand it and, consequently, are reluctant to use it.

In the following sections the narcotics selected for discussion are ones that have proved useful in the relief of acute and chronic pain in infants, children, and adolescents. Recommended dosages for narcotics are given in Table 5-5.

Morphine

Morphine, the most widely used narcotic analgesic, is the prototype for the narcotics that are used in the alleviation of moderate to severe pain and, as such, it has become the standard against which all other opioids are compared (Levine, 1983). Morphine raises the threshold for pain, allays anxiety, and often induces an euphoric state that has been likened to a kind of detachment that may increase the overall analgesic action, resulting in both physiological and psychological benefits for the child. Absorption is rapid when morphine is given parenterally, particularly after IV administration when the drug is distributed within two to three minutes (Maxwell, 1984). Oral administration is not recommended for any age group because with this method absorption is limited and variable; in comparison with parenteral administration, morphine is only one-sixth as effective when administered PO.

Morphine is capable of producing effective analgesia over a wide range of dosages, with analgesic action that has been described by Inturrisi and Foley (1984) as relatively selective. There appears to be no limit to the level of action that can be induced with morphine, although fully effective doses may cause some alteration in behavior or consciousness to the point of loss of consciousness (Inturrisi & Foley, 1984). The dose that can be used is limited, as well, by other side effects (nausea, vomiting, respiratory depression, bradycardia, allergic reactions, hypotension, increased intracranial pressure, constipation) that may appear after a single dose. If another CNS depressant, such as a sedative or anxiolytic agent, is administered concurrently, side effects such as respiratory depression are likely to be increased. Because of the likelihood of respiratory depression, morphine should not be used for children with asthma or excessive bronchial secretions; nor should it be used with those having liver impairment. Morphine is used as a preoperative medication and again as a postoperative one when the effects of surgical anesthesia have disappeared. In the latter period, a continuous-drip IV administration provides a steady level of analgesia. The drug is also effective in relieving severe pain not controllable by other less potent analgesics. Dosage must be carefully adjusted for children because they are particularly sensitive to this drug.

Morphine has been used successfully to control terminal cancer pain in children. Representative of the protocols developed for these cases is that of Rafart, Espinosa, Illa, Fabregas, and Borrego (1984). Under their medication regime, children in pain are first given nonnarcotic analgesics, such as aspirin or acetaminophen, at a dosage level of 10–15 mg/kg every 4 hours. If the pain is not adequately relieved, then combinations of nonnarcotics and narcotics are used, an example being 10–15 mg/kg of aspirin and 0.5 mg/kg of codeine every 4 hours. Should the pain persist, the child is given an oral narcotic, morphine syrup, which is similar to Brompton's cocktail and has proved to be very effective. The final step in this sequence is continuous infusion. Miser, Miser, and Clark (1980) have recommended continuous IV infusion via a constant infusion pump as a safe and effective method of relieving severe pain in children with terminal malignancy. They have reported complete pain control in a small group ($n = 8$) of children and adolescents. Although side effects, including constipation, drowsiness, and decreased respiration, were common, they were also mild. The dose required for complete pain control ranged from 0.025 to 2.6 mg/kg/hour, with dosage efficacy being jointly decided upon by the pediatric personnel, parents, and child. The same team of investigators (Miser, Davis, Hughes, Mulne, & Miser, 1983) reported similar success using continuous SC infusion with a second, larger group. Miser et al. noted the advantages that this route of administration offers for the child, the major ones being a more even and adequate control of the pain, with the need for frequent injections now eliminated, and the fact that the child can remain at home.

Methadone

Methadone is a synthetic narcotic analgesic with actions qualitatively quite similar to those of morphine despite substantial structural differences. A single dose is only marginally more potent than morphine and, like morphine, it has no obvious ceiling effect. However, with repeated doses it is several times more potent (Twycross, 1984). Adverse effects of the two drugs are also similar in kind, although differing in degree; for example, with methadone there are fewer problems of constipation and sedation. The latter characteristic is particularly useful when relief of pain without sedation is required. A further advantage is its action as a powerful cough suppressant for control of the pain-producing useless cough that often adds to the discomfort of children with cancer and leukemia.

Methadone is well absorbed from all routes of administration, although PO administration reduces its potency by about 50% in comparison with IM or SC injection, a figure that is still considerably higher than is the case with PO administration of morphine. The most important difference between the two drugs concerns the longer half-life that methadone has for a single dose: When given regularly, the half-life may increase in some patients to 2 or 3 days (Inturrisi & Verebely, 1972), which means that frequency of administration must be reduced for prolonged use. Because methadone has a longer duration of action, it can be administered as infrequently as every 6 to 8 hours without compromising its analgesic action. Berkowitz (1976) has reported that there is no consistent relationship between plasma level and degree of analgesia obtained: Analgesia is maximal between 1 and 2 hours, whereas peak plasma levels are not reached until 4 to 6 hours. When the plasma level is near its maximum, pain relief has diminished by one fourth. It is not known, however, if the time course of adverse effects is temporally related to methadone plasma level. Of the strong narcotics, methadone is considered the best choice for children with terminal cancer (Twycross, 1984).

Fentanyl (Sublimaze)

Fentanyl is a synthetic narcotic that is significantly more potent than morphine but of shorter action than that drug. Fentanyl is used mainly as a preoperative premedication in combination with other drugs. It is also used with droperidol to induce a state of detachment with analgesia during aversive diagnostic procedures, and it is the drug of choice for management of postanesthesia afitiation in the child older than age 2 who is not experiencing severe physical pain. Szyfelbein and Osgood (1984) have reported that IV administration of fentanyl was a more practical and effective procedure for the control of pain related to burn dressing changes in children than either morphine or an oral mixture of oxycodone and acetaminophen (Percocet).

Weak Narcotic Analgesics

Codeine

Codeine is generally viewed as the agent of choice for the treatment of mild to moderate acute pain when the nonnarcotic analgesics fail to provide adequate pain relief. It is similar to morphine in many respects but is much less potent because of its lesser affinity for the opioid receptors. Most of the pains for which codeine is appropriate are just as effectively relieved by aspirin but at a dosage of five times that of codeine. However, codeine is often combined with aspirin for additive analgesic effects. The small dose of codeine in many of the resultant combination drug products is viewed as questionable by some clinicians (Twycross, 1984); others (Korberly, 1985) have stated that pharmacologically the combination of nonnarcotic and narcotic agents has validity; and some (Beaver, 1981) contend that there is clinical evidence that these combinations produce additive analgesic effects and may slow the rate of tolerance development.

Codeine is widely used as an analgesic that is generally considered safer than morphine and less likely to result in serious side effects. A contributing factor is its reliable absorption, which is due to a relatively low hepatic first-pass effect (Levine, 1983). It causes less respiratory depression and is less constipating than morphine, but in comparison with other weak narcotics, it is more constipating (Twycross, 1984). Nausea and vomiting are common, and with very high doses these and other side effects increase disproportionately to analgesia. This increase imposes a clinical ceiling effect but not a pharmacological one (Twycross, 1984).

Oxycodone (Percodan)

Oxycodone is a derivative of morphine that is related to codeine. An effective oral analgesic, it is available as a narcotic combination that also contains aspirin and phenacetin in addition to homatropine. The difficulty with such combinations is that they cannot be manipulated; that is, the dosage of one of the components cannot be increased without increasing the dosage of the remaining components. Although oxycodone is less potent than morphine, it is five or six times as potent as codeine. Analgesic activity occurs within 15 to 20 minutes and peaks at 45 minutes.

Meperidine (Demerol)

Meperidine (pethidine), generally classified as one of the least potent of the clinical opioids, is a synthetic narcotic analgesic chemically unrelated to morphine but having certain of its properties. It also has some of the properties of atropine and consequently has antispasmodic action. It is not as effective in the treatment of severe pain as morphine is, but is more effective than codeine.

Meperidine is absorbed from all routes of administration but is only one-third as potent when given PO compared with SC or IM injection. With IM injection, the onset of analgesia occurs in minutes. Intravenous injection is to be avoided with ambulatory children because it may cause hypotension, dizziness, and fainting due to vasodilation. At higher doses, with any route of administration it sometimes causes tremors and twitching and so, in effect, it does have a ceiling. With equianalgesic doses, it causes as much respiratory depression as morphine, but less constipation and fewer of the other adverse side effects, and tolerance takes longer to develop (Stimmel, 1983).

Buprenorphine (Buprenex)

Buprenorphine is a potent, long-acting synthetic narcotic analgesic with mixed agonist–antagonist properties (Heel, Brogden, Speight, & Avery, 1979). Derived from thebaine, it is structurally related to morphine but is more potent and has a longer duration of analgesic action. Its side effects are similar to those of morphine but are less severe. They include mild euphoria, nausea, dizziness, drowsiness, and sweating. Buprenorphine is well absorbed parenterally as well as orally. The latter characteristic is an important consideration for patients such as burn victims or cancer patients whose condition requires pain relief by noninvasive methods wherever possible. The fact that it can be given sublingually is of particular value for pediatric cancer patients who are unable to swallow oral medication. There is no ceiling effect for analgesia, but there is evidence of a ceiling effect in the therapeutic dosage range for respiratory depression. Lewis (1986) has documented an inverted U-shaped curve; that is, at very high doses, respiratory depression is lower than it is at moderate doses.

Buprenorphine has proved useful in the treatment of a diversity of severe pain conditions in adults, particularly in respect to cancer pain. The first report in the literature of its use with the pediatric age group comes from Pothmann, Schwamm-born, Andras, Ebell, and Jurgens (1984), who used the drug with 10 patients (CA 7–19) with advanced malignancies. It was administered IM in a mean dosage of 0.41 mg and a range of 0.09–1.5 mg. There was excellent, long-lasting analgesia without serious side effects, and over a 45-day treatment period no significant dose increment was required. At the present time, buprenorphine is not labeled for use with children in the United States because safety and efficacy for this age group have not been empirically established (Benitz, 1987).

Pentazocine (Talwin)

Primarily an opioid agonist, pentazocine also functions as a weak narcotic antagonist. Consequently, it must not be used with other opioids. The effect of concomitant use would be the potentiation of the adverse reactions of both drugs, with little analgesic effect for the patient. Although it is readily absorbed from both the oral and parenteral routes, pentazocine by oral administration is regarded as a weak narcotic because most of the dose is lost by first-pass metabolism in the liver. However, when it is injected, it functions as a strong analgesic. If given repeatedly by SC or IM injection it may cause tissue damage because it is an irritant. It is an effective analgesic for the relief of moderate to severe pain, and onset of action is rapid. With lower doses, nausea, vomiting, and dizziness are common side effects. Hallucinations and other disturbances have been reported in adults at doses within the therapeutic range (Stimmel, 1983). Unlike other opioids, pentazocine may cause an increase in blood pressure and ventricular rate.

Psychotherapeutic Drugs

Depression is one of the symptoms associated with chronic pain states such as JRA, cancer, and burn injuries in children. It is often expressed through inactivity, feelings of helplessness, and social withdrawal. One group of drugs that has proved useful in the management of these symptoms is the antidepressants, particularly two of the tricyclic compounds, amitriptyline (Elavil) and imipramine (Tofranil). Children reportedly respond to these tricyclic antidepressants with improved appetite and sleep patterns and increased physical activity within the boundaries imposed by their disease. They also show an elevation of mood, a reduction in morbid preoccupation with their condition, and heightened mental alertness. Often these children report a significant increment in pain relief when imipramine or amitriptyline is added to their therapeutic regimen. Clinical personnel frequently view this increased analgesia as either secondary to mood improvement or attributable to the tricyclics' potentiation of analgesic activity, particularly that of the narcotics. In fact, this phenomenon may be a direct effect of the tricyclics. Sternbach, Janowsky, Huey, and Segal (1976) believe that decreased serotonin plays an etiological role in chronic pain and depression. The fact that amitriptyline and imipramine inhibit the reuptake of serotonin (Gilman, et al., 1985) could directly effect an increase in analgesia as well as a reduction in depression in children for whom chronic pain and depression coexist.

In a review of the pharmacological tools that have proved useful in managing chronic pain in children, Lacouture, Gaudreault, and Lovejoy (1984) concur that tricyclic compounds are effective in the management of the psychological changes that result from chronic pain. At the same time, they caution that these drugs are toxic, relatively potent, and characterized by a cluster of adverse reactions. One group of adverse reactions is the centrally mediated side effects, such as headaches, motor slowing, and lassitude (presumably due to the sedating effect of these agents), which should dimish with time. A second group is the dose-related peripheral side effects, which include dryness of the mouth, blurred vision, constipation, and tachycardia, and these may not diminish with time.

Table 5-6   Tricyclic Antidepressants

Agent (trade name)	Dosage	Route of administration
Amitriptyline (Elavil)[a]	12–15 yr: 20–50 mg	PO (preferred route); IM
Imipramine (Tofranil)[a]	1–2 mg/kg/dose q 6 hr or q h s	PO (preferred route); IM

[a]Not recommended for children under age 12.

Imipramine (Tofranil)

One of the first tricyclic antidepressants, imipramine is of great value in endogenous depression (Levine, 1983). It is rapidly absorbed when given orally and is demethylated in the liver (first-pass effect) to the pharmacologically active desipramine (Maxwell, 1984).

Amitriptyline (Elavil)

Amitriptyline has analgesic effects independent of its antidepressant effects (Foley, 1985). It is readily absorbed orally, and there is extensive first-pass demethylation to the active compound nortriptyline (Maxwell, 1984). Although it is the second most commonly used tricyclic drug, there is some dispute concerning its use with young children. Lacouture et al. (1984) provide dosages for children six years of age and up, contrary to the recommendation that it not be used with children under age 12 because of insufficient research with this age group. Recommended dosages for amitriptyline and imipramine are shown in Table 5-6.

Comment

Among health professionals there is increasing concern about the inadequacy of relief for acute pain in both the adult and pediatric populations (Angell, 1982; Bonica, 1985b; Graves, Foster, Batenhorst, Bennett, & Baumann, 1983). Research in clinical settings has provided unequivocal evidence that patients in both populations are frequently undermedicated. In their study of adult medical patients, Marks and Sachar (1973), for example, showed that three quarters of the group who had received narcotic analgesics for severe acute pain continued to experience moderate to severe pain after 48 hours of treatment. Similar results have been reported on adults in studies of postoperative pain (Cohen, F. L., 1980; Keeri-Szanto & Heaman, 1972; O'Brien, 1984; Perry, 1984b). Although in the case of children, research on this topic is limited, the available data support the conclusion that undermedication is even more marked in the pediatric population. In a comparison of the postoperative prescription and administration of analgesics following cardiac surgery in 50 children and 50 adults, Beyer et al. (1983) found that children received 30% of all the analgesics prescribed for the whole group and six of the children received no postoperative analgesics. Of the analgesics that were prescribed for the children, significantly fewer were potent analgesics than was the case with the adults. These results supported Eland's (1974) and Swafford and Allan's (1968) earlier findings on quantity and potency. In the latter study, only 2 of 60 children were given postoperative pain medication, and of 180 children in intensive care, only 26 received narcotics for pain. In the most careful study to date on this issue, Schechter, Allen, and Hanson (1986) controlled for medical diagnosis, length of stay, and type of hospital. They demonstrated significant differences in narcotic dosage between adults and children in the same diagnostic category, with adults receiving more doses per day, a discrepancy that increased with length of hospital stay. An indication of the obstacles in the way of a more enlightened attitude toward the use of analgesics in pediatric pain patients comes from a study by Perry and Heidrich (1982) in which nurses in burn units were given clinical situations in the form of vignettes describing equally severe burns in hypothetical adult and child patients. The nurses' task was to determine what analgesics should be used during debridement. Although they assessed the pain as identical in both age groups, in proportion to age and weight significantly less medication and weaker medication was their recommendation for the children despite their previous assessment of pain equivalence in the two groups.

This state of affairs is not restricted to American medical practice. In a study of Canadian drug prescription, O'Brien (1984) reported that children received more analgesics than did adults, but the analgesics that were administered to both age groups were inadequate for the alleviation of moderate to severe postoperative pain and were also given too infrequently to provide pain relief. Similar findings of grossly inadequate management of moderate and severe postoperative pain were reported by Mather and Mackie (1983) in their study of 170 Australian children. The pediatric patient with chronic pain suffers from similar mismanagement (Miser, McCalla, Dothage, Wesley, & Miser, 1987; Newburger & Sallan, 1981), which suggests that the whole pattern of underuse of analgesics has its origin outside of patient characteristics such as age or cause and type of pain.

Attitudes and Beliefs Underlying Differential Drug Treatment

Many pediatric personnel firmly believe that children feel less pain than adults do and therefore need proportionally less analgesic. This difference in pain experienced is attributed to two facets of the developmental differences that exist between the child and the adult. In the first, the neurological explanation of incomplete myelinization is used as justification for reduced dosage, despite the fact that research findings in this area are equivocal (see, for example, Haslam, 1969; Jay et al., 1983; Swafford & Allan, 1968): There is no firm evidence that children and adults do feel pain in the same way or that either group feels more or less pain. The second developmental parameter concerns the metabolism of analgesics, since differences here could justify the lesser dosages given to children. However, data on morphine kinetics from Dahlström, Bolme, Feychting, Noack, and Paalzow (1979) showed that infants and children metabolize morphine in essentially the same way as adults. The only shred of support for the differences in dosage is that children may heal more quickly and consequently experience less discomfort than adults do (Schechter et al., 1986).

Overconcern for side effects, particularly respiratory depression and the possibility of addiction, deters many medical personnel from administering these drugs at appropriate levels. This concern has exasperated Angell (1982), Portenoy and Foley (1986, pp. 182–183), and others, causing Angell to comment that in no other area of medicine has such extravagant concern for side effects so drastically limited treatment. The concern for respiratory depression, which Vere (1984) has dismissed as "paranoid worry," lacks justification: it is a rare complication that can be rapidly reversed with naloxone. As far as the addiction possibility is concerned, the data provide no support whatsoever for this belief. A recent survey of 12,000 medical inpatients who had received medicinal narcotics showed only four cases of reasonably well-documented addiction in those with no prior history of addiction (Twycross, 1984). These findings are consistent with other reports that addiction is extremely rare in hospitalized patients (Porter & Jick, 1980).

According to Bonica (1985b), a major reason for the inadequate relief of acute pain at all age levels is the improper application of the therapies that currently are available. Bonica attributes this problem to the failure to provide medical personnel with formal instruction in pain pharmacotherapy and to provide adequate sources of information in the relevant literature. In a survey of 102 doctors in training at two major New York teaching hospitals, Marks and Sachar (1973) found that this group underestimated the effective dose range of the narcotics, overestimated the duration of their action, and had exaggerated fears of addiction. Similar findings have been reported by Beyer et al. (1983), M. Cohen (1980), Graves et al. (1983), and Mather and Mackie (1983). Marks and Sachar (1973) also reported that house officers prescribed doses of narcotics for severe acute pain that were 50% to 65% of the effective dose and nurses then administered 40% to 50% of the already inadequate dosage. The "interpretation" of the analgesic medication orders by nurses is a common problem. A variation on this theme is the situation in which the nurse urges the patient to "wait a little longer if you can," totally ignoring the fact that narcotics are more effective in intercepting pain than in relieving it (Perry, 1984b).

Adding to these largely self-imposed inadequacies of ignorance and poor supervision is the fact that cues from children concerning their pain state are often difficult to interpret. Children generally do not show evidence of pain with the clarity characteristic of adults, for a cluster of reasons including the fact that they may lack verbal facility and are often intimidated by the unfavorable odds in the situation. Given the time and appropriately worded questions, most children would probably by quite forthcoming about their immediate state (Ross & Ross, 1982a,

1984b). Their nonverbal behaviors, too, are often misleading as an index of pain. Nurses, in all good faith, frequently attribute these behaviors to fear or separation anxiety. Some children deliberately hide signs of pain because they are terrified of needles (Eland & Anderson, 1977; Ross & Ross, 1982a).

An Alternate Hypothesis

The explanations listed above rest on the premise that an informational/educational gap exists that, if filled, would largely eliminate the problem of undermedication of patients in pain. In these explanations, the focus of such further education and training is on the pharmacotherapy of the analgesics. At the same time, studies in which educational content has been introduced as a means of counteracting under-medication tendencies generally have had little effect on the participants' subsequent behavior with patients in the clinical setting (Perry, 1984b). These negative findings clearly support the need for a more intensive look at the dynamics of the situation, one that goes beyond the simplistic belief that pharmacological instruction will effect behavior change. Perry (1984b) has raised the interesting hypothesis that medical personnel have an unconscious need for patients to be in pain. He is not suggesting that the motivation is merely sadistic:

> Instead, I am suggesting that a modicum of pain in the physically ill is necessary to preserve ego boundaries, to distinguish who is ill and who is not, and at an even deeper level, to provide reassurance that the patient is alive. (Perry, 1984b, p. 809)

Perry has discussed the basis for these speculations in detail (Perry, 1984a) but summarizes them as follows:

> First, in regard to pain being necessary to preserve ego boundaries, the most dramatic illustration is the disquieting experience produced in patients and staff when all pain is pharmacologically removed and, unlike general anesthesia, consciousness remains intact. For example, patients administered ketamine describe the terrifying effects of being totally pain free and "lost in space" without a sense of self. . . . patients with severe depersonalization voluntarily inflict pain upon themselves and in common parlance, we "pinch" ourselves to make sure "it's not a dream" . . . that we and our surroundings are "real."
>
> Second, in regard to pain helping to distinguish who is ill and who is not, the best evidence . . . comes from the patients themselves. For example, when postoperative patients are given a self-regulated intravenous pump to administer their own narcotic analgesics (Hull & Sibbald, 1981), they generally choose to preserve some pain, explaining that if all the pain were gone, the doctor might not know that they were still ill. . . . Furthermore, this need for pain to declare who is ill may explain why the pain caused by doctors during examinations and procedures at times seems to go beyond the necessity of professional detachment. Perhaps the overzealous infliction of pain serves some inordinate need to declare who is ill and who is not.
>
> Third, in regard to pain unconsciously offering reassurance that the patient is alive, the best evidence again comes from the patients themselves, most dramatically illustrated by . . . [burn] patients who have been . . . [given pavulon for complete muscular relaxation and narcotics] so that they lie in bed fully conscious yet unable to move or feel. . . . Once the drugs are tapered and the patients are again able to com-

municate, they recount terrifying experiences that went beyond being unsure of who they or their caretakers were; indeed, many recall wondering if they might be presumed dead by others and "buried alive" or . . . remember intense anxiety related to being uncertain themselves about whether or not they were alive. . . . Although admittedly quite speculative, one explanation for the undermedication for pain may be the deep unconscious fear of "deadening" the pain of patients and thereby removing this inherent quality of being alive. . . . These speculations may also help explain why education alone has not been sufficient in solving the documented problem of undertreatment for pain. (Perry, 1984b, pp. 809–811)

Acupuncture

Acupuncture is a therapeutic procedure that originated more than 5,000 years ago in China. Although it was used sporadically in the United States during the 19th and early 20th centuries (Millman, 1977), the major impetus for current interest in it in the United States came from publicity in 1971 concerning the dramatic postoperative pain relief experienced by newspaper columnist James Reston after acupuncture treatment following emergency abdominal surgery in China. This heightened interest was consolidated the following year by former president Richard Nixon's trip to China (Bonica, 1974). Since that time, it has been in use here for treatment of a diversity of clinical problems including migraine and tension headaches, bursitis, and other musculoskeletal problems such as low back pain.

Acupuncture is based on the theory that energy (Ch'i) flows throughout the body according to a predictable directional and temporal course along fixed major and subsidiary channels (meridians) that are connected with each other as well as with the major organs of the body. When the flow of Ch'i is obstructed or an imbalance occurs in its bipolar character (Yang [positive] and Yin [negative]), pain or disease can occur. In the treatment of pain, fine steel needles are inserted at specific acupuncture points (Hoku) and then manipulated in order to restore equilibrium to the flow of energy and thus eliminate or reduce the pain. The appropriate Hoku points for different pain conditions are identified on complex meridian maps. The traditional map described by Kao (1973) consists of 361 Hoku points on 14 meridians. Most of the needle insertions are at Hoku points at or near the site of pain, although some points are distant from it. The Hoku point for toothache and tension headache, for example, is located between the thumb and forefinger. A more detailed account of this most interesting treatment procedure is beyond the scope of the present discussion. For additional information, see Kaptchuk (1983), Macdonald (1984), and Millman (1977).

Although acupuncture has been used far more often with adults than with children, there is some clinical and empirical support for its efficacy with children. Highly qualified acupuncturists (Freeman, 1981; Lee, 1981) have reported its clinical efficacy particularly for children with migraine headaches and musculoskeletal pain, but few publications on its use with children have appeared. In an uncontrolled study, Leo (1983) successfully used electrical stimulation at acupuncture points for treating reflex sympathetic dystrophy in several children. Gunsberger (1973) has reported success with acupuncture treatment of sore throat symptomatology in children. This interesting study of 400 children was so methodologically flawed that it does not merit being called controlled, although control was intended. The procedural weaknesses included the failure to use blind ratings and inadequacies in the two control conditions. One of the latter conditions was made up of acupuncture refusers; the other had vaseline rubbed into the acupuncture point, a procedure that the children could have interpreted as treatment. The interesting finding in this study was the fact that at the 48-hour posttreatment check, 90% of the children in the two acupuncture treatment groups still reported pain relief. In a group of child and adult migraine patients, Pothmann and Goepel (1984a) used traditional acupuncture points and moxibustion (heating of acupuncture points) to treat some patients and combined these two procedures with soft laser irradiation (Robinson, 1982) and transcutaneous electrical nerve stimulation for other patients. Although they reported that 75% of the children showed substantial improvement, their study is marred by failure to provide adequate information, such as the number of children involved, and by methodological flaws. Omission of an attention-placebo group raises doubts about the treatment package as a whole and the design also does not permit the identification of the specific component(s) causally related to the improvement.

It is difficult to evaluate the findings on acupuncture because many of the studies have methodological flaws similar in degree to those of Pothmann and Goepel (1984a). Furthermore, it is difficult to assess American acupuncture fairly because many of its practitioners are singularly unskilled and underqualified. Kaptchuk (1983) has commented that to the traditional, highly-trained acupuncturists in China, much of the acupuncture that is practiced in the Western world is akin to unqualified individuals handing out antibiotics at random to those who are ill. There is no way of assessing the influence of the practitioner's level of competence on the data collected in the various empirical studies reported in the literature, but it is possible to evaluate other aspects of these studies. Vincent and Richardson (1986) have provided an excellent statement of procedural and design standards that should be used in such evaluations. Applying these standards in a careful review of the literature (primarily on adult patients), they (Richardson & Vincent, 1986) have concluded that there is evidence for the short-term effectiveness of acupuncture in relieving acute and chronic pain, with the proportion of patients helped in group studies often falling in the 50% to 75% range. In the case of long-term effectiveness, positive evidence of effectiveness exists but the data are not so strong. It is clear that acupuncture is free of complications, with few, if any, negative side effects. Reported incidents of infection from the use of dirty needles are a problem of sloppy laboratory routine rather than of inherent weaknesses in the acupuncture treatment.

Criticisms, Rebuttals, and Concessions

In a pattern common to all new treatment procedures, acupuncture has been bitterly criticized by some and enthusiastically endorsed by others as a panacea in the control of pain. One point of contention concerns the claim that there is no scientific basis for the location of the Hoku points. This claim has been soundly refuted: Melzack, Stillwell, and Fox (1977) have reported that the distribution of Hoku points is similar to that of trigger points (Travell & Rinzler, 1952). They found that every acupuncture point had a corresponding trigger point and that a close correspondence existed between the pain syndromes associated with the two kinds of points. Both kinds have widespread distribution throughout the body, and pain relief can be achieved in both by stimulation. An interesting facet here is the high correspondence between trigger points, which are firmly anchored in 20th century anatomy of the neural and muscular systems (Travell & Rinzler, 1952), and Hoku points, which are an integral part of an ancient but anatomically nonexistent system of meridians.

Because acupuncture charts vary, the possibility has been raised that it is of no consequence where the needle is inserted in relation to the specific Hoku points. There is some evidence that undifferentiated needling, loosely defined as inserting the needles anywhere, can result in pain reduction. Richardson and Vincent (1986) reported that of 11 controlled studies, five reported acupuncture points as superior to random needle insertion and six reported nonsignificant differences, but with trends favoring acupuncture points. Studies by Lewith and Machin (1983) and Co, Schmitz, Havdala, Reyes, and Westerman (1979) had similar results, the subjects in the latter study being sickle-cell anemia patients during painful crises. When degree of pain abatement is the issue, Jeans (1979) showed that acupuncture points close to those in the area of pain yielded more pain relief than did distant points, with the latter, in turn, yielding more relief than placebo. Taub, Beard, Eisenberg, and McCormack (1977) found that relief from dental pain could be accomplished by stimulating a point on the hand other than the Hoku point specified for toothache. Their results suggest that the point of effective stimulation may be a larger area in the proximity of the designated Hoku point. In a review of acupuncture treatment, Liebeskind and Paul (1977) concluded that the parameters of stimulation, such as frequency and intensity, may be more important than the locus of stimulation points.

Attempts to explain the analgesic effects that can be obtained with acupuncture fall into two groups, the first of which rests on the assumption that neurophysiological mechanisms are involved. There is strong evidence that acupuncture-produced analgesia is at least partly mediated by central nervous system mechanisms (Mayer, Price, Rafii, 1977; Pomeranz, Cheng, & Law, 1977). It is possible that the movement of the needles stimulates the large nerve fibers in the periphery of the body, that is, those that send signals via the dorsal horn to the brain to close the gate, thus blocking the transmission of pain impulses conducted through small nerve fibers. When acupuncture is performed in a body area with no sensation, as is the case when there is procaine infiltration of acupuncture points, the analgesic action of the acupuncture cannot be demonstrated (Jayson, 1981).

Another possibility is that acupuncture can stimulate the release of endorphins in the midbrain, thus preventing the perception of pain. Prior to the discovery of endorphins, experiments done in China showed that some humoral factor was involved in acupuncture analgesia. The pain thresholds of untreated rabbits, for example, were raised when they were injected with the cerebrospinal fluid of rabbits with acupuncture-induced analgesia (Millman, 1977). There is evidence from clinical and experimental studies that acupuncture analgesia liberates increased amounts of endorphins into the cerebrospinal fluid (Nathan, 1982). Further support for the involvement of endorphins in acupuncture comes from the fact that acupuncture-induced analgesia is abolished by the narcotic antagonist naloxone (Liebeskind & Paul, 1977). Recent evidence suggests that acupuncture analgesia may be mediated by two endogenous pain-relieving symptoms, one using endorphins, the other serotonin (Cheng & Pomeranz, 1986).

A third explanation lies in the possibility noted by Price, Rafii, Watkins, and Buckingham (1984) that acupuncture effects may be mediated by peripheral as well as central mechanisms. They suggest that while the initial analgesic effects of acupuncture may be centrally mediated, acupuncture could then result in peripheral changes that could facilitate a certain amount of pain relief, if not directly cause it. As an example, they point out that a patient with low back pain could develop endorphin-mediated analgesia, which allows him to move more freely. The increased movement could then have a therapeutic effect, with a consequent reduction in peripheral pathological processes contributing to the pain. It has also been suggested that psychological processes such as placebo effects, suggestion, and hypnosis, are largely responsible for acupuncture mediated analgesia. Loeser (1980) is representative of a group who attributes the reported success of acupuncture to a placebo effect and other changes such as the elimination of alcohol and medicines as part of the acupuncture treatment; the possibility that acupuncture effects a modest increase in pain threshold; or the possibility that a change occurs in response bias, that is, in the patient's willingness when under the influence of a persuasive therapist to modify his views of what constitutes pain ("not so painful") after acupuncture.

The evidence largely refutes these claims. Although it is recognized that some placebo effect is likely in the success of any mode of pain treatment, there is substantial evidence that acupuncture is more effective in pain relief than is placebo stimulation (see, for example, Reichmanis & Becker, 1977). In the review of evaluative research by Richardson and Vincent (1986), 50% to 80% of patients were helped, an immediate success rate far greater than would be expected if the acupuncture effects were entirely a function of placebo-related factors. The placebo-benefit rate set by Beecher (1959), for example, was at the 30% to 35% level for pain patients. In addition, partial analgesia can be produced in animals through acupuncture (see, for example, Bresler, 1979; Pomeranz et al., 1977), a finding that argues against a simple placebo effect. As far as hypnosis is concerned, the two methods of treatment appear to operate through different mechanisms. There is evidence that the acupuncture effect stems from the activation of the opiate-related pain modulating system (see, for example, Mayer, Price, Barber, & Rafii, 1976), whereas the analgesic effects associated with hypnosis appear to be achieved through the higher cortical mechanisms.

Acupressure

Acupressure is a noninvasive derivative of acupuncture based on the same principles but having potential for use by children. It consists of applying manual pressure to the skin at appropriate Hoku points for immediate short-term pain relief. Its apparent simplicity has resulted in the publication of a number of books and articles of a self-help nature. Representative of these publications is Dalet's (1980) book in which the specific pressure points for a wide variety of common and less common aches and pains are identified with photographs and diagrams. The nature of the pain, whether a sore throat, sunburn, tennis elbow, or menstrual cramps, is not relevant as far as the procedure is concerned: regardless of the kind of pain, the specific pressure point must be located and then stimulated. Dalet (1980) has described the procedure as follows:

With the help of the diagrams and photographs, locate the appropriate Hoku point. Although each point occupies a small area of approximately half a square millimeter, it will be immediately clear when the point has been located because it is a highly sensitive area with a markedly different feeling from that of the surrounding tissues. Now, begin stimulating the Hoku point by placing the tip of the index finger on it and pressing down forcefully. At the same time, vibrate the finger slightly to give a rapid little massage while rotating the finger clockwise. Although the length of time for relief of pain will vary for each individual, from a minute or two to several hours or even days, the effects of acupressure will remain undiminished with repeated stimulation.

We advocate that children be taught to locate Hoku points only for those pains that commonly occur in childhood. One point that has proven useful in treating lateral and bilateral tension musculoskeletal headaches is located in each hand in the web of skin between the thumb and first finger. To identify this Hoku point the child extends his hand as though to shake hands with someone; the web between the thumb and first finger then becomes clearly visible and is distinct from the fleshy part adjacent to it.

Gorsky's (1981, p. 78) description of the procedure, which, it should be noted, is not applicable to migraine headaches, is summarized as follows: For headaches on the right side, the right-hand Hoku point is used; for those on the left, the left-hand point is used; for bilateral headaches both Hoku points are used simultaneously. We will describe the procedure in terms of headaches on the left side of the head, but the general method is the same for all three locations. Using the thumb and forefinger of the right hand, firmly grasp the web of the left hand and exert pressure around the web area until locating the spot where the pressure is definitely uncomfortable. This is the Hoku point for headaches. Apply continuous pressure to this point for 15 seconds, then slowly release the pressure, and decide whether the headache pain is relieved. If not, or if it returns, repeat the procedure.

The headache Hoku point is also the pressure point for dental pain. Melzack, Guité, and Gonshor (1980) have shown that ice massage of this point provides a palliative control of dental pain. In their studies, a randomly selected group of adult patients waiting in an outpatient dental clinic were shown how to insert ice cubes into a wet gauze pad and gently massage the skin around the Hoku point of the hand (on the same side as the pain) until the area felt numb or 7 minutes had elapsed, whichever occurred first. Melzack et al. found that the majority of the group experienced a 50% or more decrease in the intensity of their dental pain.

Myotherapy

Prudden (1980) has developed another procedural variant of the basic acupuncture technique, called *myotherapy*. Central to this pain therapy is an entity known as the trigger point. This point is a highly sensitive spot in a muscle and one that is basic to the pain experience because it can cause the muscle to go into spasm (Travell, 1976). Trigger points are similar to Hoku points in that they are widespread over many parts of the body, with correspondence between some trigger and Hoku points, and pain relief is achieved by stimulating them. However, unlike the Hoku points used in other forms of pressure therapy, the trigger points in myotherapy are different in each person because they are laid down all through life by experiences such as falls, strains, accidents, the birth process, occupation, stress, and disease. A trigger point lies dormant in a muscle until the physical and emotional climate is right and then it "fires," throwing that muscle into a spasm and thus causing pain. To erase the pain, the individual is taught how to locate the sensitive spots in the appropriate muscles and then to apply intense pressure with the fingers, knuckles, or elbows. In the face and head area, 4 to 5 seconds of pressure is usually adequate; for most trigger points in other areas, 7 seconds is the norm. The relief of pain occurs because the trigger point is being deprived of oxygen (Travell, 1976). In many instances myotherapy also prevents recurrence.

Prudden's (1980) work in pain therapy is of particular interest because, in addition to developing the myotherapy procedure, she has made the only attempt that we know of in any Western country to teach children any variant of acupuncture. To determine whether children could find and erase trigger points, Prudden set up a class of first-grade children. Using a modified anatomy text appropriate for their comprehension level and teaching aids such as "Muscle Man" and "Mr. Bones," the children quickly learned the names of the muscles most important for

trigger points and the bones to which they were attached. They also had no difficulty with the myotherapy technique: According to Prudden there were no untreated cases of growing pains in the group. If the teacher did not erase the pains,
the children were able to do so. When a child in the class broke his leg, the group
studied fractures; when the leg came out of the cast, they were able to predict
accurately where the trigger points were. There is, unfortunately, only anecdotal
evidence for the efficacy of this program, but it clearly justifies research attention.

Acupressure and myotherapy appear to provide quick and safe alternatives
for selected pains, and they are less painful than certain medical techniques. As
experimental therapies, their efficacy with children has yet to be substantiated by
independent investigators. Note that they are not a substitute for medical/dental
checkups, and it is unlikely that they would be appropriate for all patients.

Biofeedback

Biofeedback training teaches the patient through an instrumental learning procedure to monitor and control physiological responses such as muscle tension, skin
temperature, and electrical activity of the brain. With the help of a computer and
electrodes attached to specific muscles or critical temperature points, the patient is
provided with continuous external feedback in the form of an electromyographic
(EMG) recording about changes in a particular response system (Melzack & Wall,
1983). The EMG measures the amount of electrical discharge in the muscle fibers
and is an index of muscle contraction or relaxation. Without this feedback, the
patient would have no awareness of these changes. The training involves two distinct steps: First, the patient learns to recognize and discriminate the relevant response system, then he learns how to produce changes in it by concentrating on
reducing or increasing the signal frequency from the visual display unit. The child
with recurrent tension headaches, for example, has instant feedback from the
EMG recordings from the frontalis muscle, which is the treatment target system
for tension headaches. He receives an easily recognized signal on the visual display unit, and this signal changes in proportion to ongoing contraction or relaxation of the frontalis muscle. The signals typically are explicit and have high appeal:
A train may go faster as muscle tension increases and slower as it decreases, or a
clown may smile more and more broadly, finally clapping as the child becomes
increasingly adept at the task, or frowning and crying as the child does poorly.

As one would expect where sensitive, electronic equipment and individually
trained clinicians are involved, biofeedback is an expensive procedure. Research
on it has been plagued by more than the usual methodological and design problems, with poorly designed research studies far outnumbering carefully controlled
investigations. There is a sufficient body of good work, however, to justify certain
conclusions on biofeedback as a method of treatment for pain. In these studies the
target population has been almost entirely an adult one. Although there is no ap-

parent reason why results from them would not also be applicable to children, we shall confine the discussion here mainly to those studies that have been done with children. Readers who are interested in the methodological problems and other shortcomings that have lessened the impact and value of biofeedback research would find it helpful to read reviews by Jessup (1984), King and Montgomery (1980), Qualls and Sheehan (1981), Tarler-Benlolo (1978), and Turner and Chapman (1982a).

Clinicians who use biofeedback training report that most children have little difficulty in gaining voluntary control of the target response system. In one study, Olness (1985) found that children ages 6 to 10 could outperform adults in controlling skin temperature. Children as young as age 3 have been able to learn pain control (Olness, 1985), the critical requirements being the ability to pay attention and understand instructions. For children with muscle contraction headaches, EMG biofeedback training is apparently beneficial, according to clinicians' unpublished reports. Since this finding has also been reported with adults, the results cannot be attributed to spontaneous remission of the headache, subject maturation, or passage of time (Jessup, 1984; Qualls & Sheehan, 1981). Thermal biofeedback training for migraine headache relief has also been reported as successful with children (Peper & Grossman, 1974), but not to the same extent as EMG biofeedback. By contrast, routine relaxation training has consistently been demonstrated to be of equal efficacy to biofeedback, with the added advantages of simplicity and greater cost effectiveness: No expensive equipment is involved, and children can be taught in groups (Setterlind, 1982; Stroebel, 1982). This finding on comparability holds up whether biofeedback is being used for specific muscle training, as in the case of frontalis muscle training, or for general relaxation (Tarler-Benlolo, 1978).

Factors in Biofeedback that Cause Improvement

A particularly intriguing and unequivocal finding concerns the fact that benefits from biofeedback therapy are not specific to the biofeedback procedure itself in tension (Andrasik & Holroyd, 1980a) and migraine headaches (Kewman & Roberts, 1980). In a creatively designed study with adult patients on what happens during treatment to cause pain reduction, Andrasik and Holroyd (1980a) compared three treatment groups (decreasing, increasing, or stabilizing frontalis muscle tension) with a no-treatment group. In a 3-month follow-up, all three treatment groups showed substantial and equivalent decreases in tension headaches and were equally superior to the no-treatment group. The equivalent decreases finding is surprising in view of the fact that two of the treatment groups were taught to increase or maintain tension, conditions that should have caused an increase in tension headaches rather than the obtained decrease. Similar results were obtained by Kewman and Roberts (1980) in a study on thermal biofeedback for migraine headaches. These findings raise the question of what mediates improvement in biofeedback training when groups such as these receive opposite treatments.

To date, no conclusive mediator has been identified for the improvement that occurs with biofeedback, although several possibilities have been proposed. Some investigators believe that personality × treatment interactions may be the key. It is known, for example, that having an internal locus of control, experiencing a reduction in anxiety, and having a strong positive relationship with the therapist are all associated with pain reduction (Jessup, 1984; Qualls & Sheehan, 1981). There also appears to be a powerful placebo effect in biofeedback that can create an exaggerated impression of its therapeutic effectiveness (Jessup, 1984). Other investigators (Holroyd, Andrasik, & Westbrook, 1977) view cognitive processes as the decisive mediators of the biofeedback effect. Meichenbaum (1976, p. 203) has suggested that

> One of the consequences of biofeedback treatment may be to change the client's perceptions, attributions, appraisals—his internal dialogue about his ability to control, first his physiological response, and then his cognitions, feelings and behaviors.

This theme of control is a common one in patient reports. Perceived increased control over bodily processes may well be the unifying element that explains the efficacy of biofeedback as well as other behavioral–cognitive strategies for decreased pain reactivity in both adults and children (Thompson, 1981).

Unlike most medical treatments that children undergo, biofeedback training requires the child to become actively involved and to assume some responsibility for coping with his pain. The concrete nature of the training, for example, seeing a train on the visual display unit, is particularly appropriate for children who are at the concrete operations stage (Piaget & Inhelder, 1969). These children often report that the images displayed in the training situation facilitate their efforts to reproduce the training behaviors in other settings:

> Every time I started to wriggle I just said, "Now, relax, so the train goes slow, you dummy" and when it got to people going up for communion when I usually start getting in trouble I just kept having train-talks to myself and after church my mom gave me a special smile . . . and I had this real good feeling. I never had that good a day before in my whole life. (Boy, CA 9, hyperactive, Ross & Ross, 1982b, p. 275)

In biofeedback training the child with tension or migraine headaches is shown visually that if he grits his teeth or clenches his jaw the tension in the frontalis muscle increases and that *he* can reduce this tension by relaxing the appropriate muscle. It is our opinion that biofeedback is effective here not because the child actually relaxes the appropriate muscle but because he learns that he *can* do it. This idea would explain the apparently contradictory results in the studies by Andrasik and Holroyd (1980a) and Kewman and Roberts (1980) discussed earlier. We believe that a critical factor in the efficacy of biofeedback is that it enables the child to look objectively at his tension or migraine headaches (or other biofeedback-treated problem) for the first time. The detached and unemotional presentation of information from the visual display unit combined with the relaxed, nonthreatening environment is a setting conducive to insight. Coupled with this is the quality and significance of the child's relationship with his therapist, a warm, nonthreatening, no needles, no lectures relationship that offers many opportunities for discussion and further bolsters the child's self-confidence. In this setting, the child learns to recognize first the physiological cues to his headaches and then the psychological cues associated with them. He is then equipped to focus on the precipitating antecedents of the headaches, which might be family problems or peer problems, such as being bullied at school. Usually the child can learn how to avert the headache at the antecedent stage of the sequence. In the process, he becomes more objective about looking at others as well as looking at himself. Biofeedback teaches the child that he can control aspects of his own behavior to an astonishing degree. One result may be an increase in his internal locus of control (Stern & Berrenberg, 1977), a finding that led Conners (1979, p. 149) to comment that

> It may well be that one of the most important implications of the striking degree of self-regulation possible with biofeedback is an increase in the child's sense of autonomy and self-sufficiency in a world where his general helplessness is all too frequently fostered by malign environments and a history of inability to control events around him.

Another result is the feeling of competence that is generated by the child's knowledge that he can control his body's responses. Often this ability is interpreted as a kind of magic, particularly at the early and middle childhood levels. Some children conclude that they have extraordinary powers that other children lack. This strong positive feeling is especially beneficial for those who secretly believe that something is wrong with them for having headaches. Following their success in the biofeedback training, children show this confidence in comments such as the following: "I can do anything now." "I'm not going to have any trouble with math." "I'm Superman." A clinical example of the confidence and other benefits discussed above is contained in the following comment by a boy age 8 (Ross & Ross, 1985) who was then undergoing biofeedback training for recurrent tension headaches:

> Well, at first it was scary like in *The Mad Magician*—like you can *see* a headache or not a headache. Now when I start to get uptight I can *see* what's happening and I get right in there fast like *Action Front*. And what is real good is it's *me* that has to do the stopping. I'm *real* good at it. . . . Steve [therapist] says a hotshot like me can beat a headache any day.

It is this cluster of additional benefits that makes biofeedback the treatment of choice for children over relaxation therapy despite their equivalence in effect on headaches, and the clear advantages in cost and time of relaxation therapy.

Relaxation

The ability to relax is a valuable skill for the child who is in the throes of treatment-related or spontaneous pain, in a state of tension induced by the anticipation of impending painful procedures, or confronted by environmental or social stressors. For some children this ability appears to have been acquired on their own, although it would be difficult here to separate out the influence of observational learning (Bandura, 1969). An 8-year-old boy describing how he coped with burn treatment said

> I told myself to go soft all over and start rolling in deep snow.

When asked who had taught him to do that, he replied with some surprise that he had always done it. Many children report relaxing when they have a headache (Ross & Ross, 1984b):

> I just sink. (Girl, CA 9)

> You just be like a cloud and it goes. (Boy, CA 8)

Self-induced relaxation has the immediate effect of providing the child with a feeling of self-control over the situation at hand. It allows him to think more clearly and increases the probability that he will mobilize himself psychologically for whatever action may be appropriate. Over the long term, this habit pattern should act toward attenuating or preventing nonproductive states of high levels of tension that, if frequent or prolonged, are associated in adulthood with headaches, elevated blood pressure, cardiac dysfunctions, and other stress-related conditions.

During the past 15 years there has been a proliferation of clinical research and vocational interest in relaxation training, but primarily for adults. The increased interest has been due in part to the conviction that the general autonomic relaxation that occurs with biofeedback was the reason for the efficacy of that technique. Direct relaxation training offered the important advantages of greater cost effectiveness and the possibility of group training. As the efficacy of this simple, safe, and usually immediately effective form of therapy has been established, interest has expanded to include individual training of children with medical problems such as asthma (Gardner & Olness, 1981), burn treatment (Elliott & Olson, 1983), chronic arthritic pain in hemophilia (Varni, 1981), dental treatment (Nocella & Kaplan, 1982; Parkin, 1981), migraine (Diamond & Franklin, 1975; Werder, 1978), and skeletomuscular pain (La Greca & Ottinger, 1979). The clinician or researcher who wishes to teach children how to relax should refer to the excellent training procedure developed by Cautela and Groden (1978).

One of the best studies in the relaxation literature is that of Richter et al. (1986) on relaxation treatment for migraine in children and adolescents. They

found progressive deep muscle relaxation and cognitive restructuring of dysfunctional thought processes to be equally effective in reducing frequency and overall
headache activity. Of note in this study was the credibility of the attention-control
group treatment in which the stress reduction training procedure used was structurally identical to the procedures used in the two experimental groups. The foregoing study was conducted in the clinical setting. The efficacy of relaxation training has also been demonstrated in the school setting (Larsson & Melin, 1986) in a
study of adolescents with tension and combined tension and migraine headaches.

The benefits of relaxation training have been so decisive in these clinical conditions that the potential benefits of teaching relaxation as a preventive strategy
have also been explored, within the format of group instruction. Of relevance here
are two school programs developed by Setterlind and his associates (Setterlind,
1982; Setterlind & Uneståhl, 1978) in which large groups of elementary and high
school students learned the relaxation response. The first and more comprehensive
of these was a 6-week program in which 294 students in Grades 6 through 12 were
given relaxation training for periods of 7 to 12 minutes, three times a week during
physical education classes. Table 5-7 shows the content and sequence of the program. From observational reports and the children's descriptions of the relaxation
feeling (heaviness, warmth, and lightness of body; a sinking down feeling, a float-
ing away sensation, and complete detachment), it was apparent that the majority of
the children had learned successfully to relax. In addition, almost all of them had
positive attitudes about the use of relaxation.

The next step involved a comparison of the following four modes of presentation of the relaxation training: taped instructions, oral instructions, personal relaxation to music, and personal relaxation without music. This time, 303 children in

Table 5-7   Content of the Relaxation Programs

Phase
1   Gives experience of what relaxation is and is not through shortened versions of Jacob-
son's method of progressive relaxation through conditioning processes. (Programs 1
and 2)

2   Learning relaxation through conditioning processes. (Programs 1 and 2)

3   The passive concentration on particular muscles or muscle groups will after some
training elicit a tonus decrease in the intended muscles or part of the body by the
effect of the "reversed ideomotoric tendency." (Programs 3 and 4)

4   Learning of a "trigger" (a specific stimulus or signal) which alone can elicit relaxation. (Program 5)

5   Presenting different methods of deepening the relaxation such as imaginative training, techniques of breathing and meditation. Individual choice of a technique. (Programs 6 and 7)

6   Self-training without instruction. (Program 8)

Note. Adapted from Setterlind, 1982, pp. 4–5.

Grades 4 through 6 took part. The lessons were shortened to between 5 and 7 minutes and were given two to three times a week for the first 3 weeks, after which they tapered off, with a shift in emphasis away from class instruction to personal control. The results showed oral instruction to be clearly superior to the other modes of presentation. In addition, several interesting sex differences occurred. Girls were consistently more positive in their feelings about relaxation and more often reported being less easily frightened and less often sad; boys, on the other hand, reported two somatic improvements—fewer headaches and stomachaches. Overall, the results were so strong that relaxation training is now a regular part of the physical education program in Swedish schools.

Quieting Reflex

Another relaxation procedure easily learned by children is a 6-second exercise called the quieting reflex. Developed by Stroebel (1982), it was designed for immediate use in counteracting the fight-or-flight syndrome activated by most stressful experiences. The quieting reflex, unlike many relaxation routines, can be used in any setting, thus effectively eliminating the temporal gap between stress arousal and reversal that occurs when a quiet room is required for the relaxation procedure.

The first step for the child involves being aware of the stress and identifying it to himself by a statement such as "I am really scared and upset about having a shot." Next, he must decide whether his body will be a help or whether to bypass it (because of an increased cardiac rate or trembling, for example) and let his mind struggle with the problem that is causing stress. In the third step, the child learns to smile inwardly with his eyes and his mouth ("smile on the inside where only you know that you are smiling") in order to reverse the tendency of eyes and mouth to go into a grim, tension-filled set. The final step requires the child to inhale smoothly (with no gulping) to the count of three while imagining that the air he is inhaling comes through holes in the soles of his feet. The effect of this imagery is a sensation of flowing warmth and heaviness rising through the body. Then as the child exhales, he lets his body go slightly limp starting with his jaw and continuing down through shoulders, feeling as he does so, the wave of warmth and heaviness flowing down to his feet. He is now ready to resume his normal activity. The goal is to have the child practice the quieting reflex whenever he is annoyed, worried, or otherwise stressed. It will become an automatic skill for approximately 80% of the children if they use it consistently for several months. A classroom program was developed by Stroebel (1982) and has been used successfully with over 600 school districts. Its brevity, simplicity, and immediacy of effect give it considerable appeal as a technique.

Relaxation training is safe, simple to administer, and free of any known adverse effects on personality and cognitive abilities. It falls short of the criterion of the "ideal" analgesic because although it is often effective immediately, its input is usually not long lasting. Typically, it has to be repeated at least twice a day for optimum results.

Comment

The 1980s have been notable for the application of intervention procedures, such as variants of relaxation, to the reduction of pediatric pain. Most school-age children and adolescents can acquire a reasonable proficiency in the use of these procedures and, once they have, are able to use them independently of adult help. Anecdotal reports of the success of these procedures in the clinical setting far exceed the experimental evidence of their efficacy; however, there is increasing empirical support for their use. These and many of the cognitive procedures that are discussed in Chapter 6 are proliferating without any serious attempts being made to identify the underlying mechanisms of effect. An essential refinement now should be to establish whether specific factors intrinsic to each of the procedures can account for their success or whether one or more factors common to all of them are responsible for it.

6
Management
Behavioral and Cognitive Interventions

Behavioral Interventions

Operant Conditioning

Operant conditioning is concerned with observable actions and is based on the premise that such overt behavior is governed by its consequences. Those that strengthen or weaken behavior are called *reinforcers,* and for optimum effects, reinforcers should be delivered immediately following the emission of the target behavior. When behavior is followed by a positive reinforcer, such as praise or reward, the behavior is likely to increase in frequency. If the reinforcer is negative, the behavior is likely to decrease in frequency. Such a decrease also occurs when neither positive nor negative reinforcers follow the behavior. When this latter sequence is repeated over a period of time, the process is termed *response extinction.* There are various schedules for the delivery of reinforcers: Every response may be reinforced; a fixed number of responses may have to occur for each reinforcer, a schedule that is referred to as *periodic* reinforcement; or in the case of *aperiodic* reinforcement, the number of required responses may vary between reinforcers, but not on a particular schedule. The different schedules have specific purposes or results. For example, reinforcement of every behavior (or "trial") is essential in the early stages of intervention for establishing a specific behavior or behavior pattern. From then on, the target behavior is best maintained by aperiodic reinforcement, with periodic reinforcement being significantly less effective in building maximum resistance to extinction (Ferster & Skinner, 1957).

Three requirements are essential in using operant conditioning in the modification of behavior. First, the behavior to be elicited, increased, and maintained, or lessened or extinguished, must be identified and operationally defined. Next, the appropriate reinforcers, whether positive or negative, must be determined. This step ideally should be done on an individual basis for single-case treatment; it is difficult to achieve in group operant conditioning because what is reward or punishment for one child may have little or no effect on another. The third requirement is that the person monitoring the operant conditioning procedure must have sufficient control over the social environment to ensure that the appropriate consequences do occur when the behaviors to be modified are emitted.

The observable behaviors in respect to pain consist of verbal and nonverbal responses emitted by the child in response to aversive stimulation. The child may vocalize complaints or requests for help, emit paralinguistic vocalizations such as screams or moans, assume postures such as hunching or curling up to minimize the pain, or exhibit facial expressions such as frowns, grimaces, or winces. When these pain behaviors occur, people in the vicinity are likely to respond with sympathy or other kinds of positive attention involving physical proximity, all of which serve as positive reinforcers of the pain behaviors. If medication is prescribed, the consequent pain reduction becomes the reinforcer of the pain behaviors. Note that the reinforcement sequence is likely to be bidirectional: An appreciative response from the child may constitute tertiary gains for the caregiver, thus causing the latter's behaviors to recur and persist.

While responding to pain behaviors with solicitous behavior is usually desirable in the early stages of trauma, continuing with such responses may not be in the child's best interests over the long term. Instead, it may be preferable to respond positively only when the child is engaging in what Varni (1983) has called "well" behaviors, defined as positive or adaptive responses to the child's problem that maximize his return to nonpain behavior. Ignoring the child's pain behaviors at this point does not mean that no sympathy or concern should be shown for the child's complaints of discomfort. What is important is that this concern not be contingent on pain behaviors that result in secondary gains for the child, because these gains have an extraordinarily powerful effect on his subsequent pain behavior.

An example of the powerful influence of secondary gains has been reported by Sank and Biglan (1974) in the case of a 10-year-old boy with recurrent abdominal pain. This child reported a continuous low level of abdominal pain along with daily severe pain episodes usually lasting up to 20 minutes but occasionally stretching to several hours. He had a low rate of school attendance (37.5%) and when absent was given privileges and social proximity with his mother, along with medicine and temperature checks that supported his claim of pain.

As a first step in the operant conditioning sequence, Sank and Biglan had the child record over a 7-day baseline period the frequency and duration of all severe pain episodes and rate their intensity on a 10-point scale. Sank and Biglan then developed a reinforcement and shaping program to decrease the frequency of severe pain episodes and intensity of pain ratings, while increasing school attendance. Reinforcement consisted of points that could be exchanged for items or events on a reinforcement list. Points were given on a half-day basis for no severe pain episodes, lower pain ratings, and school attendance but the child could attend school only if he had not had a severe pain episode in the previous half day and his pain intensity rating was below a certain criterion. When a severe pain episode was reported, he was required to stay in bed for the rest of the half day and could read only school books, whereas previously he had had story books, television, and radio, as well as freedom to get up if he wished. The temporal criteria were gradually increased, meaning that he had to go for longer periods and do more for points. At the end of the treatment, the child had had no severe pain episodes during the previous 15 weeks, his daily pain ratings were low, and his school attendance rate had risen to 86%.

Miller and Kratochwill (1979) have reported similar results with this type of recurring pain. Positive results have been reported for a number of other studies for various pain conditions including migraine headache (Ramsden, Friedman, & Williamson, 1983) and painful treatment procedures such as those in insulin-dependent diabetes (Lowe & Lutzker, 1979).

Operant conditioning frequently has been one of several treatment procedures in multimodal interventions. Consequently, in demonstrating the efficacy of operant conditioning, it is difficult to separate out its contribution to outcome from that of the other components of the multimodal intervention procedure. One of the best "pure" demonstrations of efficacy in the pediatric pain literature and a model of methodological rigor was the single-case study in which operant conditioning was the only intervention used to modify the pain behavior of a severely burned 3-year-old child who was hospitalized for 10 months (Varni, Bessman, Russo, & Cataldo, 1980). Because of scar contractures and consequent decreased range of motion in both knees, it was essential for the child to wear Jobst stockings and knee extension splints to prevent further contractures while undergoing a series of plastic surgery operations. The child exhibited a cluster of pain behaviors that interfered to a significant degree with her rehabilitation and prevented constructive interactions with pediatric personnel. These behaviors included crying that ranged from sobbing to screaming, verbal pain behaviors of both a specific ("my leg hurts") and nonspecific ("ouch") nature, and nonverbal pain behaviors such as grimacing and rubbing her legs. Data on these responses were obtained in three hospital settings: the clinic room and her bedroom, where in both places she wore the knee extension splints, and the physical therapy center where she was undergoing treatment designed to improve her range of motion and independent ambulation. (In the latter setting, data on another response, number of steps descended, were also collected.) Baseline assessment of her pain responses revealed that these responses increased in both intensity and frequency as a function of adult attention and demand situations. They were noticeably infrequent when no adults were present or when adults were present during an ongoing activity of interest to the child.

Because the baseline assessment sessions showed clearly that the pain behaviors were under the control of environmental social factors, treatment focused on rearranging the existing reinforcement contingencies. Varni et al. (1980) used an intrasubject multiple baseline design across clinic, bedroom, and physical therapy settings in combination with a reversal design to assess the efficacy of the behavioral program. Multiple baselines were begun simultaneously in all three settings, with treatment beginning first in the physical therapy situation while baseline assessment continued in the other two settings. Treatment then followed in the clinic and finally in the bedroom. A further assessment of the program's efficacy was made by using brief reversals back to baseline conditions in the clinic and physical therapy settings. In all three settings tangible rewards in the form of food and social rewards were used for not exhibiting pain behaviors, and social rewards were used for "well" behaviors such as helping to put on splints in the clinic. Emission of pain behavior was put on an extinction schedule and the schedules of tangible reinforcement for all tasks were gradually extended in time, but social reinforcement was provided continuously in all settings. The therapeutic efficacy of the program is documented in Figures 6-1 and 6-2, but other clinically important changes also occurred. Behaviors that previously had disrupted treatment and isolated the child from other children dropped out and she became positive about her accomplishments. In addition, she used "well" behaviors in seeking attention.

Comment

Clinical reports and empirical evidence suggest that operant conditioning procedures are generally effective in strengthening target responses and weakening pain behavior responses. With a minimum of training, these procedures can be implemented by pediatric personnel, mothers, teachers, or other competent adults in virtually any setting and for a diversity of behaviors. Despite these positive features, operant conditioning is the target of considerable criticism, much of it ill advised. One criticism concerns the possibility that instead of feeling any less pain, the patient has merely learned to complain less. The fact is that operant conditioning procedures do not have as their main objective the direct modification of pain. Instead, they are designed to lessen excessive expressions of suffering (constant crying, groaning) and related behaviors (hindering treatment by resistance, school absenteeism). Indirect modification of amount of reported pain may occur; for example, the child may report pain as less severe because he becomes more amenable to treatment, but since expressions of pain are not proof that there is pain, a reduction in their frequency cannot be interpreted as diminished pain. This issue reverts back to the thus far unresolved problem of identifying acceptable pain criteria. In summing up their rebuttal to the criticism that operant conditioning (and other behavioral methods) have little effect on pain but, instead, teach a stoic attitude toward it, Fordyce et al. (1985, pp. 120–121) state that

> This criticism represents a misunderstanding of the goals of behavioral treatment. . . . The problem arises from confusing the hypothesis that pain *behaviors* can be learned and unlearned with the notion that *pain* can be learned and unlearned. Behavioral treatments for chronic pain are intended to reduce the *disability* associated with chronic pain problems . . . but decreased pain per se has never been a primary goal for these rehabilitation methods.

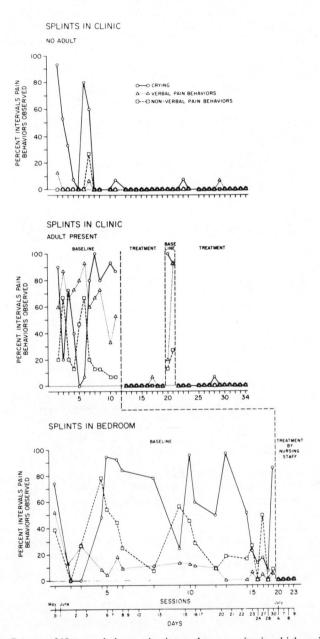

Figure 6-1 Percent of 10-second observation intervals per session in which crying, verbal pain behavior and nonverbal pain behavior were noted while the child wore leg splints in each of three settings: in clinic room alone (top graph), in a clinic room with an adult (middle graph), and in her bedroom (bottom graph). The vertical broken line indicates when treatment (reinforcement for nonpain behavior) or a return to baseline was initiated. The date abscissa indicates the distribution of sessions across days. (Reprinted, by permission, from Varni, J. W., Bessman, C. A., Russo, D. C., & Cataldo, M. F.: Behavioral management of chronic pain in children: Case study. *Archives of Physical Medicine and Rehabilitation,* 1980, *61,* 375–379. ©1980, Archives of Physical Medicine and Rehabilitation.)

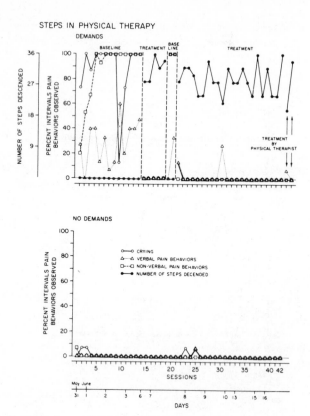

Figure 6-2 Number of steps descended and percent of 10-second intervals in which crying, verbal pain behavior and nonverbal pain behavior were noted when either demands or no demands were being made on the child to participate in physical therapy. The vertical broken line indicates when treatment or a return to baseline was initiated. The date abscissa indicates the distribution of sessions across days. (Reprinted, by permission, from Varni, J. W., Bessman, C. A., Russo, D. C., & Cataldo, M. F.: Behavioral management of chronic pain in children: Case study. *Archives of Physical Medicine and Rehabilitation*, 1980, *61*, 375–379. ©1980, Archives of Physical Medicine and Rehabilitation.)

A second criticism concerns the lack of evidence for the relative efficacy of operant conditioning compared with other behavioral interventions such as biofeedback or relaxation training, and even questions if the positive results are anything more than a placebo effect. The latter possibility seems remote since one would have to have a placebo as powerful as all the procedures used in operant conditioning, including tangible and social reinforcers and behavioral extinguishers. The question of relative efficacy is far more interesting because any discussion on this topic should recognize the importance of long-term follow-up data in making such comparisons. Such data are not often collected in operant conditioning research, although informal reports generally show that the changes effected in a child's repertoire are maintained. The basic problem in long-term follow-up is that social reinforcement may subsequently occur in the child's environment quite apart from the earlier operant conditioning reinforcement procedures, thus making it impossible to attribute long-term gains to any specific source.

Although operant conditioning techniques do not require sophisticated or expensive equipment, programs such as Varni et al.'s (1980) are often criticized as being expensive in terms of personnel and time. This short-sighted view disregards their effective prevention function of avoiding a major problem at a later date by setting a child on a more socially acceptable path. Objections have also been raised that no attempt is made to find out what the patient thinks, that the focus solely on behavior bypasses the important topic of subjective pain. In rebuttal, it should be obvious that a focus primarily on behavior is reasonable since it is the behavior that is the target for change. In a number of studies (see, for example, Miller & Kratochwill, 1979) the patient has provided self-ratings of his pain, but this procedure should be viewed with caution. Behavior therapists are sometimes reluctant to assess patients' perceived pain levels because this procedure may reinforce an awareness of pain by drawing the child's attention to it.

Clinicians frequently express a strong preference for operant conditioning over cognitive approaches and, in doing so, imply a clearly defined dichotomy between the two. In fact, as Turner and Chapman (1982b) point out in their excellent critical review article, there are definite areas of overlap between the two. Although Turner and Chapman focus on empirical research on chronic pain in adults, the issues and problems that they discuss concerning operant conditioning are equally relevant to its use with children.

Film Modeling Procedures

Film modeling procedures have been extensively and effectively used with young children in a diversity of settings, the goal being to transmit new behaviors and eliminate maladaptive response patterns through the process of observational learning (Thelen et al., 1979). The finding that modeling procedures have proved to be particularly effective in reducing or eliminating fears and avoidant behavior (Bandura, 1969) has resulted in their use in clinical settings to reduce fear and to prepare children for potentially painful medical and dental interventions. Some attention has been given by investigators to incorporating in the film presentations model attributes with proven efficacy for facilitating acquisition of the film model's behaviors. Models having perceived similarity to the observer increase observational learning (Bandura, 1969), so many of these films have models of the same age, sex, and race as the child observer. The pattern of response behavior that the model exhibits is another model parameter of relevance to the clinical pain situation. In this instance the model has sometimes been a *coping* model, who initially exhibits fear in the stress situation but overcomes it and behaves with confidence as the sequence draws to a close, or at other times a *mastery* model, manifesting confidence, competence, fearlessness, and positive affect throughout the sequence. Meichenbaum (1971) has reported that initially anxious coping models who finished the task competently were more effective in reducing anxiety and avoidance behavior than mastery models who showed no fear or concern.

Representative of these film model presentations is the 16-minute film *Ethan Has an Operation* (Melamed & Siegel, 1975) that has been used extensively (see, for example, Elkins & Roberts, 1985; Penticuff, 1976; Peterson & Ridley-Johnson, 1984). In this film a 7-year-old Caucasian boy is shown entering the hospital for an elective herniectomy. Some scenes depict the routine hospital procedures from admission to discharge, hospital personnel are shown explaining to Ethan those medical procedures that are potentially frightening, and Ethan describes his feelings and fears. His narration and behavior are typical of a coping model in that he acknowledges some initial anxiety but gradually overcomes this and copes with the demands of the situation competently and confidently.

Slide and audiotape combinations have also been used. Ginther and Roberts (1982) developed a 10-minute presentation to reduce fear and fear-related behaviors in children prior to their first visit to a dental clinic. They had four experimental conditions with two models, a 10-year-old Caucasian girl and a 7-year-old black boy, each portraying a coping role and a mastery role. In each condition the model was portrayed having his or her teeth examined, cleaned, and x-rayed, followed by a fluoride treatment. An interesting feature of the coping model condition was the modeling of coping strategies. The narrations gave factual information concerning dental procedures, personnel, and equipment, differing across the four tapes only in respect to coping and mastery.

In the above studies, the outcome variables were concerned with the child observer's subsequent performance. Film model presentations have also been used with nonpatient children in classroom settings, the goal being to increase their medical knowledge and improve their attitudes toward pediatric personnel (see, for example, Elkins & Roberts, 1985; Klinzing & Klinzing, 1977). Essentially a preventive approach, the outcome variables in this case are concerned with the acquisition of learning in the form of information designed to reduce fears related to common medical events.

The overall findings from the research on the use of film models in eliminating fears relevant to the medical/dental setting can be summarized as follows. Whether the observer has prior experience in the specific pediatric setting may influence the efficacy of the film model presentation: Children who are undergoing medical/dental experience for the first time generally benefit from the film presentation (Klinzing & Klinzing, 1977; Klorman, Hilpert, Michael, La Gana, & Sveen, 1980; Machen & Johnson, 1974; Melamed & Siegel, 1980; Vernon, 1973), whereas those with prior experience in the setting benefit less or not at all (see, for example, Klorman et al., 1980; Melamed et al., 1978). However, Ginther and Roberts (1982) reported no reduction in children's dental fears regardless of level of prior dental experience. In this study, there were no differences due to model type, a finding that raises critical questions regarding the efficacy of mastery versus coping models as well as the theoretical distinction between the two types. Results consistent with those of Ginther and Roberts (1982) have been reported by Zachary, Friedlander, Huang, Silverstein, and Leggott (1985) on stress-relevant and irrelevant film models in the dental setting. In terms of design and discussion of the issues surrounding the use of coping and mastery models, these two studies are the best in this medical/dental literature. Coping models in school programs (see, for example, Penticuff, 1976; Roberts, Wurtele, Boone, Ginther, & Elkins, 1981) have been effective in reducing nonpatient elementary school children's medical fears. In the Elkins and Roberts (1985) study, the observers' initial level of fearfulness concerning medical events influenced the extent to which they benefited from the model presentation: The more fearful children decreased their medical fears below baseline, but no significant changes occurred for the less fearful. Age differences were a factor, with a more marked increase in medical knowledge occurring in the older children than in the younger ones. Film-mediated participant modeling has proved more effective than standard film modeling in transmitting information and reducing anxiety and disruptive behavior during dental treatment in children and adolescents who were highly fearful of dentists (Klingman, Melamed, Cuthbert, & Hermecz, 1984). Age differences were also evident in the use of a film model with insulin-dependent diabetic children learning to self-inject insulin: The older children in a group of 6- to 9-year-olds performed best (Gilbert et al., 1982). Of relevance to the topic of film modeling in medical/dental settings are the excellent critical reviews by Siegel (1987) on dental fears, Thelen et al. (1979) on film modeling in general, and Siegel (1986) on the status of assessment procedures related to medical procedures and hospitalization.

The sparse and disappointing findings on film models are in marked contrast to the impressive evidence of the efficacy of film models in a diversity of nonclinical situations (see, for example, Thelen et al., 1979). In view of this evidence, it is clear that the limited success in demonstrating the efficacy of film model presentations for modifying fears and avoidant behavior in the clinical setting should be attributed to procedural shortcomings rather than to limitations inherent in the use of models to effect these behavioral changes. Consider, for example, the following aspects that appear to be overlooked in most of the studies.

Timing Research by Peterson and Ridley-Johnson (1984) and others (Roberts et al., 1981) suggests that the greatest reduction in medically related fear occurs in the long-term follow-up rather than directly after exposure to the model. Yet in most of the film model studies, the child's exposure to the film intervention occurs almost immediately prior to the event, which means that he has little time to assimilate the film material.

Single-Trial Exposure   The fears of even the young child are generally deep rooted, yet a 10- or 15-minute presentation is expected to reduce these fears and at the same time provide a barrage of new information. The highly successful results obtained in the phobia studies (Bandura, 1969) were never the result of single-trial exposure to the feared stimulus.

Individual Differences   No attempt is made to assign subjects to subgroups on the basis of characteristics known to influence receptivity to film model presentations. Instead, entire groups of children participate, and while in some studies child (and parent) consent has been obtained (see, for example, Elkins & Roberts, 1985; Ginther & Roberts, 1982), in others everyone in the presurgical setting (Melamed & Siegel, 1975), classroom (Peterson & Ridley-Johnson, 1984), and camp (Gilbert et al., 1982) apparently participated automatically since no mention is made either of obtaining consent or of children who chose not to participate. It is likely that a certain number of children in these various groups would have preferred not to have prior information about the impending aversive procedure or possible hospitalization at some later date. That some children do not want this prior information is evident from interview data (Ross & Ross, 1982a; Ross, S. A., 1984). It is possible that children who do not benefit from preparatory film model interventions are similar to the "avoiders" (Cohen & Lazarus, 1979), who when given preparatory information prior to surgery did relatively worse than similar patients not given such information. To disregard such individual differences is poor methodology, not to speak of the ethical considerations involved.

Similar elements could have been operating in the study by Ginther and Roberts (1982) of exposure to the model and of coping models versus mastery models, the particular variable of interest being the child's self-efficacy expectancies. These expectancies represent the child's estimate of his potential for being able to perform or behave in a certain way in a specific situation. There is a real possibility that they may interact with the type of model, thus influencing outcome scores. For example, a child with high self-efficacy expectancies about how he will manage in the hospital is not likely to be influenced by a coping model, but he should be highly receptive to a mastery model. This situation is analogous to that of the child who is an advanced figure skater not being interested in watching a beginner. Conversely, the child with low expectancies may be convinced by the mastery model that he could never be like that, so he very sensibly gives up.

The problem here really concerns the interpretation of the principle of similarity between model and child observer. Age, sex, and race are gross indications of similarity. Further refinements on the similarity continuum are essential if researchers are to comply with this principle when evaluating the efficacy of such variables as type of model. A true assessment of coping versus mastery models would involve a test for a level of self-efficacy expectancies $\times$ type of model interaction effect.

In addition to the procedural problems described above, an overview of the film model research in the pediatric setting shows a lamentable lack of imagination and enterprise on the part of investigators in their narrow focus on a single child undergoing some intervention and functioning as a coping or mastery model. Consider the following research possibilities:

Other things being equal, perceived similarity to the model unquestionably facilitates observational learning. However, no research attention has been given to the possibility that *dissimilarity* could have a powerful effect. Suppose a 10-year-old boy sees a 6-year-old girl (age and sex differences) functioning bravely, that is, as a *challenge model* (Ross, D. M., 1987). Might this not be more effective in spurring him on to reproduce her behaviors than the sight of another 10-year-old boy?

Observational learning research has focused on models exhibiting desirable behaviors. There is a strong possibility that models exhibiting nonreinforced *excessively negative* behaviors prior to or during brief minor pain procedures could instill in the child observer intense motivation to avoid behaving "like that," thus paradoxically exerting a powerful *positive* influence on the observer. The child who observes a same-sex, same-age or older model have a tantrum, stamp his feet, thrash around, and so on may be so repulsed by this exhibition that he resolves to distance himself from the model by exhibiting behavior that is the antithesis of the model's behavior. The clinical setting would provide an excellent opportunity for testing this *repugnant model* (Ross, S. A., 1987) hypothesis.

There is some evidence to suggest that multiple models have more powerful effects in naturalistic settings than do single models (see, for example, Apley, 1975; Craig, 1980; Edwards et al., 1985). Why not have multiple models in the film presentation rather than relying on a single model? One of several advantages would be that fears could be voiced and rebutted.

Children with hospital experience generally do not benefit from the film presentation prior to their next experience in hospital. Why not have multiple viewings? If one starts with the premise that the child's fear of painful medical/dental procedures results from prior aversive classical conditioning, then extinction of these conditioned fears would require a series of nonreinforced exposures to the feared stimulus (the medical/dental setting). Repeated or extended exposure to the film in the absence of medical/dental treatment should thus reduce the fears of the child with previous experience.

Psychotherapy

Of the diversity of therapies available for the pediatric population, the group therapies have an advantage over the individual therapies in that they acknowledge the increasingly important role of the peer group to the child and incorporate its supportive element in the therapeutic process. Although many group therapies have been used with considerable success in the clinical setting with children and adolescents who must undergo painful treatment or who experience chronic or recurring pain, there are relatively few published reports of such use. Of these therapies, play therapy, group therapy, and family therapy are discussed in the following sections. Family therapy is included because the influence of the family is consonant with our social ecology approach to an understanding of children's pain.

Play Therapy

The value of play as a factor in the socialization of the child has long been recognized. It is a source of pleasure to the child and at the same time serves a number of other useful purposes. It is a natural medium of communication and as such stimulates intellectual growth and facilitates emotional development. By providing a nonthreatening outlet for anxiety and fear it helps the child resolve some of his uncertainties and cope with the frustrations and disappointments that are almost inevitably a part of most children's experience (see, for example, Bruner, Jolly, & Sylva, 1976; Erikson, 1963; Piaget, 1951). Play also often offers important therapeutic benefits for behavioral problems and for problems within the realm of medical care (see, for example, Adams, 1976; Erickson, 1958; S. Freud, 1920; Ginott, 1958; Piaget, 1951). In the medical setting, the therapeutic use of play has a unique position in management because of the diversity of problems and situations amenable to modification through it. It offers the child an opportunity to forge a link to life outside the hospital and serves to remind him of his place in this other world. When impending painful procedures are required, play therapy has been used to familiarize children with frightening instruments and procedures prior to treatment and has also been beneficial for those procedures regarded by adults as routine but by children as a source of considerable concern (Ellerton, Caty, & Ritchie, 1985). Simulating routines in a play context can help the child accept that pediatric personnel are not being deliberately and unnecessarily unkind and that they are not being punitive. Tucker (1982, pp. 58–60) has given an interesting account of the use of play therapy to help a 3-year-old child adjust to painful procedures by having her play the role of "doctor" with a doll. Note in the following incident (Thompson & Stanford, 1981, p. 84) how a 5-year-old boy with a fractured leg was able only through play therapy to express his anger and reveal his anxiety about not being home for Christmas:

> Barry had been too cooperative since his arrival . . . on Thanksgiving Day. . . . and had been in traction for nearly three weeks. His uncomplaining adjustment to the immobilization caused staff to wonder if he weren't suppressing his anger and fears.
>   As Barry molded figures from the Play-Doh, the child life worker, whom Barry had grown to accept, asked Barry to tell him about the figures. Becoming increasingly agitated as he molded and kneaded the substance, Barry formed the figure of a boy. Taking a knife, he slashed the boy apart, saying, "The doctors did that to him!"
>   "Oh, why did they do that to him?"
>   "Because they're mean and they don't like him," was his reply. Smashing the fragments of the boy into a wad, Barry molded something that looked like a stocking. Again he destroyed it with a knife.
>   "That's Christmas! The doctors took it away 'cause they don't like the boy!"

Play therapy is particularly beneficial for the child whose condition or treatment involves protracted pain so that he is fearful that the pain will never end, he will lose control, or his parents have deserted him. To facilitate open-ended dialogues with the child about such feelings, Linn (1977) has developed an engaging puppet procedure. The use of painful procedures is more readily accepted by the child if he understands the necessity for them. To convey the idea that the child's well-being is dependent on the procedures being used, Rae and Stiber (1976) incorporated plants in their play therapy routines, with the plants being completely dependent on the child for life-supporting needs. Care should be taken with this approach to avoid having the child abdicate his input as unimportant.

Play therapy also enables the child to shift from the role of the passive recipient to that of the pediatric professional who administers the painful treatment. In this vein Peller (1952, p. 73) has commented that

> . . . the child can inflict upon another person what has previously been done to him. The change from a passive to an active role . . . mitigates the traumatic effect of a recent experience and it leaves the player better equipped to undergo the passive role again . . .

An excellent example of such a change occurred in a very young child participating in an ego-oriented play therapy program (Adams, 1976, p. 420):

> When we first brought Karen, age two, to the play session, she was very frightened and cried, "No needles, no needles," thinking that the materials would be used on her. We found that verbal reassurances would not reach her, and that she was too threatened to be approached directly. Without talking, I sat a little distance from her, drew up a syringe, and injected it into the little girl puppet's arm, making crying noises and offering reassurance that it would just hurt a minute. Deliberately casual, I left the supplies within Karen's reach and went to another child. I also placed within her reach some less threatening items such as bandages, a tongue depressor, and a stethoscope. When I looked over later, Karen was busily applying eight bandaids to the puppet's arm and playing with the tongue depressor. By the end of the next session, she had advanced to the stethoscope and would listen to her own heartbeat, laughing. . . . Within four sessions, she was no longer threatened by the syringes and needles and had learned how to manipulate them. . . . Outside of the group, she became cooperative when getting an injection, even participating by wiping the spot with alcohol herself.

The fact that Karen performed each procedure many times is consistent with Piaget's (1951) description of a child's repetition in play being a means of assimilating reality to the ego. The repetition stops when the child has acquired sufficient mastery of the anxiety-arousing experience (Nagera, 1978).

In addition to these isolated examples of play therapy in action, there are some excellent reports of play therapy programs (see, for example, Adams's [1976] comprehensive report of a structured therapeutic group play program for preschool children to early adolescents); as well as reports on therapeutic techniques (Linn, 1977; Petrillo & Sanger, 1972; Rae & Stieber, 1976; Steele, 1982); theoretical statements (see Ginott, 1958, on play group therapy); and guidelines for non-directive play therapy (Axline, 1969), an approach that has been widely used to help children withstand adverse conditions through insight and self-understanding.

Comment Although play therapy and its variants have had extensive use over a long period of time in the clinical setting, empirical validation has been minimal. Much of the literature on the topic consists of accounts by experienced clinicians of case studies and descriptions of interventions used in the medical setting with reported success. One problem here is that play therapy is conducted in a treatment setting rather than in a research-oriented one. Empirical evidence in the form of observational data could have been obtained, for example, in the Adams (1976) case study quoted above. From a set of baseline observations it would have been a straightforward task to rate increases in compliancy and reductions in upset during intrusive procedures after completion of the series of play sessions. But this kind of data collection requires additional trained staff.

Furthermore, design refinements involving control groups, as opposed to each child serving as his own control, cannot be justified because withholding play therapy treatment from those in the control group would be unethical. To allow the misery to continue in the face of ongoing treatment when the probability is high that the children involved could benefit from play therapy cannot be justified even when such therapy is to be delayed only temporarily during the data collection periods. Having each child act as his own control would make rapid data collection impossible: It would be necessary to build up a pool of baseline and posttherapy data on children all of whom exhibited similar behaviors, such as fear and withdrawal, to a specific target or situation. Since most pediatric settings service a variety of problems, such a pool would likely take a long period of time to accumulate. In addition, for each subset of children (that is, each subject pool) specific rating forms would have to be developed and data on their reliability obtained. Until an acceptable research framework of this sort is in place, it is far better to continue the careful reporting of individual cases than to rush into methodologically unsound "research" and what is worse, to publish it.

Group Therapy

Group psychotherapy is one of the most commonly used treatment modalities for child and adolescent patients in a medical setting. It is of great value in this setting because the child often feels abandoned by his parents and the adolescent feels lost without his friends. The group therapy situation provides patients in both age groups with a reasonably close approximation of a real-life peer group that functions as a source of social support and, in addition, meets needs that are specific to their hospitalization. The homogeneity of the group in respect to type of problem provides the comfort of seeing that there are others like the patient, that he is neither unique nor alone. Those with visible disfigurement such as facial burns or baldness from chemotherapy, those who must endure continuing treatment such as dialysis, and those with fears about impending painful events such as surgical intervention are particularly responsive to the comfort of the group and the freedom to voice fears and concerns without criticism. The discussions allow the participants to place their problems within the perspective of peers rather than adults and discuss them in these terms. The procedure of sharing experiences related to the pain of disfigurement with a group having similar experiences is a very effective one, particularly since the participants see themselves as knowing how it is in a way that they feel adults cannot know.

In the typical group therapy configuration, a therapist meets with a homogeneous group of at least five and usually seven or eight children. Frequently the group is a closed one, with the same participants from the beginning to the final session. However, the open-ended group, with a constantly rotating membership, offers the advantage of a modeling effect in that the group sees members who are ready to cope with the problem "graduate." If these children then return for one meeting to talk about their experiences, they can be a source of hope to the current group members. Depending on the type of problem, the frequency and number of meetings vary greatly: If the problem has an element of urgency, such as impending surgery, several daily meetings may suffice; if it is one of physical disfigurement, 20 or 25 meetings held twice a week for an hour at a time may be required.

Prior to the first meeting, the therapist sometimes interviews each child in a very informal manner; but, in any case, he reads up on the child's history and, if possible, fills in background by talking to pediatric personnel. In the first meeting the therapist is moderately directive: He identifies issues for discussion, provides interpretations when necessary, and structures the content of sessions to address the problems that have brought the group together. In the beginning, the group is a group in name only, that is, a cluster of individuals brought together through the volition of others. The therapist's task is to make the group cohesive (Yalom, 1975), and this goal is achieved when its members have a sense of belonging and acceptance along with a feeling of solidarity, loyalty, and mutual support, so that their membership becomes important to them. In this connection it is interesting that high-cohesive groups have a better record on attendance, punctuality, member activity, and stability than do low-cohesive groups. The therapist keeps the group on track, knows when to interfere and when to allow confrontations to proceed, and continuously monitors the effect and impact of the discussion on the group as a whole as well as on specific members, so that antitherapeutic situations do not arise (Slavson & Schiffer, 1974). In the security engendered by the therapist, the child can take risks without disastrous repercussions; he feels secure and safe in the knowledge that he will not be judged, found wanting, and rejected; and he can allow himself to enjoy close contact with the others in the situation.

Group Therapy for Chronic Problems   Magrab (1975) held weekly meetings for pediatric patients in a dialysis program with the goal of allowing the children to air their feelings and grievances, form strong peer affiliations, and begin to develop a sense of normal living as opposed to feeling so different. A similar program, for children with renal disease, has been reported by Korsch, Fine, Grushkin, and Negrete (1971). In the area of muscular dystrophy, two programs have been described: In one, Bayrakal (1975) obtained significant improvement in the attitudes and functioning of severely disabled adolescents. Her goal was to relieve chronic feelings of apathy, depression, and low self-esteem, and to achieve this she used a relatively inactive, analytic group-oriented approach. Her group progressed through a series of stages before they could openly express their anxiety and hopelessness (realistic feelings in view of the overwhelmingly stressful reality with little hope that children with muscular dystrophy face). By the time they had reached that point the group was truly cohesive, with the members able to engage in highly realistic discussions of their plight and how to attack their problems.

In a second study on group therapy with muscular dystrophy patients, Adler (1973) reported significant improvement in emotional state and interpersonal behavior in a group of young children in a camp setting. It should be noted that for neither of these studies do we wish to imply that the therapy sessions became a solution to the participants' problems or constituted a happy ending. Rather, the sessions offered a comforting setting for attempting an appraisal of the problems to be faced with the help of the perspective of others with similar problems. Irwin and McWilliams (1974) have reported a successful long-term group therapy program for preschool children with cleft palate and Colman, Dougher, and Tanner (1976) had similar results with their group therapy program for children in this age group who had multiple physical handicaps.

Positive effects have also been reported for the use of group therapy with children facing relatively immediate problems. Schowalter (1971) reported that in his group of adolescents facing surgery, details of the surgery occupied much of the therapy sessions; although there was a tendency to focus on the frightening aspects, overall the effects were positive. A very helpful procedure used with this group consisted of having the participants record their hopes, fears, and expectations for the surgical intervention and then, in the postoperative phase, dictate how the actual experience compared with their expectations. One possible variation on this procedure would be to select good tapes in which the respondent is clearly a coping model whose joyous postoperative statements show clearly that his original fears proved to be unfounded and to expose the therapy group to these accounts as a convincing way to correct extreme fantasies and misconceptions.

Although there are many good review articles (see, for example, Meissner & Nicholi, 1978) and texts (for example, Wolberg, Aronson, & Wolberg, 1977) on group therapy, empirical studies, especially in the medical setting, are rare. In the cluster described above, for example, only Adler's (1973) study was a controlled one. It would be a real contribution to the pain literature to develop a framework for collecting data in the group therapy situation that would enable therapists to report empirical results and at the same time take into account the realities of the setting. One goal here would be to define and refine a cluster of procedures that could serve as a base from which to develop age- and problem-related strategies for use in group therapy sessions.

Family Systems Therapy

In family systems therapy the family is viewed as an interrelated homeostatic system in which the members are functionally interdependent (Jackson, 1957). The assumption made is that certain types of family organization are related to the development of physical symptoms, such as pain, and that these symptoms can play a major role in maintaining equilibrium in the family. The symptoms fulfill the emotional needs of other members of the family although not necessarily all of them: Sometimes there is one key member whose needs must be met if family stability is to be maintained. If the symptom meets that person's needs then the family is able to function harmoniously providing the symptom is maintained. Family systems therapy focuses on changing the structure of the family organization so that a new homeostasis is reached that does not require any member of the family to asssume a sick role. It assigns to the family the role of a small, powerful, intricate, interdependent, social transactional system with its own unique rules and problems. When the system is ignored, treatment is likely to be undermined because the family tends to resist changes in its members (Framo, 1979; Watzlawick, Weakland, & Fisch, 1974).

A symptom may appear in the form of acute, perhaps fairly serious, pain for no apparent reason and be unnecessarily prolonged because of its role in maintaining family harmony. It may subsequently evolve into a recurring pain problem that eventually merits chronic pain status, all as the result of a process of reinforcement that may be deliberate on the part of some family members but is usually in the realm of the subconscious. The following is an example of such a sequence (Buckman, 1973):

> The patient was an 11-year-old girl with frequently recurring abdominal pain with no evidence of an organic base. At age six she had an attack of appendicitis that coincided with her father's decision to divorce her mother despite the latter's opposition. The child was terribly upset and implored her parents to stay together until she came home. Both parents were devoted to the child and concurred with this request. The curious thing about the parents was that they rallied to any kind of crisis, functioning harmoniously and cooperatively. The effect of the child's appendectomy was to temporarily postpone the divorce proceedings and interpersonal conflict. The pediatrician was puzzled by the child's unusually prolonged convalescence. Harmony reigned for several weeks thereafter, the child returned to school, and the father again initiated the discussion of a divorce. At that point the child experienced some abdominal discomfort that the pediatrician viewed as mild, having made at the mother's request a house visit that he considered unnecessary. The child was pampered unnecessarily for a week and was absent from school. Once again the parents united in the face of this pseudo-crisis and all was well. In the next three years this sequence was repeated

many times until finally the girl was experiencing attacks twice a month, to the detriment of her school attendance record. The father was increasingly concerned about his daughter's semi-invalid status, had some inkling about what was going on, and sought therapeutic help.

The symptoms described in this case take on new meaning when they are considered within the context of the family: They represent only the visible part of the total problem. Often the basis for what appears to be solely the child's problem can be traced to one or more other family members. Zimmerman and Elliott (1984) have reported the case of a 16-year-old girl with hereditary angioneurotic edema who had developed a negative cycle of pain behavior resistant to both medical intervention and a stress management program. An analysis of the behavior patterns within the family strongly suggested that the girl's pain behavior was being maintained by reward contingencies. A combination of family therapy and behavioral management procedures was instigated and subsequently was successful in eliminating the pain behavior.

In this approach, the therapist brings the family together for interviews once or twice a week. These meetings typically provide a wealth of first-hand information that enables the therapist to analyze patterns of interaction within the family and identify the processes that are causing the child's problem. Over a series of sessions the therapist is able to detect behavior patterns such as overt verbal communication that is at odds with nonverbal communication, secondary gains that the child's pain may provide, and tertiary gains. Quite often the management plan that is then devised gives only minimal attention to changes in the child. Generally it is one or both parents who must modify their behavior.

Within this family systems framework, Minuchin et al. (1975) have proposed a comprehensive model of the development of psychosomatic illness in children. They suggest that the following elements play an important role in the development of a chronic pain problem in the child. A certain physiological predisposition or vulnerability must exist on the part of the child, coupled with such maladaptive transactional characteristics in the family as overprotectiveness, enmeshment, rigidity, and lack of conflict resolution capabilities. The child then becomes the means for conflict resolution: The onset of his pain problem may be precipitated by a threat to family harmony and the symptom is then maintained for the new stability that it provides for the family. It is obvious that this model has important implications for the development of chronic pain conditions with a psychogenic base and ultimately, perhaps, for the chronic pain syndrome. There has been a proliferation of clinical reports of its use. Liebman, Honig, and Berger (1976) reported the first application of family systems therapy with children presenting with recurrent abdominal pain and Allmond, Buckman, and Gofman (1979) have written an excellent text on the efficacy of family systems therapy in specific case studies. Although family therapy for children has been criticized (Masten, 1979; Schomer, 1978), the general consensus is that it is as effective as individual therapies and in some respects involves fewer risks (Fox, 1976; Gurman & Kniskern, 1978). Bierenbaum and Bergey (1980) suggest that pediatric personnel should have family therapy training and they have presented an interesting account of the rationale in support of this view. Although empirical data on the validity of family systems therapy are sparse, it appears to have considerable potential for families such as those described by Dunn-Geier et al. (1986) in their study of adolescent copers and noncopers. Under the guise of concern, mothers of the noncopers in fact prevented their sons from coping.

Talking Through

Most of the procedures discussed in this chapter are not markedly influenced by the personality of the professional or parent who is implementing them. Given a certain level of competence, the procedures will be effective in the face of considerable differences in ability and training across users. This is not the case for the technique of talking the child through. The purpose of this technique is to distract the child during an ongoing painful treatment by keeping up a running line of chatter that draws his attention despite his concern with the treatment. Some professionals seem to have the particular combination of skill, personality, and presence needed to carry it off successfully, whereas others do not. It is difficult to teach because there is no set routine with content and steps following an orderly sequence. However, there are certain characteristics of the interaction that appear as a common theme when the technique is used by those having the requisite talents. In all instances, the child (or, for that matter, the adult) knows, likes, and trusts the professional. The topic of conversation is one that is familiar to the child or has high appeal for him. Once the professional begins the talking through routine (which coincides with the onset of the sequence of treatment), there is an insistent quality about his comments that focuses the child's attention. Often there is a novelty factor that is highly attention directing; for example, the topic is treated in an unusual way or the ideas are outrageous. In any case, the topic always has positive affective and cognitive valence whatever its other attributes, whether funny, interesting, or stimulating. There is frequently a second person assisting the professional who contributes by asking appropriate questions, making suitable comments, and feeding the professional the right lines. The interaction between these two combines to produce an unbroken stream of verbiage, with virtually no pauses. The professional may ask the child questions, but rarely waits for an answer and, of course, sometimes the patient is unable to answer, for example, when he is at the dentist.

Although children have no label for this technique, they are able to describe its sequence quite accurately. One child, for example, said that her pediatrician recited limericks whenever he was doing anything painful, often paused before the last line to ask what she thought it should be, and supplied a choice of several. She said that even though it was hurting, she could not completely concentrate on either the hurt or the limerick, so that she felt "all mixed up about the whole thing," a description that could reflect a strong state of distraction.

In the following quote (Miller, S. W., 1980), note how well the resident uses the talking through procedure with a 10-year-old boy:

> Hey, sport, I'm sorry—you gotta have another Groan Marrow [child smiles weakly in spite of his obvious anxiety]. Now this isn't a fun thing but it won't take long and I have an idea that might help. Remember when your mom had the baby and your dad just talked her through [Lamaze]? Okay, now I'll talk you through. So, to start with you're pregnant [child expostulates], now *no arguing,* this would make a good TV show and I'm the script writer and you're just the star so you don't have *any say* [doctor works busily getting child ready]. Now, put your knees up like this—by the way, how often are you having pains? Here comes the bad news, sport, you're having triplets. No good saying you aren't, start breathing like your mom did [demonstrates and they do it together]. You have to come up with six names [child asks, "Why six, why not 12, how do you know what sex the babies are?"]. Okay, here's the coach [nurse enters wearing baseball cap].
>
> Doctor explains that expectant father is *totally irresponsible,* having triplets and hasn't thought of any names. As he inserts the needle, he and the nurse both start suggesting funny and generally inappropriate names. Child is laughing, crying, and criticizing names but the whole procedure goes as smoothly as can be expected. Nurse and child continue arguing about names of baseball players, with nurse suggesting names of other sports greats who have nothing to do with baseball. Doctor throws in a name and the nurse tells him indignantly that that was a racehorse. They all start laughing.

Partial Control with Self-Pacing

Implicit in many of the developmental tasks of childhood is the expectation that the child will assume increasing responsibility for his general behavior. Being in control is both a challenge and a source of reward for the child. Although the control-related demands sometimes exceed his capabilities and motivation, still, he typically is reluctant to relinquish control gains once they have been achieved. In the pediatric setting, one problem for the child, and even more so for the adolescent, is the loss of control that occurs in areas of functioning that the child takes for granted as his domain. The injustice of this situation is particularly galling for the child when it is obvious to him that allowing him to make a decision or choice would not interfere in any way:

> There were all these pajamas and some were clowns and some were big bears and I wanted bear pajamas and she never even asked which, she just gave me the clowns. (Boy, CA 7, Ross & Ross, 1982a)

When faced with treatment-induced pain, loss of control has major impact on the child because it thwarts his instinct to terminate immediately aversive stimulation of any kind. That he cannot do anything about the pain may result in feelings of helplessness, with detrimental results. Over the long term he may even be reluctant to seek professional help for pain until its intensity leaves him no other option (Remen, 1980).

One partial compensation for the loss of control in an aversive treatment situation involves allowing the child to decide how long he can endure ongoing pain before he asks for and receives a temporary halt. Allowing the child limited control of the aversive stimulation is called *self-pacing*. This procedure is the clinical analogue of the experimental pain tolerance model in which an experimenter administers a noxious stimulus to a subject and terminates it when instructed to do so by the subject. (It is this facet of the laboratory study of pain that has made investigators [Beecher, 1959; Wolff, 1984] reluctant to accept laboratory-induced pain as the equivalent of iatrogenic pain on the grounds that there is a notable lack of fear and anxiety in the laboratory setting).

Of all the pediatric personnel, dentists, as a group, have made the most concerted effort to remedy the effects of loss of control by providing signal procedures that the child can use when he needs a brief respite from the pain (Neal, 1978). Although there are anecdotal reports of improvement in children's behavior as a function of this self-pacing procedure (Neal, 1978) and empirical evidence that aversive stimulation can be more tolerable if the subject controls its onset, termination, or intensity (Averill, 1973; Thompson, 1981), there is no consistent evidence from empirical studies in dentistry (Corah, 1973; Lindsay, 1984) that children (or adults) benefit significantly from such control procedures. A similar state of affairs exists in the medical area, where there are anecdotal reports (Bradshaw, 1985; Neal, 1978; Waechter, 1971) of increased ability to tolerate the sudden onset of intense pain as well as its duration when self-pacing is used, but little empirical data.

The apparent increase in tolerance that occurs in self-pacing is attributed to the child's knowledge that he has some control over the aversive stimulation. Also plausible is the possibility that the child's knowledge that he is no longer completely helpless causes a lessening of tension and fear, with a consequent reduction in perceived pain intensity. Whatever the explanation, pediatric medical personnel agree that self-pacing allows painful treatment procedures to be completed more smoothly and, after an initial period of frequent checks by the child to verify that his command does temporarily halt the proceedings, they take less time to complete. From the child's point of view, those who have experienced self-pacing strongly advocate its use:

> I said, "How about a hurting break?" And he [interne] said, "Hey, man, are you serious?" And I said, "Sure. Even when ladies are having babies they get a little rest in between the bad pains." And they [pediatric emergency room personnel] all laughed and he said, "O.K., you get a 60-second break whenever you need it" and then it was *much, much better,* like you wouldn't believe it. (Boy, CA 10, emergency room burn treatment, Ross & Ross, 1985)

It is equally clear from children's accounts of their experiences with aversive medical treatment that self-determined pauses or even aperiodic pain breaks at critical points in the procedure would have increased their duration of tolerance.

> If he would stop every little while so I could take a big breath and sort of let go of the hurt, I could be still a lot more and it probably wouldn't hurt so much. (Girl, CA 8, burn treatment, Bush, 1982)

> If I could've just got my breath, it would have been O.K. (Boy, CA 8, undergoing bone marrow tap with Mizzy Gun, Ross & Ross, 1982a)

Cognitive Interventions

Hypnosis

Hypnosis is an altered state of consciousness, or condition, that occurs when appropriate suggestions are used to elicit distortions of perception, memory, or mood (Orne, 1980). This state differs from both the normal waking state and the stages of sleep in that it has some of the characteristics of certain meditative states. The lighter levels of hypnosis are sometimes difficult to distinguish from related states such as muscle relaxation, distraction, and certain cognitive activities, for example, daydreaming (Olness & Gardner, 1978). Hypnosis is not in itself a therapeutic intervention; that is, no patient is treated with hypnosis. Although a patient under hypnosis might experience reduced tension and a consequent attenuation of pain, merely entering the hypnotic state cannot be equated with treatment of that pain. Hypnotizability is the ability to experience the suggested distortions of perception, memory, or mood. There are marked individual differences in hypnotic responsiveness that at one time were attributed to variations in hypnotists' skill. In the 1970s Morgan and Hilgard (1973) introduced the concept of hypnotic responsivity, which shifted the emphasis to the patient's hypnotic capacity, his ability, skill, or talent to respond to suggestion. Placing the locus of control within the patient changed the face of hypnotherapy and focused research attention on patient correlates.

A major component in hypnotizability appears to be the individual's capacity for imagination (Hilgard & LeBaron, 1984). A second component is chronological age. Early research on norms has suggested that hypnotizability is limited in preschool children, increases markedly in the middle childhood years, and decreases somewhat in adolescence before stabilizing during adulthood into a gradual decline (Morgan & Hilgard, 1973). Recently, however, a body of clinical data has accumulated indicating that children of preschool age (Gardner, 1977; Kuttner, 1984, 1986; Kuttner, Bowman, & Teasdale, 1987; LaBaw, 1973; Olness, 1985) do respond positively to the therapeutic use of hypnosis. In none of this research does sex appear to be a factor. In a scholarly review of the empirical research and procedures used to arrive at hypnotizability norms, Gardner and Olness (1981) have noted a number of methodological and other problems. Samples have tended to be drawn from predominantly middle socioeconomic status populations, with large standard deviations despite the unifying effects that might be expected as an offshoot of such sample homogeneity. The problem of simulation in some subjects has had certain contaminating effects, as have the use of inappropriate induction techniques and tests with construction flaws. In summing up their conclusions about hypnotic responsiveness in children, Gardner and Olness (1981, p. 34) state that

> First, most studies err on the side of underestimating children's hypnotic talents. Second—and this conclusion derives from the first—the lack of solid evidence concerning children's hypnotic responsiveness does not imply that we should abandon our clinical efforts to help children through hypnotherapy.

Clinically, hypnotizability can be evaluated with standardized tests such as the Stanford Hypnotic Clinical Scale for Children (Morgan & Hilgard, 1979). This scale, which can be administered in 20 minutes, comes in a modified form for ages 4 to 8 and a standard form for ages 6 to 16. The items in both forms are appealing to children, are designed to ensure some success at all ages, and also provide information facilitating the subsequent choice of hypnotherapy techniques. Some support for the validity of the scale comes from correlations of .67 with the longer Children's Hypnotic Susceptibility Scale developed by London (1962) and based on items from Weitzenhoffer and Hilgard's (1959) Stanford Hypnotic Susceptibility Scale, Form A.

Hypnotizability can also be evaluated clinically by rating the child's responsiveness to suggestions following induction. Hilgard and LeBaron (1984, p. 7) describe induction procedures as simple procedures "designed to provide a gradual transition from our usual generalized reality orientation to the limited orientation characteristic of hypnosis." Two that are frequently used with children are eye fixation and arm levitation. In eye fixation, the child is asked to relax in a comfortable chair and then focus his attention on a target, such as a face painted on his thumbnail or a coin held between his thumb and forefinger. The hypnotist then suggests feelings of sleepiness that become strong enough for the child's eyes to close. In arm levitation, the child is first asked to focus on his hand, which is resting comfortably on the side of the chair, and then is given the suggestion that the hand feels light and is about to rise from its resting position. Imagery is used to reinforce the lightness feeling: The hypnotist may, for example, describe a soft breeze that tosses the hand up in the air like a leaf. As the child's hand rises, suggestions designed to encourage general relaxation continue. The hypnotist then tells the child that when the hand touches his face, he will know that the hypnotic condition has been established and the hand will return to the arm of the chair. The child's reaction to this kind of instruction shows the hypnotist how responsive he is and thus provides an index of hypnotizability (Hilgard, Crawford, & Wert, 1979).

Although physical relaxation is used in both of these techniques, it is not a necessary condition for inducing hypnosis (Orne & Dinges, 1984).

The choice of an appropriate induction technique depends on the needs and preferences of the child as well as on the experience, creativity, and preferences of the therapist. In a preinduction interview, the therapist should obtain a substantial body of information about the child, including his likes and dislikes, and at this time should also clarify his ideas and misconceptions about hypnosis. It is essential that the child have a comfortable, trusting relationship with the therapist and feel safe with him. Treatment should not require passive submission but instead should emphasize the child's involvement and control in the situation and be permissive enough to allow the child to participate actively and enthusiastically. Of course, the child should also be physically comfortable so that related distractions do not draw his attention from the hypnotist's suggestions (Hilgard & LeBaron, 1984).

Hypnotherapy

When hypnosis is used in combination with various forms of medical or psychological treatment, the intervention is referred to as *hypnotherapy*. It is a treatment modality with specific therapeutic goals and with techniques that are used while the patient is in the state of hypnosis at least for part of the time. The therapeutic intervention is implemented by either the therapist or, in the case of self-hypnosis, the patient. In either case, the goal is to increase the child's feeling of control over a behavior or problem. Although the need for external help may sometimes be eliminated, usually the child continues with such help but in a changed form (Gardner & Olness, 1981). Hypnotherapy has appeal for children, and they generally accept the idea more readily than adults do. Response to treatment is frequently rapid, and few risks and side effects, if any, are involved. With pain problems in children, hypnotherapy is aimed at eliminating or alleviating specific symptoms such as the pain of burn dressing changes or bone marrow aspirations. Gardner and Olness (1981) have labeled this target *symptom-oriented hypnotherapy*, although most clinicians use the more general descriptor *hypnotherapy* for pain problems.

In order to be considered a suitable candidate for hypnotherapy, the child must be responsive to hypnotic induction methods and be able to establish rapport with the therapist, particularly in respect to a trusting relationship. He must also have adequate motivation to cope with the problem, which must be one that is amenable to treatment by this therapeutic mode. Parents and other adults important to the child and involved with him must view hypnotherapy in a positive way: Gardner and Olness (1981) report that most parents are positive and those that initially have misgivings about hypnotherapy can, with help, overcome their resistance to it. Finally, the use of hypnotherapy must not cause indirect harm to the child by superceding other treatment modalities: medical, surgical, and psychotherapy approaches take precedence over it. Used properly, hypnotherapy can alleviate much otherwise unapproachable pain; it also can help maintain the functional ability and dignity of many patients who would otherwise be dependent on high doses of medication with possible dulling of consciousness. At its best it can be a powerful means of controlling pain; at its worst, it probably causes no change in the patient's condition.

Keeping in mind Gardner and Olness's (1981) cautionary statement that there are very few cases in which complete certainty exists that the reported positive results are due entirely to hypnotherapy, let us consider specific findings in the hypnotherapy literature. It is clear from surgical reports that hypnotherapy can suppress pain in at least some patients (Orne & Dinges, 1984). The best single predictor of success in pain reduction is the amount of pain reduction that occurs when this intervention is first attempted, with the next best predictor being measured hypnotic responsiveness (Wester & Smith, 1984). There is documentation of hypnotherapy's use as the sole anesthetic in surgery for appendectomy, tooth extraction, caesarean section, cardiac conditions, and hysterectomy (for reviews, see Finer, 1980; Hilgard & Hilgard, 1975). With children and adolescents, hypnotherapy is also an effective analgesic for pain resulting from treatment procedures such as burn debridement (Bernstein, 1965; Gardner & Olness, 1981), bone marrow aspiration (Hilgard & LeBaron, 1984), and dentistry (Bernick, 1972). It has been used as well to alleviate pain associated with illness and other conditions, for example, cancer (Gardner & Lubman, 1983; Zeltzer & LeBaron, 1982), sickle-cell anemia (Gardner & Olness, 1981), hemophilia in children and adolescents (Olness & Agle, 1982; LaBaw, 1975), juvenile rheumatoid arthritis (Cioppa & Thal, 1975), ongoing surgical (Andolsek & Novik, 1980) and postoperative pain (Bensen, 1971), itching (Gardner & Olness, 1981; Mirvish, 1978; Olness, 1977), reflex sympathetic dystrophy (Lewenstein, 1981), leukemia (Gardner, 1976; Hilgard & LeBaron, 1984), and insulin injections (Gardner & Olness, 1981). It has also been used for hip pain having no organic basis (Sarles, 1975) and as an adjunct to psychotherapy in recurrent abdominal pain (Williams & Singh, 1976).

There are many reports of the successful use of hypnotherapy with preschool children. Among them is one by Kuttner (1984; see also Kuttner et al., 1987) in which hypnotherapy resulted in the immediate and enduring attenuation of anxiety and distress and minimized the effect of pain in preschool children undergoing bone marrow aspirations. The favorite-story technique was the hypnotic method used with these children. In this technique, the child's favorite story is first identified and then used during the painful procedure. In addition to having considerable distraction potential and a number of positive and reassuring associations for the child, it can be adapted and interwoven with procedural and sensory information about the ongoing painful treatment. For example, one child insisted that he be told when the needle was in place, so this information was incorporated into the hypnotic trance in the following way:

And Goldilocks sat down to eat baby bear's porridge. It tasted so yummy and made her feel so comfortable and now the poke is over and the water [cerebrospinal fluid] is being collected. But Goldilocks didn't stop eating . . . and guess what . . . soon there was no more porridge . . . and now she started to feel good and sleepy. (Kuttner, 1984, p.7)

The favorite-story technique can also become a metaphor for courage and the use of coping skills:

One day while she was sweeping the floor Cinderella said, "Oh I wish I were brave and not scared of all of my sisters." Well as soon as she said "I wish" a Magic Fairy suddenly appeared in the room and said, "Cinderella, you are a wonderfully brave girl. You have handled some tough things so I am going to reward you for your courage. You can have your wish come true!" What do you think Cinderella wished for? . . . That's it, to go to the King's Ball. Cinderella took a deep breath in and sighed it out. She felt marvellous because she knew she'd soon be having fun and all the hardships would be over.

This technique is one of a variety of therapeutic interventions, including self-hypnosis and distraction procedures, depicted in an outstanding videotape produced by Kuttner (1986). The sequences capture the extreme anxiety that children and adolescents experience while undergoing painful cancer-related treatments. This videotape presentation should be mandatory viewing for all pediatric professionals who are working with children undergoing any painful treatment.

In their excellent general text, Gardner and Olness (1981, p. 253) provide the following description of a case study in which hypnotherapy was beneficial to a terminally ill child with cystic fibrosis:

Steven T., a 10-year-old boy, also in the end stages of cystic fibrosis, was referred to us for hypnotherapy because of depression and decreased tolerance of medical procedures including postural drainage and intravenous infusions. He would resist and cry, asking the medical staff members why they continued these painful treatments when they knew as well as he did that he was going to die anyway. In the first hypnotherapeutic session, Steven quickly learned self-hypnosis to control pain and to decrease his anxiety about being unable to get enough air during postural drainage treatments that resulted in prolonged and violent coughing. He was also able to clarify that he really did want continued treatment, since he wanted to live as long as possible, and he asked that the nurses ignore his pleas when his frustration resulted in "temper tantrum" behavior. He immediately developed a strong positive alliance with the therapist.

Although the efficacy of hypnotherapy for the control of clinical and experimental pain has been demonstrated, the theoretical basis for it is still a subject of controversy (Hilgard & LeBaron, 1984). Several theories have been proposed, including psychoanalytic ego theory (Gill & Brenman, 1959) and role theory (Sarbin, 1950). Hilgard (1977) has formulated the neodissociation theory of hypnotic analgesia, sometimes referred to as the theory of alternative cognitive controls, based on empirical evidence that highly hypnotizable individuals who report analgesia overtly are often able to reveal a covert facet of their pain that is equal to that of the waking state pain with respect to intensity, but is singularly lacking in the affect that normally would be present. For an interesting case report of this phenomenon, known as "the hidden observer," see Hilgard and LeBaron (1984, pp. 162–166). Hilgard has hypothesized that hierarchically ordered cognitive systems may become reordered while the individual is in the hypnotic state and that one result of these changes is that the significance and awareness of the pain message is changed.

Self-Hypnosis

In hypnotherapy, the therapist, with the consent of the child, assumes some of the executive functions of the child and uses suggestion to influence the direction of therapy. Although the child is participating in a fantasy during it, one small sector of his mind functions as a monitor that observes and processes the hypnotherapeutic procedure. In self-hypnosis, the child assumes the executive function and serves both as hypnotist and patient, with the monitoring self now shifting from the previous role of observer to the much more active one of initiator of executive action (Hilgard & LeBaron, 1984).

Although children have little difficulty in learning to function in the dual role of hypnotherapist and patient, for a variety of reasons some resist learning to use self-hypnosis. Immaturity, lack of motivation to do it themselves, not wanting to sever ties with the therapist, and parental interference are among the reasons for their negative reactions. With the exception of immaturity, all of these can be overcome. Once the technique has been learned, the quality of the patient/therapist relationship appears to be a crucial factor in maintaining self-control over pain, and periodic contact must be sustained if the child is to maintain the degree of pain relief possible with self-hypnosis (Gardner & Olness, 1981). A major problem is ensuring compliance to daily practice of the procedure. In an evaluation of self-hypnosis for a cluster of problems, Kohen, Olness, Colwell, and Heimel (1984) found that relatively few children maintained their self-hypnosis practice for more than a few months. This drop-off occurred even in children using the procedure for pain control and is particularly surprising in this group since one would logically predict high motivation to sustain practice of a pain-reducing skill. In any case, the practice problem underscores the importance of continued contact with the therapist.

The technique selected for training a child in the use of self-hypnosis for pain control varies, depending on the type of pain and characteristics of the child (Gardner & Olness, 1981). Assuming therapist skill and child motivation, most techniques are effective and there is no empirical evidence for differential efficacy of those in use. Gardner (1981) has reported a three-step procedure that can be learned in one session. In the first step, the therapist uses various induction and then deepening methods. In the latter phase of this first step the child is guided toward an increasing involvement in his imagination and is helped to disassociate further. Usually, the emphasis is on imagery and ideomotor techniques that give the child an outward and visible sign that hypnosis has been induced. A demonstration by the therapist that the child can independently come out of hypnosis and return to the alert state completes this step. Next, the therapist and child discuss which induction procedure was most helpful and the remainder are abandoned. The child then describes in detail the one selected and demonstrates going into hypnosis and returning to the alert state. Problems are clarified, discussed, and resolved. In the final step, the child covertly repeats the previously selected induction procedure. During this period neither participant speaks. The child indicates by a nod that he is in a trance and then returns to the normal waking state. Any other problems or ideas are discussed and at this point the child is now ready to use self-hypnosis independently. Self-hypnosis can be learned even by children who obtain low scores on hypnotic responsivity assessments. According to Hilgard and LeBaron (1984), the degree of success in self-hypnosis corresponds to that achieved by the child in hypnotherapy.

The child who practices self-hypnosis for pain control achieves a sense of mastery over his pain that induces a feeling of self-efficacy (Bandura, 1981) that is additionally therapeutic. There is generally less need for medication or other help from adults, and this too decreases the child's feeling of helplessness in the situation. Typically, he becomes skilled at self-hypnosis and this success increases his receptivity to learning other self-control techniques, such as coping strategies, as well as his confidence in his ability to use them effectively. Furthermore, the knowledge that a means of pain control is always available to him is tremendously reassuring and, consequently, anxiety reducing and relaxing.

A substantial body of clinical reports and empirical data attest to the efficacy of self-hypnosis for pain control in children and adolescents (see, for example, Bernick, 1972; Gaal, Goldsmith, & Needs, 1980; Gardner & Olness, 1981; Hilgard & LeBaron, 1984; Kohen, 1980; McGrath & de Veber, 1986; Olness, MacDonald, & Uden, 1987).

Cognitive Coping Strategies

Before beginning this discussion of the *cognitive* category of coping strategies (CCS), it should be noted that there are other coping strategies that children use prior to and during pain events (see, for example, Gaffney, 1983; Ross & Ross, 1982a, 1985; Siegel, 1987) and that they are frequently used in combination with CCS. For instance, during the event children have reported using physical resistance and escape as a means of terminating the noxious stimulation or have sought social support to help in enduring it. Our focus here, however, is on CCS, those covert techniques that influence pain through the medium of the child's thoughts. Despite unequivocal evidence that many children use these strategies (Brown et al., 1986; Ross & Ross, 1982a; Savedra, 1977) and increasing recognition of the importance to children of coping successfully with pain (Beales, 1983; Stoddard, 1982), there are relatively few instances of pediatric personnel spontaneously teaching children and adolescents to use CCS in clinical pain situations. In the Ross and Ross (1982a) study, for example, only 13 such instances were reported: Seven of these involved pediatricians working with children with leukemia and the remaining six involved orthodontists. Yet there is unequivocal clinical (Peterson, 1983; Ross, D., 1984) and empirical evidence (see, for example, Jay, 1987; McGrath & de Veber, 1986; Peterson & Shigetomi, 1981; Siegel, 1987) that children and adolescents can be taught to use these strategies for the attenuation of pain.

When the child uses a CCS (or other coping strategies) he is, in effect, assuming some responsibility for his own well-being. Competence in the use of CCS is associated with feelings of confidence and mastery that should exert a strong positive influence in the pain situation. Bandura's (1981) self-efficacy theory is relevant here. According to this theory, the child's perception of his capabilities in a specific situation affects his fear reactions. The child who feels helpless in the face of impending or ongoing pain typically experiences significantly more anxiety (Seligman, 1975) and consequently, more anxiety-heightened pain, than does the child who is confident that he has some control over the pain event. This does not mean that the child who uses coping skills feels *no* pain. His knowledge of his coping efficacy should diminish his anticipatory anxiety as well as his fearfulness during ongoing pain, thereby reducing the amount of pain experienced, but coping skills seldom eliminate pain completely.

Although any of the pediatric group could teach these strategies, it is generally an advantage if the person selected is not the one inflicting pain. Preferably, his schedule should also allow him to be present in the role of supportive coach on the first few opportunities that the child has to use CCS in the pain situation. A person with child life training would be ideal because typically he would have the child's trust and have the requisite time to help the child practice the new skills. The general procedures for introducing the concept of using CCS are discussed first, followed by a description of several kinds of CCS and the recommended strategies for teaching them.

General Procedures

Begin by asking the child if there is anything that he does all by himself that helps when he is in pain. Do not be surprised at an affirmative answer: Hilgard and LeBaron (1982), for example, reported that in a group of children and adolescents with leukemia (n = 24), seven were already using CCS on their own during bone marrow aspirations and were able to achieve marked pain relief during this very painful procedure. If the child already effectively uses some form of coping strategy, mention that there are others. Pursue teaching these only if he shows interest. Similarly, if he uses no coping strategy, continue only if he shows interest when you tell him about coping strategies. Before we move on to describe the specific procedures for teaching the child each strategy, it should be noted that in addition to the case in which the child shows no interest in being taught CCS, there are other circumstances in which no such attempt should be made. If a child is seriously ill, depleted, or exhausted, any nonessential demand is inexcusable. If the child is an avoider (Cohen & Lazarus, 1979), a characteristic evidenced in such behaviors as not wanting advance information (Ross, S. A., 1984), teaching him CCS or other coping strategies may be unethical as well as futile since it could result in his experiencing more upset during the event than if he had been left to his own resources (Harris & Rollman, 1985). Now proceed with the following steps:

1. Explain that attention to one activity limits the amount of attention you have for another. Use everyday examples to transmit this idea. You might ask the child if he has ever had either of these experiences: He is so absorbed in an activity or book that he does not hear his mother calling or notice noise around him; or he is playing a game, is injured to the extent that he should notice the hurt, but he does not notice it until after the game. Gearing the explanation to the child's cognitive level, explain that attention is a finite characteristic, that we have a limited and fixed capacity for focusing on stimulus events. To show a young child that attention is limited, use blocks or other tangible objects to represent attention; for an older child or adolescent, verbal explanation should suffice. You might use these hypothetical situations: He is listening to X when Y starts to talk, too; he cannot take in what both are saying. Can he hear A in the room when talking to B on the telephone? The point to make is that to a great extent the child is in charge of a scarce resource that he can allocate in any way he chooses. He can move it around and he can also put it in a "safe" place where there is no pain.

2. Point out that you are more aware of feelings if you give them all your attention. Use as examples hunger, noise, and then pain. Most children have had the experience of being so interested in some ongoing activity or event that although it is far past their usual mealtime, they are completely unaware of hunger until the event ends, at which point they suddenly realize that they are very hungry.

3. Explain that you will show him some ways to keep his attention off ongoing pain or any other aversive, unavoidable experience. Emphasize the unavoidable aspect here: If the pain or other aversive experience is avoidable, steps should be taken to terminate it. Tell the child that you will describe several procedures and he can pick the one that he would like to try first. For older children and adolescents use the term *strategy* for this explanation and define it as "a plan of action for handling pain," or "a skill for managing pain." Note that the inclusion of several strategies is a principle of Meichenbaum's stress inoculation procedure (1977) and that preferences often are indicative of strengths. It is important to match the child's strengths to the appropriate strategies in order to have the optimum child $\times$ strategy fit. Children differ in cognitive ability, and these differences will affect their strategy preferences. Some children generate rich fantasies in seconds, whereas others have great difficulty in doing so. Mention the idea that knowing

several CCS is a good idea because they may have differential efficacy for different types of pain experience. As Meichenbaum (1977) has noted, having a particular weapon in one's arsenal may be less important than having a variety of weapons. Explain that some of these ways of not thinking about ongoing pain are very good for a short pain, such as a shot that is over in seconds, or for a series of short pains with intermittent periods of no pain, as in some dental procedures. Different strategies may be needed for a long, continuous pain (McCaul & Malott, 1984). In addition, the goal of coping may differ across aversive situations. In certain situations not breaking down and crying may be the goal rather than minimizing the pain experienced.

4. Find out what nonschool activities the child participates in that would require practice on his part, perhaps baseball, dancing, basketball, or playing a musical instrument. Point out that it is virtually impossible to succeed at any of these without practice: First, skills and subskills are practiced in isolation, for example, dribbling practice off the court, then the skills are used in the setting where they really count. Practice is also needed in school activities if the child is to become proficient at the various tasks such as reading. Similarly, the child must practice his pain-coping strategies in relevant nonpain situations if he is to use them effectively in a pain situation. If the child is at a boring event (a speech, performance, movie) that he cannot leave, he can practice not attending to the proceedings by thinking of something else. Help the child identify other similar situations in which he finds himself and stress that he should use these opportunities to practice his CCS in order to be able to mobilize the strategies when he really needs them. Research by Brown (1984) with adult migraine headache patients suggests that intensive practice is of critical importance to the efficacy of CCS.

With respect to practice, it is important to stress that the child can use the CCS anywhere and at any time. Research with college students (Spanos, Hodgins, Stam, & Gwynn, 1984) and hospitalized adults (Copp, 1974) suggests that for some unknown reason, these groups are reluctant to use coping strategies across situations. Spanos et al. found that college students in experiments involving pain refrained from using CCS unless given explicit permission to do so, and this finding held up even when there was neither implicit nor direct mention that coping strategies were forbidden. In Copp's study, patients who at home had successfully used various procedures for relieving their pain were reluctant to use them in the hospital setting. These findings suggest that considerable emphasis should be placed on encouraging the child to practice attention diversion and the other CCS in a variety of situations. The ultimate goal is to facilitate the generalizing of CCS across aversive situations.

Successful demonstrations of the efficacy of CCS in relatively low stress situations are of immense importance to the child's outcome expectancies in the pain situation. Bandura (1981) has distinguished between self-efficacy and outcome expectancies, with the former referring to the child's belief in his ability to use a CCS, which should be firmly established during training, and the latter referring to his assessment that the CCS will result in reduced stress, which can be acquired only through successful use.

Attention Diversion

Point out to the child that by focusing his attention elsewhere during a painful procedure or other aversive event he will have less attention for the pain and, as a result, it should not hurt so much. Mention that some children have even reported that the pain stopped, but you cannot promise that this will happen. All that you can say is that it should not hurt so much if the child uses attention diversion. To do this, the child sets a task that can be done right in the pain situation and pursues that task with single-minded devotion. The chosen task should be a "hard" one, because distraction techniques that require more attentional capacity will be more effective (McCaul & Malott, 1984). It may depend on either external or internal cues or on a combination of these. When the task involves external stimuli, the child focuses on some feature of the immediate environment. In an emergency room he might count the acoustic tiles on the ceiling or the number of times pediatric personnel make a certain response that occurs frequently. One child, for example, reported counting the number of times the doctor who was working on him blinked. When attention diversion is internal, the task is independent of the immediate setting. The child may make himself say the alphabet backwards three times, recite a poem covertly, or sing songs to himself, before allowing himself even to think about the pain. In external/internal combinations, the child uses some feature of the immediate setting but imposes an additional interpretation on it:

> Our dentist has this music, see, and I say to him to turn it up real loud because I really think that kind is mink [good]. Then I pretend that I have to really *learn* the music, like the tune, or something terrible will happen to me. And I keep telling myself to listen, listen, listen, and after awhile sometimes I almost don't know I'm getting drilled. (Girl, CA 11, Ross & Ross, 1982a)

> I counted everything in the [examination] room if it was shiny or not shiny and I made it like a game, like the shinies team against the not shinies team and the shinies won. You have to count real fast so you can't think about what they [emergency room personnel] are doing. (Girl, CA 9, traffic accident victim, Ross & Ross, 1982a)

Use role-play to demonstrate the use of attention diversion in a pain situation. Have the child practice by first seeing if he can shut out or diminish noise or any other aversive situation in real life.

Attention diversion has been used in three studies with leukemic children undergoing bone marrow aspirations. In these studies the stimuli or activity were supplied by the experimenter rather than generated by the children. In a particularly well-designed experiment, Kuttner (1984) demonstrated the successful use of external attention-diverting stimuli (toys, bubbles) in reducing distress in preschool and, particularly, in school-age children. Jay et al. (1984) used internal attention diversion (simple breathing exercises) as part of an ingenious and successful multicomponent treatment package for children. In a study of children and adolescents undergoing cancer chemotherapy, Redd, Jacobsen, and Die-Trill (1986) used videogames: The introduction and withdrawal of the opportunity to play these games produced significant changes in the form of reduction and exacerbation, respectively, in conditioned nausea. These tasks all involve active participation on the child's part. By contrast, passive attention diversion requires only that the child watch the stimulus. Orthodontists (Lemchen, 1987) report that television programs so enthrall children that they appear almost oblivious to discomfort. The disadvantage here is that the child is dependent on others for attention diversion, whereas once he has learned this strategy himself he can use it independently of adult help.

Self-Instruction

In this strategy the goal is to teach the child to coach himself, a concept that is readily grasped by most children. Self-instruction works best when the child has some foreknowledge of what is coming, when the situation has a known procedural structure.

1. Start by asking if the situation is one in which the child knows ahead of time what the pain will be like, for example, dental treatment, injections, and burn dressing changes generally follow a prescribed sequence.

2. Point out that unless the pain is very, very quick, he should not think about the pain treatment as a *whole* thing. Instead, think of it in parts (one child thought of it as steps where he had to get to the top). Thinking in terms of parts is helped by the fact that in many painful treatments the pain is intermittent rather than continuous. The task for the child then becomes one of getting past (or coping with) one painful part at a time. This is a variant on quota setting (Dolce, Crocker, Molettiere, & Doleys, 1986).

3. The child must talk continuously to himself, giving advice ("Just relax"), encouragement ("You're doing great"), and reassurance ("You're past the worst part"). He must concentrate on this internal self-instruction. Some children combine this strategy with attention diversion:

> I just don't think about this machine. And if I think about it I get real mad at myself and I say "Fritz, you stop that thinking, you hear me," and then I close my eyes tight and I think only about TV, and then I watch it and if I start thinking about the machine I just say, "Stop thinking, you dumbbell." (Boy, CA 7, dialysis treatment, Ross & Ross, 1982a)

In two successful treatment packages for children undergoing dental treatment, Siegel and Peterson (1980, 1981) used calming self-instruction, and Nocella and Kaplan (1982) used positive self-instruction of a reassuring and confidence-building type, for example, "If I get scared or worried I tell myself this is a good dentist, I'm doing good, I can handle this, I'm doing terrific."

Transformative Imagery

Context Transformation   Unlike the previous strategies, no attempt is made here to ignore the pain. Instead, the child focuses on transforming the pain situation into another more exciting or more desirable context. A child having venipuncture might see himself as a policeman shot in the arm while pursuing criminals, but continuing on bravely despite his injury. The pain is still present, but in the new context it becomes easier to take.

> As soon as I get in the chair I pretend he's the enemy and I'm a secret agent and he's torturing me to get secrets and if I make one sound I'm telling him secret information and I never do. I'm going to be a secret agent when I grow up so this is good practice. (Boy, CA 10, at the dentist, Ross & Ross, 1982a)

Use the following steps in teaching this strategy:

1.   Talk about pretending, about how when something awful happens you sometimes pretend that it did not happen.

2.   Ask the child if he is good at pretending. Assuming an affirmative answer, ask about his most recent pain experience. Tell him that it often helps when in pain to pretend that you are somewhere else and something else is going on.

3.   Suggest some other exciting or pleasurable contexts for that specific pain, for example, a sports competition, saving someone from a dangerous situation, or scouting the enemy's strength before an important battle. Make sure the new context is appropriate for both the type of pain experience and the child.

4.   To help the child imagine himself in a new context, have him first decide what the context is to be, then pretend that he is turning the television on and when the picture comes on the screen, the action starts. Use role play for these sequences. As one component of the successful treatment package referred to earlier, Jay et al. (1984) used context transformation with leukemic children undergoing bone marrow aspirations. Some children used spy and adventure themes; others used favorite-place fantasies.

Stimulus Transformation   The general procedure for this strategy is the same as that for context transformation, but the target is the instrument that is causing the pain (needle, dental drill, having bands tightened on teeth). The goal is to transform the instrument into something better, more exciting, and more positive. The child must be convinced that he can look at *any* procedure or instrument and almost always think of it as something other than it is. Given encouragement, most children are imaginative and have little difficulty with this task. Once the child has the idea that almost any procedure can be viewed as something else, he should be helped to think of other ways of viewing the instruments used in painful procedures. For example, in Ross and Ross (1982a) one 8-year-old leukemic boy saw the needle used to draw blood as "a silver knight slaying the wicked enemy" (cells indicative of leukemia). Another 6-year-old boy undergoing radiation treatment viewed the equipment as "a friendly robot, I call him Robert Robot and I talk to him the whole time and he watches over me." A 9-year-old girl thought of chemotherapy as "a flood that washes away all the things that are causing the good people a lot of trouble." An 11-year-old undergoing orthodontistry thought of the brace-tightening procedure as "like being poured into a beautiful mold, like he (the dentist) is a magician and he's forcing me to become beautiful." The child must be helped to think of specific substitutions that have high credibility for him. If the stimulus is a spontaneous pain, for example, a stomach ache, the child might imagine that there is an unhappy dragon twisting and pushing around in his stomach trying to get out. He visualizes the dragon getting smaller and smaller until it shoots out when the child coughs and goes away, never to return. If the pain is menstrual cramps, it could be imagined as a multiknotted rope around some valuable object that should be loosened one knot at a time.

Incompatible Imagery The strategy of incompatible imagery involves having the child imagine that he is in some pleasant setting engaged in an activity that is inconsistent with pain. The task is to dwell in minute detail on all facets of the imaginary setting:

> I went back to the very first day at our beach house and I started with the smell—you know that smell you get from the sea—and I got dressed and I walked in the sand and I put one foot in and I got it wet. (Girl, CA 9, Ross & Ross, 1982a)

The method is similar to that in the other imagery strategies: The child first identifies the contextual change, then turns on the imaginary television set and "sees" the setting, and starts going over every part of the experience. Note that the pain is not in the scenario at all. The imagery involved is all positive and highly detailed and everything is pleasant. There is no challenge to the pain, instead, the imaginary place displaces the whole pain situation and pushes it out of the child's attentional focus. Varni et al. (1981) used incompatible imagery in combination with relaxation to demonstrate decreased pain intensity and analgesic dependence in a 9-year-old hemophilic boy with recurring hemorrhages and consequent arthritic pain. In this case, the patient imagined himself in a warm, pain-free setting. In a study of needle-phobic children in a dental setting, Ayer (1973) used imagery that was congruent with compliance with the demands of the dental treatment but incompatible with the dental setting itself: The children imagined that their mouths were open because they were barking dogs.

One dimension of imagery that merits research attention with children is the relative efficacy of stimulus versus response elements in incompatible imagery. In his work on fear-related imagery, Lang (1977, 1979) has emphasized the importance of vivid imagery. His conceptualization of vivid imagery requires that the detailed mental picture include the child's actions as if he were actually in the setting (response element) as opposed to just imagining the setting (stimulus element). The 9-year-old girl's strategy quoted above is a good example of the response dimension in imagery. The fact that many of the coping strategies that children report involve activity (response) rather than passivity (stimulus) on the child's part suggests that response element strategies might prove more effective for this population.

Thought-Stopping

Thought-stopping is a coping technique designed to help individuals who have persisting and unpleasant thoughts about specific events or conditions to eliminate or reduce the frequency and intensity of these thought sequences (Bain, 1928). Representative of the substantial number of papers that have appeared on thought-stopping, particularly with the advent of interest in behavior modification, is the following description by Wolpe and Lazarus (1966, p. 132) of a standard thought-stopping procedure: The patient is first helped to relax his muscles, and while in this relaxed state, he is told to engage in his unpleasant thought sequence for a specified period of time, such as one minute. At some point in this temporal sequence the therapist sounds an auditory signal and simultaneously shouts, "Stop," whereupon the patient is told to terminate the unpleasant thought sequence and start actively thinking about some previously identified pleasant topic. Typically, the patient finds that he has successfully substituted the pleasant topic. The therapist helps him practice his thought-stopping and substitution until he feels competent at it. He is then told to use the procedure of shouting "Stop" if he is alone, or saying it subvocally if he is with others, whenever he thinks of the unpleasant topic.

Although this procedure has been used successfully with problems such as fear of heart attacks (Wolpe & Lazarus, 1966), it has two marked disadvantages. The technique does not effect any change in the quality of thoughts that the patient has about the event or condition. For example, if prior to therapy he engaged in exaggerated fantasies about the possibility of having a heart attack, he would probably continue to have the same kind of fantasies, albeit less frequently and intensely. Second, the patient is not given any information in the course of learning this technique that would help him to cope effectively should the feared event, such as a heart attack, occur.

Recently, D. Ross (1984) developed a thought-stopping procedure that eliminates both of these disadvantages and is appropriate for use by children. Originally designed for those who experience high and persistent anxiety about appointments with the dentist, it has also been highly effective with leukemic children in clinical settings. The goal for these children was to reduce the anticipatory anxiety typically experienced about impending painful procedures because it heightens the pain experienced during treatment. The procedure went as follows.

The nurse first helped the child assemble a set of positive facts about the impending pain procedure. For venipuncture these might include "Having a needle put in my arm doesn't take long; I have good veins; the girl who comes to do it is nice; the doctor needs to know how my blood is to help me get better." Next, the nurse helped the child to think of some reassuring facts, for example, "The rest doesn't really hurt once the needle is in, and if I think hard about something else while it's being done, it won't hurt as much." These facts were then condensed so that the child could easily memorize the material: "A needle in my arm is quick. I have good veins. The girl who does it is nice. The doctor has to know how my blood is. It won't hurt as much if I think hard about something nice." For those children who had difficulty with memorizing, the nurse wrote the facts on a small card and went over them with the child until he had committed them to memory. He was then told that whenever he thought about the impending pain event he must stop what he was doing and recite the entire set of sentences subvocally, if others were in the room, or aloud if he was alone. He was then to return to his previous activity, but *every* time he thought of the venipuncture he was to stop and say it all again. Note that each child's set was designed specifically by and for him, making the content of the statements a highly individual matter. Although the example here was for leukemic children, the thought-stopping procedure is applicable to a variety of anxiety sources. All that is necessary is to follow the steps of assembling positive facts and reassuring facts, condensing and memorizing them, and then repeating them each time the anxiety-arousing thought occurs.

Although there have been no formal trials of the thought-stopping procedure, clinical and parental reports indicate that it is potentially a viable solution to the often severe and long-term anticipatory anxiety that many children experience prior to impending aversive events. The foregoing reports obviously do not constitute well-controlled data, but they are nevertheless encouraging. The next steps should be to conduct studies to provide empirical confirmation of the procedure's efficacy; specify the effective factors; establish the application potential, particularly with respect to age; and identify any limitations in the technique.

We attribute the reported efficacy of this procedure partly to a change in the child's feelings from helplessness (Seligman, 1975) in the face of the coming event to confidence that there is some action that can be taken. However, the major reason for the procedure's efficacy concerns changes that occur in the child's feelings of anticipatory fear and anxiety. The patient with persisting and unpleasant thought sequences about a specific event has fear responses whenever he thinks of it. Typically, these fear responses are strengthened by the exaggerated fantasies that he engages in whenever the topic occurs. By giving him a set of rational information that he must recite whenever he thinks about the event, positive responses are consistently being substituted for his fear responses. As a result, the fear responses are gradually weakened. Furthermore, having material to recite or read over and over again is very boring, so much so that children often have reported a feeling of exasperation at "having to go through all that again." The overall effect of such monotony is to further weaken the fear responses. Meanwhile, with each repetition the child is actively presenting himself with a set of information of a positive nature, all of which he knows to be true and related specifically to him.

His cognitions about the situation are almost inevitably changed and his fears diminish to a considerable extent.

The feelings of calm engendered by this procedure may extend into the treatment event if it does not involve continuous or intense pain. The children in the dental situation, for example, were, according to their parents and dentists, unusually calm not only prior to the session but also during it when caries were filled. For the leukemic children, thought-stopping was highly effective only up to the onset of the actual treatment; during painful procedures there was little apparent carryover of effect. For the latter children, the great benefit lay in the anxiety-free periods that preceded painful treatments.

Comment

The pain management literature has focused almost exclusively on the optimal approach for reducing anticipatory fears about impending aversive events and on procedures to facilitate coping and minimize discomfort during these events. A serious omission in this literature concerns the predicament of the child or adolescent who has difficulty coping with the aftermath of the event. In this instance the child is unable to keep himself from actively reconstructing the pain experience and, in addition, frequently dreams or has nightmares about it. Although sometimes he is unable to verbalize his distress, more often he is prevented from doing so by his parents under the misguided assumption that the child will then forget about it. Reports from clinicians (Peterschmidt, 1984; Remen, 1980; Waechter, 1971), from parents who initially had had strong reservations about permitting their children to be interviewed because it would "bring it all back" (Ross & Ross, 1982a), and from the children themselves (Adams, 1976; Bruce, 1983; Ross & Ross, 1982a, 1985) all attest to the need to "let it all out" and the relief that ensues from doing so. In the following account (Rosenbaum, 1984, p. 190) a boy in late adolescence faces for the first time the pain experiences he had had as a child of six:

> So many times I have satisfied the questioners' curiosity [about a massive scar on the hip]. Yet never did I satisfy myself with an answer. I thought I had gotten over my operation and 8 months of rehabilitation which was over a decade ago. . . . I decided to write my personal essay on my painful experience. . . . I relived the pain and loneliness of hospitalization which I had locked within me for over 10 years. My recollection of the operation was horrifying. My life was once again disrupted. My work, ambition, and motivation reached the lowest ebb. I tried to avoid writing my personal essay. When I did start writing I felt pain in my hip. . . . I realized that it was time that I confront the pains of my operation even though a decade had passed.

Reasons for Efficacy of Cognitive Coping Strategies

Although there is a paucity of empirical evidence for the efficacy of CCS with clinical pain in children and adults (see Tan, 1982, for an excellent review), there is substantial anecdotal support from both age groups. Why these strategies work remains unknown. One explanation rests upon the pain attenuation that occurs as a result of the successful use of the CCS and consequent enhancement of self-efficacy (Bandura, 1981). A second possibility is that the feeling of action mediated by the use of the CCS eliminates feelings of helplessness in the pain situation along with the heightened pain that ensues from such feelings (Seligman, 1975). Implicit in the latter explanation is the assumption that it is action per se rather than the nature of the action that is important. Anecdotal evidence opposing this explanation comes from reports by children (Ross & Ross, 1982a) that if one strategy proved ineffective, another was tried. In addition, McCaul and Malott's (1984) finding that distraction does not work for severe pain suggests that having something to do may not be the crucial variable. An alternate explanation attributes the efficacy of CCS to their distractibility function: By focusing completely on one set of generated events, the patient has less attention left for other events such as the pain.

These explanations are somewhat glib in that they tend to seize upon the obvious in the CCS situation. That there are pitfalls in this kind of reasoning is particularly apparent in the case of somatization (Tan, 1982). In this strategy, the individual focuses on his ongoing pain (or on the body part being subjected to aversive stimulation) in an intent but detached way that Tan (1982, p. 206) has described as analytical, "as if preparing to write a biology report." Anecdotal reports of this strategy have attributed its success to the detachment's effecting a psychological separation of the individual from his pain, with a consequent attenuation of discomfort. Although this facile explanation has a certain appeal, it lacks a theoretical as well as a factual base. The work of Bailey and Davidson (1976) on factor analysis of pain descriptors leads to a markedly divergent explanation for the efficacy of somatization. Noting that the general assumption that pain descriptors primarily relate to intensity has never been subjected to empirical test, Bailey and Davidson factor analyzed ratings of pain descriptors. Although the first factor identified was an intensity factor, it was not, as one would expect, a large single intensity factor. A comparison of the pain descriptors with Melzack and Torgerson's (1971) categories showed that intensity was distributed in an affective-evaluative rather than a sensory factorial space. This finding caused Bailey and Davidson (1976, p. 323) to speculate that

> If the patient's verbal self-report can be shifted away from affective-evaluative adjectives (for example, by suggesting that he focus on the sensory qualities of the experience instead), then in effect the patient would not be attending to the intensity domain of the pain experience and his pain tolerance would increase.

It follows from this hypothesis that the success of somatization may be a function of attention to qualities of the pain experience other than intensity, rather than to a nebulous separation process.

An Intriguing Possibility

The fact that children are able to use cognitive processes to attenuate their discomfort suggests that at some point in the future it may be possible to devise psychological or physiological techniques to trigger the pain-modulating system. The significance of such a breakthrough for pain management is evident in the following statement by Liebeskind and Paul (1977, p. 54):

> We think it likely that all mammals possess a set of powerful and endogenous centrifugal mechanisms of pain control within the brainstem. Lower animals may have little access to these systems except under the most dire circumstances. . . . In man, however, it may be that there are better developed pathways of access . . . to these brainstem systems. Thus, our cognitive capacities to think, to believe, and to hope enable us, probably all of us under the appropriate conditions, to find and employ our pain inhibitory resources. The important challenge in the years to come for behavioral scientists involved in pain research will be to explore and ultimately bring under control those precise circumstances and techniques that will reliably enable people to make use of these resources when needed.

7
Pediatric
Pain Problems
Primary Dysmenorrhea,
Burns, Migraine,
and Intrusive Procedures

In this chapter we show how the medical and psychological intervention procedures described in the previous two chapters are used in the management of four different types of pediatric pain. Our choice of types was guided by two criteria: They had to range from those treated mainly through medical intervention to those in which psychological intervention plays the primary role, and they had to be representative of the great variety of pain conditions. Using Varni's (1981) categories of pain associated with physical injury or trauma (e.g., burns, fractures, excessive cold, accidents), pain that occurs as a result of disease (e.g., leukemia, arthritis, hemophilia) or psychophysiological activity (e.g., headaches, abdominal discomfort), and pain from diagnostic and treatment procedures (e.g., ear examination, surgery, other intrusive procedures), we added a fourth category: pain that is associated with normal physiological, age-related function, such as cutting teeth, growing pains, or dysmenorrhea. From these categories we chose dysmenorrhea, burns, migraine, and intrusive procedures. Dysmenorrhea was of interest because it is specific to adolescence in relation to the pediatric population. As an area, burns are greatly in need of research interest and methodological change, with Kavanagh's (1983a) work standing out in a generally passive field. Recent findings on migraine have propelled it from the benign category into one of more urgency, with the evidence now that chronic migraines can cause brain damage and cognitive impairment. The last type, intrusive procedures, was selected because these procedures are a major source of misery for the whole gamut of the pediatric population. Some notable pain problems, such as dental problems, recurrent abdominal pain syndrome, accidents, arthritis, hemophilia, and leukemia, were bypassed because there are already many excellent papers on their management.

Primary Dysmenorrhea

Painful menstruation, dysmenorrhea, has been categorized as primary (idiopathic), occurring in the absence of any significant abnormality; and secondary (organic), having a known organic base. It is the most common menstrual dysfunction in adolescence, with prevalence figures ranging from 45% to 60% (Neinstein, 1984). It is also the leading cause of recurrent short-term school absenteeism among adolescent girls (Klein & Litt, 1981) and a major reason for periodic absenteeism from work. Ylikorkala and Dawood (1978) have estimated that 140 million school and work hours across relevant age groups are lost anually because of dysmenorrhea. Secondary dysmenorrhea should be suspected if the pain occurs for the first time with the onset of menarche or after the age of 20 (Neinstein, 1984). The most frequent of the organic problems are endometriosis, which is not as rare in adolescence as is commonly believed (Goldstein, deCholnoky, & Emans, 1979; Renaer, 1984), and pelvic inflammatory disease. It is primary dysmenorrhea, however, that is the focus of interest here.

Onset and Etiology

For any particular menstrual period, the onset of primary dysmenorrhea typically occurs prior to the beginning of menstrual flow or coincident with it. During the first few hours blood flow is usually slight but the pain may be severe. With increasing blood flow, the pain tends to diminish. Its pattern varies, but it is most often characterized by sharp, colicky, suprapubic, sometimes debilitating pain that radiates to the lower back and thighs. The pain may be accompanied by a cluster of symptoms such as nausea, vomiting, headache, irritability, and diarrhea, which may last for several hours, a day, and occasionally, several days. Beginning in late adolescence, primary dysmenorrhea generally diminishes in intensity and frequency with increasing age and in most cases disappears after the first pregnancy (Gantt & McDonough, 1981).

There is controversy about whether primary dysmenorrhea coincides with menarche or appears shortly in the next few periods or whether it is delayed until ovulation occurs. Neinstein (1984) is representative of a group favoring the latter view on the grounds that dysmenorrhea is a disorder of the ovulating female and consequently cannot occur until cyclic ovulation has begun, one or more years after menarche. He states that "primary dysmenorrhea usually starts 6 to 12 months after menarche, most commonly begins between the ages of 14–16, and peaks around 17–18" (Neinstein, 1984, p. 461). Similarly, Klein (1980) has noted that the prevalence of primary dysmenorrhea is most strongly correlated with increasing gynecological age. This view is hard to reconcile with questionnaire data (Ruble & Brooks-Gunn, 1982) as well as with anecdotal reports from mothers, school nurses, and adolescent girls themselves that this condition often occurs soon after menarche. In commenting on this inconsistency, Ruble and Brooks-Gunn (1982) have offered alternative explanations: Some girls at all stages do exhibit signs of ovulation (Vollman, 1977), so those reporting primary dysmenorrhea at or very shortly after menarche could be early ovulators; or cultural beliefs and stereotypes concerning the symptoms experienced may influence self-reports of menstrual cramps.

Although the pathophysiological mechanism of primary dysmenorrhea has not been unequivocally established, a small but convincing cluster of empirical evidence suggests that it (as well as dysmenorrhea in general) is largely the result of prostaglandin-mediated uterine hyperactivity. The empirically based rationale for this theory is as follows. Most cases of primary dysmenorrhea are characterized by an excess of myometrial activity during menstruation (Gantt & McDonough, 1981). A smooth muscle stimulant that is found in menstrual fluid comprises the prostaglandins E_2 and $F_2\alpha$ (Pickles, 1957; Pickles, Hall, Best, & Smith, 1975), both of which stimulate the myometrium (Neinstein, 1984). These prostaglandins are synthesized locally in endometrial tissue and appear to be under the influence of progesterone. Levels of prostaglandins, especially $F_2\alpha$, are higher in the endometrium of patients with primary dysmenorrhea (Dawood, 1981) as well as in cases of secondary dysmenorrhea associated with endometriosis, submucous fibroids, and the use of intrauterine devices, whereas anovulatory cycles are characterized by lower prostaglandin levels and more often than not by an absence of dysmenorrhea. Bygdeman, Bremme, Gillespie, and Lundström (1979), among others, have shown that excess uterine activity and pain can be precipitated with intravenous or intrauterine injections of prostaglandin E_2 and $F_2\alpha$. Finally, prostaglandin inhibitors diminish dysmenorrhea either by inhibition of prostaglandin synthetase activity or by direct antagonistic action on prostaglandin receptors (Klein, 1980; Neinstein, 1984).

Other etiological factors have also been postulated. One theory (Renaer 1984) speculates that primary dysmenorrhea is caused by intermittent pressure of the uterine contents on the richly innervated uterine isthmus and that the discomfort persists until the distention of the isthmus diminishes to a point permitting the free passage of menstrual blood and endometrial debris. Empirical support for this "obstruction" theory comes from investigations by Youssef (1958a, 1958b) demonstrating the role of the timing of isthmic tone in primary dysmenorrhea.

Role of Psychological Factors: Maternal Input

In view of the dominant role often arbitrarily accorded to psychological factors in the menopause, it is ironic that these factors are almost entirely overlooked in the case of primary dysmenorrhea. Traditionally, its treatment in the literature has been predominantly as a medical problem with pharmacotherapeutic solutions. Although we agree with Renaer (1984) that the basis for the occurrence of primary dysmenorrhea is generally physiological and that it is not essentially a psychogenic disorder, it is naive in the extreme to brush aside the possibility that a complex interaction of physiological and psychological factors may be involved in its etiology. Psychological factors can exacerbate or attenuate pain to an astonishing degree and must be carefully considered in the assessment and management of most painful conditions, including primary dysmenorrhea. It is a gross oversimplification, for example, to view reports of mother–daughter concordance for primary dysmenorrhea (Widholm & Kantero, 1971) as evidence solely of genetically based physiological similarities such as elevations in prostaglandin concentrations; concordance could also be attributed to maternal handling of the daughter's menarche or to the influence on attitudes toward menstruation from live and symbolic peer models, the media, and other informational sources. As one of a cluster of potentially important psychological determinants that warrant investigation on the clinician's part, we shall consider some of the possibilities inherent in the variable maternal input.

The potential effect of maternal input on the preadolescent's perception of menstruation should not be overlooked since it is the mother who is often the primary informant about the approach of menarche. Some mothers present this topic as the end of a carefree era, an ordeal that encompasses physiological discomfort and psychological distress, a burden that women must bear, and a period of sickness, all of which constitute a viewpoint likely to elicit feelings of apprehension and anxiety. Typically, such mothers offer misinformation ("If you go horseback riding during your period, you will have a hard time next month") that serves to heighten a sense of general unease. Furthermore, these mothers often focus undue attention on the adolescent's menstrual periods by emphasizing how the adolescent must plan around them, monitoring them unnecessarily, and encouraging their use for such secondary gains as absenteeism from school or being excused from physical education classes.

Compare this pattern with that of the mother who views menarche as the beginning of an exciting period of critical importance to fertility and the menstrual period itself as one of physiological activity that imposes few restrictions, an event that is the adolescent's responsibility although the mother is always available. In a hypothetical situation in which two adolescents exposed to such differential maternal input situations have the "same" degree of physiologically based pain in a specific menstrual period, it is highly likely that the effect of such cumulative maternal input would exacerbate the pain perceived in the former situation and minimize it in the latter. It should also be noted that mothers' attitudes to menarche are often consonant with their attitudes about other areas having high-stress potential for their daughters and these stressors should not be overlooked in management of the problem.

Evaluation of the Adolescent

A careful menstrual history should be taken to obtain detailed information about the onset, pattern, and character of the pain as well as its effects on daily activities.

Primary dysmenorrhea has been categorized as Grade I if the pain does not interfere with participation in everyday activity, Grade II if the pain causes the patient to avoid activity such as school or parties due to discomfort, and Grade III if it involves severe discomfort so that the patient prefers to stay in bed. It is important to establish which of these grades or what range is most representative of her typical painful period. The Menstrual Symptom Questionnaire (Chesney & Tasto, 1975a) may be useful for this, and it is suggested only because the items describe symptoms, such as premenstrual lethargy, that the adolescent girl might not realize are relevant to her menstrual history. The test was developed for the express purpose of validating Dalton's (1982) hypothesis that there are two forms of primary dysmenorrhea, the congestive form, having symptoms of tension, heaviness, depression, headache, and breast pain; and the spasmodic form, characterized by sharp, colicky, suprapubic, sometimes debilitating pain that radiates to the lower back and thighs. In addition to having different symptoms, these two forms were also believed to differ in etiology in that they were characterized by imbalances in different hormones. Dalton concluded on these grounds that both sets of symptoms could not occur in the same menstrual cycle. Although there is no empirical evidence for either the theory or the constructs of spasmodic and congestive dysmenorrhea, the hypothesis has generated considerable interest (see Parlee, 1973, for a review, and Webster, 1980, for a critique of efforts to demonstrate the validity of the constructs).

Following a physical examination with an emphasis on pelvic pathology (e.g., endometriosis or uterine abnormalities) and any laboratory tests indicated by the history and examination, the patient should be intensively questioned on her information about menstruation, beliefs concerning the etiology of dysmenorrhea, the typical pain and the most painful period ever, how she handles it, and what goes on in her life immediately prior to her period and during it. In this phase a wide-ranging true–false questionnaire would be of immense help, but at the present time no such instrument has been devised. The patient's mother should be interviewed separately to ascertain her views of the problem and beliefs. In addition to the clinician's assessment of the mother's influence in the case, he should be alert to the possibility of marked discrepancies between the mother's and daughter's perception of the information that the mother had given to the daughter.

After gathering all the data, the clinician then decides which of three categories is most consonant with the patient's case:

Class I—Primary Dysmenorrhea A: primarily physiological determinants
Class II—Primary Dysmenorrhea B: important psychological determinants as well as physiological ones
Class III—Secondary Dysmenorrhea: pelvic pathology

The following section describes a treatment regimen for Primary Dysmenorrhea B consisting of pharmacotherapy combined with psychological intervention.

Treatment Regimen

Pharmacotherapy

The goal of pharmacotherapy is to reduce the immediate discomfort of dysmenorrhea. Although mild to moderate dysmenorrhea (Grade I) may respond to rest, heat (hot water bottle), and relaxation, the more severe grades (II and III) require measures strong enough to reduce such uterine activity as spasms. These effects may be accomplished with aspirin therapy administered prior to onset of menstruation. Aspirin is not effective when it is taken at the onset of cramps because it only inhibits prostaglandin synthesis, it does not exert an antagonistic action on prostaglandin receptors. When started 3 days prior to the expected onset of menstruation, aspirin (600 mg four times a day) has been reported to be effective in alleviating incapacitating dysmenorrhea in some adolescents (Klein et al., 1981), although there was also some evidence of increased menstrual blood loss. From our point of view, another disadvantage of aspirin therapy is that it forces the adolescent to start thinking of the onset of her period three days prior to it. For a patient with recurring dysmenorrhea this pain anticipation is neither desirable nor beneficial, and for the one with menstrual irregularity, it would be unquestionably detrimental.

Other prostaglandin inhibitors, such as mefenamic acid (Ponstel) and naproxen (Anaprox), also antagonize prostaglandin at receptor sites, which means that they can be administered when the onset of menstruation is impending and continued as needed for 1 or 2 days. This attribute makes them useful for the patient with menstrual irregularity. Recommended dosages (Neinstein, 1984) for drugs that are approved by the U.S. Food and Drug Administration for mild to moderate pain (ibuprofen and mefenamic acid) or specifically for dysmenorrhea (naproxen) are as follows:

Naproxen sodium (Anaprox): 550 mg initially, then 275 mg every 6 to 8 hours
Ibuprofen (Motrin): 400 mg three to four times a day
Mefenamic acid (Ponstel): 500 mg initially, then 250 mg every 6 to 8 hours

Although double-blind crossover studies have demonstrated the efficacy of mefenamic acid and naproxen, these drugs are not without risk. Potential side effects range from headaches to more serious side effects such as aplastic anaemia. In fact, it is the opinion of some investigators (see, for example, Klein et al., 1981) that widespread use of these drugs should be delayed until further testing demonstrates their safety. Potent analgesics containing opium derivatives such as codeine should generally be avoided. In some patients, however, combination preparations with codeine may be used sparingly for severe cramps of short duration.

Hormonal treatment may also be used. If the adolescent girl wants to use contraceptives, oral contraceptives will alleviate primary dysmenorrhea by suppressing ovulation, which in turn prevents endogenous production of progesterone and possibly affects prostaglandin liberation from the endometrium. This treatment is effective, simple, and generally well tolerated (Cholst & Carlon, 1987). When the drug is stopped each month, painless withdrawal bleeding occurs (Klein, 1980). Low-dose contraceptives such as Modicon, which contains 0.5 mg of norethindrone and 35μg of ethinyl estradiol, should be prescribed initially. If the lower dose fails to provide relief, a combination pill containing 50μg of ethinyl should prove effective. In younger adolescents it is wise to avoid ovulation suppression because of its possible effect on an immature axis (MacKenzie, 1980).

Jessop (1987) advocates the daily use of Vitamin B_6 and magnesium, the goal being to reduce the sensitivity of the nerve cells that react to the prostaglandins with a resultant decrease in the intensity of dysmenorrhea. According to preliminary research (Abraham, 1978) Vitamin B_6 diminishes the probability of strong uterine contractions and promotes relaxation of the uterine muscles. The magnesium facilitates the penetration by the vitamin of the membranes of the uterine cells. The treatment regimen that has proved successful consists of 200 mg each of Vitamin B_6 and magnesium per day for three months.

Psychological Intervention

The physiological dimension of primary dysmenorrhea has been the main focus of management procedures for the alleviation of this condition. There has been considerable interest in relaxation using direct teaching of relaxation procedures as well as in biofeedback. The rationale for this approach is as follows. There is evidence that during menstruation it is the dysrhythmic character of the contractions rather than their amplitude that is a correlate of severe pain. The pain sensation is a function of the combination of elevated uterine muscle tone and these dysrhythmic contractions that compress the blood vessels in the uterine smooth muscle tissue, with a consequent myometrial hypoxia (Filler & Hall, 1970). The lack of oxygen in turn inhibits the metabolism of the toxic chemical substance that is a by-product of the contraction so the pain receptors become irritated and they discharge, causing the diffused and deferred pain that results in abdominal cramps and also pain in the lower back and legs.

On the basis of Filler and Hall's (1970) conclusions, Heczey (1975) hypothesized that Luthe's (1963) autogenic relaxation exercises could produce responses incompatible with uterine tensing. Heczey's rationale was that if the uterine myometrium could be brought under voluntary control, its relaxation would correct the elevated muscle tone and painful contractions. Because muscle relaxation results in vasodilation and a subsequent rise in temperature, Heczey (1980) used a telethermometer to provide signals for uterine relaxation training. He demonstrated the efficacy of autogenic training facilitated by vaginal thermal biofeedback, with continued improvement shown (with patient compliance to daily relaxation exercises) in the first 2-month follow-up. Subjects who were given autogenic training in either individual or group sessions also improved but not to the same degree as subjects did with the autogenic relaxation-biofeedback combination. In addition to these manipulations, all participants were exposed to a reeducation program designed to correct negative misconceptions about the menstrual experience. Kohen (1980) has reported the successful use of relaxation/mental imagery with adolescents undergoing pelvic examinations.

Relaxation also played a part in the first published account of the use of behavior therapy for primary dysmenorrhea in which Mullen (1968) described the successful use of systematic desensitization with a 37-year-old woman. In order to desensitize this patient to anxieties relevant to menstrual symptomatology, she was required to engage in anxiety-provoking imagery of increasing intensity while she physically relaxed. In this case study and in a subsequent controlled investigation that included a no-treatment control condition (Mullen, 1971), systematic desensitization proved effective in reducing menstrual discomfort. Similar results were obtained with college students by Tasto and Chesney (1974) and Chesney and Tasto (1975b) with a treatment package that combined deep muscle relaxation and imagery consisting of scenes of menstrual pain reduction. It is unfortunate that none of these studies included a muscle-relaxation-training-only condition, since the combination program cannot be regarded as an empirical test of relaxation training. Once a patient has mastered the relaxation response, she can use it when confronted with any stress-producing situation. If she can then learn to identify stressful situations that are functionally related to her primary dysmenorrhea, she can use them as cues for initiating the relaxation response.

Meichenbaum (1977) has advocated a sequence in which a patient confronted with a stressor first reassures himself that he can cope with the situation by physical relaxation or some other coping skill, then implements the coping action, and finally rewards himself covertly for doing so. Although this procedure clearly has relevance for the self-management of primary dysmenorrhea, there are no reports in the literature of its use for this purpose. A similar disregard has been shown for other cognitive procedures, such as self-hypnosis and attention-diversion, that would appear to have considerable potential for reducing the subjective intensity of primary dysmenorrhea.

Regardless of the specific form of treatment selected, a program of patient reeducation should also be initiated. Inaccurate information and misconceptions concerning menstruation should be cleared up and the patient reassured that primary dysmenorrhea is not symptomatic of reproductive abnormality. As Iacono and Roberts (1983) have pointed out, there is also no empirical basis for either a dysmenorrhea personality or personal maladjustment as a causative factor in this condition. It may be necessary to use counseling with the mother in order to terminate or modify her input. One gynecologist started this process by insisting that the mother not mention anything about her daughter's periods for the next 3 months. The patient should also be reassured that the problem usually diminishes with time. In respect to this pattern, we offer the following hypothesis: The role of psychological stress as a major contributor in primary dysmenorrhea has been largely ignored or downgraded. There has been little or no concern about the mother's role as a possible source of misinformation and negative attitudes. This omission ignores the potential of the cumulative effects of generally stressful interpersonal relations in the home, a long-term stressor that becomes a part of the girl's life. The apparent diminishing with time of primary dysmenorrhea often coincides with the adolescent's separation from the household to attend college, work, or marry. It is our hypothesis that this separation from a long-term stressful situation is, for some adolescents, as important etiologically in the diminishing of primary dysmenorrhea as are the age-related physiological developments.

Burns

Although the number of burn injuries and burn-related deaths is not known (Wagner, 1977) it is clear from the available statistics that children are at high risk for burn injury. It is estimated that every year in the United States, 600,000 children under the age of 15 suffer burns, and of this group, 1 in 6 requires hospitalization (Welch, 1981). In fact, burns are responsible for more hospitalization days in children than any other injury (Warden, Kravitz, & Schnebly, 1981), and in North America (Snyder & Saieh, 1984) they are the second leading cause of death in children under age 15. For every death, three other children suffer serious disability. In approximately 75% of the cases, the child has caused his own burn (Breslin, 1975), a statistic that assumes great importance when one considers the additional burden of guilt.

The incidence of burns in the pediatric population is not evenly distributed across age groups. Instead, certain subgroups have been identified as at increased risk. Infants and children under age 3 represent a disproportionate number of burn cases. Sex differences in risk status do not occur until age 9, but from then until age 15 boys suffer three times as many burns as girls do, possibly because boys are more likely to play with materials of an inflammable or explosive nature. Children from low socioeconomic families are also at increased risk for burns (Libber & Stayton, 1984; Savage & Leitch, 1972). However, the commonly reported relationship between increased risk for burns and disturbed homes (see, for example, Bernstein's [1976] report that 80% of the children in a Boston burn unit were in this category) has been disputed. After reviewing the methodology of studies on disturbed homes, Wisely, Masur, and Morgan (1983) concluded that there was no firm empirical support for this variable as a predisposing factor. It is clear, however, that familial influences other than disturbances may be operating in the burn risk situation, for example, a lack of parenting ability or parental safety precautions or a tendency to overestimate the child's capabilities.

Medical Aspects and Care of Burns

This section provides a brief overview of the medical aspects and care of burns. More detailed accounts are beyond the scope of this book but can be found in a number of sources including Artz, Moncrief, and Pruitt (1979), Bernstein and Robson (1983), and Wagner (1977).

Burn injuries are categorized on the basis of histologic depth and other variables into first-, second-, and third-degree burns (see Table 7-1). Temporal progression of the injury and treatment within each of these categories follows a three-phase sequence (Welch, 1981).

Emergent Phase

The emergent phase covers the 72 hours immediately following the occurrence of the burn, with the treatment goal being to reduce the burn-related physiological shock. To this end the major focus of treatment is on the maintenance of the child's resuscitation and adequacy of the airway so that sufficient oxygenation can occur; maintenance of circulation, by remedying fluid losses, and body heat; and, while underlying tissues heal, prevention of infection by applying topical antibacterial agents, performing frequent burn dressing changes (BDC), and carrying out wound debridement. The infection problem can be a very serious one. After a severe burn the skin either no longer exists or is so badly damaged that it cannot perform its normal protective function against bacterial invasion. Furthermore, the warm, moist crust of dead tissue under the eschar that forms over the burn is an ideal environment for bacterial growth (Robson, 1983). Infection is a particular problem in children because their skin is relatively thin so that the bacterial invasion process occurs more rapidly than it does in older adolescents or adults. Should noncontained infection occur, it can result in slower healing of the wound and also graft rejection (O'Neill, 1979). If partial-thickness (second-degree) burns become infected, they may convert to full thickness, with subsequent treatment becoming more difficult and prolonged. Any event that prolongs treatment is particularly detrimental because children have a tendency to become increasingly intolerant of the pain the longer the treatment continues.

Physiological pain experienced during this phase is related to histological depth of the burn, but not on a one-to-one basis. Superficial second-degree burn areas result in the most pain because free-nerve endings are exposed. In the case of deep second-degree and third-degree burns, all layers of the skin are involved and the free-nerve endings have been largely destroyed so there may be less pain. Often the child is in a state of emotional shock and disintegration that tends to take two forms. One is a dream-like state in which he may talk lucidly but later have no memory of this period; the other, more common form, is an acute traumatic reaction with symptoms that include insomnia, emotional lability, exaggerated startle reflexes, and nightmares. Sometimes a major (Thorazine) or minor (Mellaril) tran-

Table 7-1 Burn Categories in Children

	First degree	Second degree (partial thickness)	Third degree (full thickness)
Criteria	*Minor* unless child is under 18 mos. or has experienced severe loss of fluids	*Minor*: less than 10% of body in children, less than 15% in adolescents *Moderate*: 10–30% in children or less than 15% with involvement of face, hands, feet, or perineum; minor chemical or electric *Severe*: more than 30%	*Minor*: less than 2 percent *Moderate*: 2–10% with any involvement of face, hands, feet, perineum *Severe*: more than 10% and major chemical or electric
Cause	Flash flame, excessive heat exposure, sunburn	Contact with hot liquids or solids, flash flame to clothing, direct flame, chemical	Contact with hot liquids or solids, flame, chemical, electricity
Skin Surface	Dry, no blisters, edema	Moist blobs, blisters	Dry with leathery eschar until debridement, charred blood vessels visible under eschar area
Pain Level	Painful	Very painful	Controversy re amount of pain: Wagner (1984) says little or no pain; Kibbee (1984) says moderate to severe pain
Histologic Depth	Epidermal layers only affected	Epidermis, papillary, and reticular layers of dermis; may include fat domes of sub-cutaneous layer	Down to and including subcutaneous tissue; may include fascia, muscle, and bone
Healing Time	2–5 days with peeling, no scarring but may have discoloration	Superficial burns: 5–21 days with no grafts. Deep burns with no infection: 21–35 days. If infected, burn converts to full thickness, equivalent to third degree	Large burn areas require grafting that may take many months. Small areas sometimes heal from edges after a few weeks

Adapted from Wagner (1984, p. 304).

quilizer is administered if the child is significantly out of control or experiences the toxic delirium that is sometimes referred to as burn psychosis (see Elliott, Miller, Funk, and Pruitt, 1987, for a brief but useful discussion of this phenomenon). By the end of the emergent phase the patient has usually recovered from the physiological and initial emotional shock of the experience.

Acute Phase

The acute phase begins at the end of the emergent phase and continues until complete skin coverage of the burn site has occurred. It has the highest mortality rate of the three phases and is also the most painful. The child is not, however, in a chronic pain state; rather, he is acutely ill for a long period. With superficial partial-thickness injuries, this phase is over within 21 days, but second-degree burns of deeper thickness extend this period to 5 weeks, or longer if there is infection. With third-degree burns this phase lasts until the wounds are covered with autografts (skin taken from the patient's body) or homografts (skin from a donor). The major objectives at this time are first to remove all eschar as soon as possible and start covering the wound area with autografts or homografts and second, to avoid complications or, if this is not possible, to initiate early aggressive treatment of them. The onset of complications tends to be sudden, so that the patient may be doing well one day and have a severe complication arise the next day.

Sources of Treatment-Related Pain   Burn dressing changes are made twice a day and involve several steps. The dressings must be removed, and if they do not come off easily they have to be soaked off with a 0.5% silver nitrate solution. When the dressings have been removed the next step is tubbing or tanking: The child is placed in a large hydrotherapy (Hubbard) tank in which the burn wound areas are soaked, washed, and rinsed, followed by piecemeal debridement. This latter and final step involves removing all loosened eschar by means of scissors or hemostat. If two or three experienced burn unit personnel work together, the dressings can be removed in about 15 to 20 minutes from a 70% burned patient (Wagner, 1977).

Every 3 hours the dressings must be soaked with a 0.5% silver nitrate solution to keep them moist: This helps the pain and makes the dressings easier to remove. Twice a day the child must do active range of motion exercises to prevent the development of contractures and consequent loss of function. All of these treatment steps may take about 45 to 60 minutes for each session. Every 5th or 6th day an additional step is added in which autografts or homografts are applied after debridement in order to protect the wound. This process is repeated until burned areas are fully covered and graft areas have healed.

Throughout the acute phase the child's pain must be assessed regularly, since the pain experience is highly individual. It is essential to acknowledge the child's reports of his pain and to convey confidence that improvement is possible. At the same time, pediatric personnel must avoid responses, such as consistently reward-

ing the child's catastrophizing and complaints, that are likely to elicit pain behaviors (Fordyce, 1976). The goal should be to demonstrate sympathetic concern
for the child's plight and encourage adaptive coping behavior. As the child settles
into the acute phase, he develops an awareness about the extent of his burns that is
likely to arouse anxiety. At this time emotional support in the form of helping the
child toward self-acceptance should be initiated. If the burn pain is to be optimally
managed, it is essential to reduce the anxiety, and one way to do this is to ensure
that the child has confidence in the burn unit personnel. He must know, for example, that they will give him pain medication when he needs it and that they believe
his accounts of the degree of pain he is experiencing. When pain medication is
requested but withheld, the child may see this as a lack of concern or even an
indication of malevolence on the part of the staff. Should the child feel uncertain of
this support, his anxiety will increase along with a concomitant increase in pain.

Rehabilitation Phase

This phase follows the acute phase and lasts until the child's potential in terms of
function and appearance has been achieved. The specific concerns at this time are
to restore maximum possible function in joint surfaces that were scarred, provide
continued emotional support, and equip the child with the skills that he will require to combat the stress associated with his return to school and the peer group.
It is almost useless to rely solely on discussions with the child's teacher or talks to
his classmates as a way of easing the transition for the child (Cahners, 1979). A far
more effective approach is to combine the latter approach with teaching the child
skills for coping with the barbaric behavior that he is unfortunately likely to meet
should he have any visible disfigurement or physical disability. Instruction in such
skills as coping with teasing (Ross & Ross, 1984d) should be an integral part of the
rehabilitation phase activities.

After the initial discharge, it will be necessary to continue physiotherapy over
the long term in order to counteract the effects of scarring over the child's joints
and the consequent retardation in his growth and development. Emotional support
should also be maintained in helping the child master the various social hurdles
that he will face, without damage to his self-esteem. In any such interventions, it is
essential that the child's cognitive level be considered.

Medical Setting

Major burns are beyond the capabilities of the general hospital setting and are best
handled in a children's burn unit with a well-established multidisciplinary approach that acknowledges the emotional as well as the physical problems associated with children's burn injuries. Placing pediatric burn patients in adult burn
units is unsatisfactory. Children require special help in coping beyond that of adult
needs: In fact, often the psychological damage and subsequent management of it

are more important to the child's prognosis than is the extent of the organic injury. From a practical viewpoint, children need a steady stream of visitors (parents, siblings, teachers, peers) and this is disrupting in the adult burn units. In respect to sibling and peer visitors (and, unfortunately, some adults), a briefing routine should be set up to prepare these visitors for the child's appearance and to prevent damaging reactions to it.

Burn Team

The care of the child with burns is a team task in which physicians head a multi-disciplinary group of exceptionally broad range. In addition to the burn unit nurses, the staff includes a physiotherapist whose responsibility it is to maintain function in muscles and joints and respiration; a social worker who acts as a link with the child's family, some of whom may be a source of helpful information concerning the child's special needs; a dietician who must meet the severely burned child's vital need for adequate nutrition in the face of his strong inclination to turn away from food; and a teacher who provides a link with the child's "other" life. A child life worker should also be a member of the team because the most effective psychological support may come from someone who is not involved in any phase of the child's direct physical care but is a constant positive presence. Psychiatrists and psychologists complete the team roster (Morris & McFadd, 1978). For interesting accounts of the roles of psychiatrists in burn management see Bernstein, Sanger, and Fras (1969), Nover (1973), and Sykes (1979).

Traditional Burn Treatment Procedure

The child is usually, but not always, given drugs an hour before the BDC (Perry & Heidrich, 1982). They may be narcotics such as morphine, meperidine, or fentanyl; nonnarcotic analgesics such as aspirin and Tylenol; or tranquilizers (Valium or Mellaril) (Sykes, 1979). When narcotics are the choice, they are administered intravenously because intramuscular injections are not as readily absorbed and may also have a cumulative effect when remobilization of fluid occurs, with consequent respiratory difficulty. The problem with the narcotics is that they may cause vomiting or nausea, which in turn creates problems for fulfilling the nutritional needs of the burned child. In any event, analgesics are adjuncts to other forms of intervention: The complexity, severity, and potential duration of problems confronting the pediatric burn patient require the use of a variety of intervention procedures.

In addition to the guidelines concerning drug treatment, the traditional approach involves an assortment of other recommendations specifically for management of the BDC procedure. Nurses are customarily told to "stay in control" and also to use distraction techniques. It is not clear how these directives could be handled simultaneously with the ongoing dressing change demands, nor are the kinds of distraction specified that are feasible in this situation. Some children prefer that the staff keep talking and use objects to distract them, whereas others require silence in order to hold on to their shaky self-control:

> They [BDC] should be done fast, quick, and soft, with no talking. (Girl, CA 7, Wagner, 1977)

> I needed all I got to get through it and when they [burn personnel] talked to me it was hard because it takes some of me to listen to them. I wanted to say, "Shut up." (Boy, CA 8, Ross & Ross, 1982a)

Similar vague recommendations are usually made that the child should participate actively and as much as possible in the BDC process. What this entails is not clear. Burn unit personnel are also advised to encourage the child to verbalize his feelings. The problem is that often the child fears and hates the team that performs the BDC, a reaction that eliminates any possibility that he would confide in them, particularly since his comments would probably be of a critical nature. If the child is one of the group of approximately 75% of burn cases responsible for causing the burns (Breslin, 1975) he may be overwhelmed with guilt, prefer to see his pain as just punishment for his sins, and decide that as part of the punishment he should remain silent. As Bernstein (1976) has pointed out, this behavior occurs at great psychological cost to the child. The psychiatric members of the burn unit *must* help the child deal with the guilt, however, because otherwise it will function as a significant deterrent to the adjustments that are of critical importance to the child's psychological survival. Supportive psychotherapy is readily available for adolescents and older children during hospitalization (Seligman, Macmillan, & Carroll, 1971), with play therapy for younger children. Play therapy may be of only limited use because the child often is unable to make physical contact with play objects because of occlusive dressings and immobilization. Other approaches are clearly needed. Parental presence is also considered to be of some help during BDC and at other times, but this source of comfort may be limited by the fact that the parent not only cannot stop the pain but often is unable to make physical contact with the child because of isolation procedures and other treatment-related restrictions.

In view of the limitations inherent in these recommendations, it is not surprising that the BDC procedure becomes a twice-daily obstacle of major proportions even when the recommendations are followed as well as possible by skilled burn teams. Although differences in reaction to the whole process are partly related to the child's level of cognitive development, his behavior, despite age differences, generally consists of the following kinds of responses. He is negative to all tactics of the pediatric personnel, such as time-outs and incentives, and cannot be distracted; and he is physically aggressive to the nurses (bites, claws, scratches) and verbally abusive (swears, calls them names) (Walker & Healy, 1980). These behaviors jeopardize the treatment schedule and also generalize to all pediatric personnel so that the environment becomes one of all-encompassing threat to the child. In light of this, the fact that the child screams, cries, and pleads for mercy even during nonaversive events (Elliott & Olson, 1983) is completely rational. From week to week the child may become increasingly more obstructive to all treatment and in the struggle may inadvertently damage his burn wounds (Kavanagh, 1983a). He often refuses to eat, withdraws within himself, is angry, has temper tantrums in which he breaks everything that he can throw, and perceives the treatment as punishment. These markedly regressive behaviors occur most often in children and adolescents who are psychologically immature. Note that *limited* regression is an adaptive response in that it allows the child to adjust to a dependent situation. What we are talking about here is the child or adolescent who is virtually unmanageable because of excessive irritability, insatiable demands and complaints, and disruptive physical behaviors.

To a large group of pediatric personnel in the burn unit arena, these reactions by the child are seen as the inevitable result of unmodifiable and continuing pain coupled with the knowledge, for many children, that permanent change of an undesirable sort has occurred. Two notable exceptions have been reported in the literature in the form of specific changes that could be made in the traditional treatment process (Beales, 1983) and presentation of a new burn treatment model (Kavanagh, 1983a).

An Expectancy Approach

On the basis of careful observations over a 6-month period in a pediatric burn unit and extensive interviews with the patients, Beales (1983) contends that the traditional treatment system creates fear, anxiety, and expectations of pain. The children, two thirds of whom were boys, were from 4 weeks to 15 years of age and had burns ranging from minor ones that nevertheless required a few days in hospital to life-threatening burns needing extensive surgery and a long-term hospital stay. Beales analyzed the problems that occurred in terms of possible causes and then made recommendations for improvements.

A major discrepancy was apparent between the children's cognitions concerning optimum treatment and the actual treatment. The children's idea of recovery from a burn wound was to keep it still and leave it undisturbed. The BDC procedure and physiotherapy violated these cognitions. Beales thought that the children should be helped to see the treatment as desirable rather than as physical assault and that in this reeducation process the cognitive level of the child should determine the approach. (Leavitt [1979] gives an excellent example of sensitive and skilled management of burn trauma and treatment pain carried out in accordance with the cognitive level of an adolescent boy.) The use of physical restraint during BDC terrified the children and heightened their feelings of helplessness. Here the recommendation concerned having the child help in the procedure in order for him to have a feeling of at least partial control in the situation. The effects of other children's behaviors were often negative; for example, modeling of pain occurred when the children could overhear screams, and the "veterans" on the ward frequently gave exaggerated accounts of what was to come. This negative input usually made the newer patients expect the worst. Although input from other children can undoubtedly have a psychologically detrimental effect on the child, there is no question that the presence of same-age peers is preferable to isolation (Kueffner, 1976).

Although Beales (1983) has made no suggestions on this point, there are some possibilities for counteracting these peer effects. It might be possible to put the newer patients together in a room or have a child life worker present as a buffer for long periods of time when new patients arrive on the ward. Beales found that having instruments set out on a loaded trolley and in place for several minutes before the BDC occurred raised anxiety and apprehension, the simple solution being to keep the trolley covered until the last minute. The sight of burn damage when the bandages were off was tremendously upsetting for all the children, but particularly so for the adolescents. The slow rate of healing, which was quite apparent, was also discouraging for them. Here, too, the suggestion was to keep the wound out of sight as much as possible. One solution to this problem would be to prevent the patient from observing the wound by giving him a task that involves an incompatible response. For example, tape-recorded tasks having high appeal and, of course, content appropriate to the patient's cognitive level could be used. This suggestion should be particularly useful in keeping the child's burn wound out of his line of vision at those points when it is impossible to keep the wound covered and it is preferable to having him close his eyes. The distraction practices that Beales did observe were not well prepared and consequently were ineffective. As one would expect, the children became familiar with the BDC procedure to the point where they could anticipate the worst parts and thus showed great fear prior to the onset of the heightened pain. Often the burn personnel's conversation functioned as conditioned stimuli that indicated that difficult parts were approaching, leading the child to expect severe pain. Beales recommended that conversation be modified to eliminate such cues. We advocate that the burn personnel have a code covering such events, with periodic changes in it to prevent the child from decoding the messages.

Kavanagh's Burn Treatment Model

Kavanagh's (1983a) model represents a radical departure from the traditional treatment procedure. The rationale for it is based on learned helplessness theory (Seligman, 1968, 1975) that has great relevance for both the clinical context of BDC and the children's reactions to them (Beales, 1983). Seligman believes that what determines the stressfulness of an aversive event is not its intensity but, instead, whether or not it is predictable and controllable. Unpredictable and uncontrollable aversive events, especially those of an intense, frequent, or prolonged nature, lead to experimental neurosis, a confluence of cognitive/affective/somatic disturbances. The symptomatology of experimental neurosis includes agitation followed by lethargy and depression, feeding disturbances, chronic anxiety, passivity, withdrawal, and difficulty distinguishing aversive from nonaversive experience. All in all, Seligman's description is a textbook picture of the burned child's behavior under the traditional treatment procedure. Note that we are not saying that this child has a neurosis: what we are saying is that there is a remarkable similarity between Seligman's experimental neurosis description and case reports of the behavior of burned children when their injuries are handled within the traditional treatment approach. The following case study of a traditional treatment (Kavanagh, 1983a, pp. 613–614) illustrates this point:

Despite a supportive burn unit team who encouraged the mother to be with her 5-year-old daughter whenever possible, offered distractions in the form of movies and other diverting objects, were verbally soothing and encouraging, administered liberal dosages of pain and anxiety medication prior to dressing changes, and were themselves competent, quick, and confident, the patient exhibited all of Seligman's experimental neurosis behaviors. The child had 40% third-degree burns that had resulted from match play. Observations of her behavioral response to her burn injury and its treatment over an 8-week period showed the following behavior patterns.

Week 1: Anxious, whiney, very angry, and somewhat depressed.
Week 2: Described by mother as agitated and angry and by staff as "hostile." High level of protest for all procedures.
Week 3: Protests increase and pain tolerance decreases during BDC. Not so depressed but is very demanding and anxious, and refuses to eat. Screaming is uncontrollable during BDC, and incentives, time-outs, and withdrawal of privileges have no effect.
Week 4: High anxiety now during BDC. Eating problems continue, demanding and whiney, and screams for nonaversive events.
Week 5: Problem behaviors all continue with vigorous protest and screaming during BDC. Mother's presence has no effect.
Week 6: Angry and very negative, fighting with younger patient, screaming for everything. High anticipatory anxiety but more cooperative during BDC.
Week 7: Although healing is almost complete, protest and screaming during BDC. Striking out physically at staff, labile mood, eating problems persist.
Week 8: Continues to be anxious, angry, and somewhat depressed. Hyperactive, hyperverbal. Temper tantrums. Eating problems.

Although the burn unit routine depicted in this case study could be regarded as having some degree of predictability, in Kavanagh's (1983a) model predictability is markedly increased: The burn unit nurse wears a special uniform such as a bright red apron and, in order to focus the child's attention on the BDC, she provides as much sensory and procedural information as possible both prior to and during each step. (Note that these methods contradict the procedures advocated in almost all textbooks on burn pain.) From the beginning of the BDC the child is encouraged to actively participate by making decisions, such as where to start or when to have a break, and to help with specific steps, such as removing dressings or washing wounds. Keeping well within the bounds of safety and under the nurse's close supervision, a child as young as age 2 can take on this active role, and for the older child, the expectations concerning what he can do increase. If a child resists, the nurse encourages him to do some small task and persists with this expectation, with gradual daily increases in the demands. Throughout all of this increased control on the part of the child, the nurse remains in charge: She sets time limits for the child's tasks, with the cautionary comment that she will have to finish them if the child is too slow, and sets up prearranged rest periods by having the child at his own speed count to 10 before having a break. The counting periods are not used as distractions because during them the child is encouraged to watch what is happening and comment on how the wounds feel and look. All the while, the nurse is giving information on what is being done, how the wound is progressing, and what the next step will be.

Active participation by the child in the BDC procedure precludes the use of heavy medication. Kavanagh recommends that narcotics be either used conservatively or discontinued. The case that follows (Kavanagh, 1983a, p. 616) describes the reaction to the Kavanagh procedure of an 11-year-old boy with first- and second-degree burns on his abdomen, groin, penis, and left upper thigh.

> Rick was initially approached in the standard way. During that time his major problems involved dressing change anxiety and pain and persistent vomiting. His combative behavior during burn care exhausted the patience of the staff and interfered with adequate debridement. . . . By the ninth hospital day, Rick was receiving 65 mg of Demerol intramuscularly and 5 mg of diazepam (Valium) by mouth prior to burn care, and additional intravenous Demerol after burn care for continuing pain and anxiety.
>
> On the fifteenth hospital day . . . the [Kavanagh] experimental approach to dressing change . . . was implemented. A positive response was seen immediately. For the first time, sedation after dressing change was not required. Rick's tolerance of the dressing change continued to improve over the next two days, at which time he was discharged. . . . During these last 2 days, dressing change premedication consisted of Tylenol and 10 mg of Valium by mouth, or nothing. The patient's pre-dressing change anxiety had disappeared . . . and he appeared happy and relaxed between dressing changes. Rick's behavioral progress was maintained during a second hospitalization.

Kavanagh makes it quite clear that this new model is not a panacea. The BDC procedure continues to elicit protests and anger. However, the anger does not reach the level of unresponsive rage characteristic of many children undergoing traditional treatment procedures, and the protest does not interfere with the ongoing procedures. Although many children do experience some degree of anorexia, with tube feedings required, the persistent vomiting or diarrhea usually accompanying the BDC procedures tends not to occur. There is grief, but not incapacitating withdrawal; as recovery progresses, anxiety and pain appear to diminish somewhat rather than plateau or increase, and wound healing typically progresses without complications. Compared with the traditional approach, the overall impression is that with this model the child is better able to tolerate the whole procedure.

In support of her model, Kavanagh readily acknowledges that the extensive and detailed case study data that have been collected are anecdotal. However, the data are consistent with experimentally documented trends in her other work (Kavanagh, 1983b) that provide some empirical support for the model. This support is weakened by methodological shortcomings in choice of dependent variables and the excessive number of statistical procedures used, as well as by the use of very small groups. These shortcomings are readily remedied and should not obscure the potential value of this treatment model.

A replication of Kavanagh's participation versus diversion study at the Shriners' Burns Institute in Boston (Lasoff & McEttrick, 1986) has confirmed her original hypothesis and has also provided evidence of a reduced need for pain medication in the participation group. Furthermore, follow-up data showed that children in the participation group had returned to school and resumed normal or near normal social activity whereas those in the diversion group were characterized by school absenteeism and social withdrawal.

Psychological Intervention

Although many of the burned child's responses to the wounds and their treatment clearly have a psychological base, scant attention in the form of either theoretical or empirical interest has been paid to this aspect of the treatment problem. One of the few general statements on psychological aspects of pain management of the burned child has been made by McGrath and Vair (1984), and empirical studies have ranged from multitreatment packages through single-treatment evaluation to minor changes directed at a narrow range of behavior change. Group size has been small and methodology frequently less than rigorous, an exception being the methodologically sophisticated example of the use of operant conditioning with a 3-year-old burn patient (Varni et al., 1980) described in Chapter 6. Despite the various weaknesses and omissions of many of the studies, it is clear that definite advantages could accrue from incorporating the psychological approach in the management of pediatric burn patients.

As an adjunct to pharmacotherapy, Wakeman and Kaplan (1978) reported some success with hypnotherapy in a controlled prospective study involving three age groups, one of which included children and adolescents (CA 7–18). Those in the experimental group learned to use self-hypnosis whereas those in the control group received supportive psychotherapy, with the dependent variable being percent of maximum permissible analgesic per day. For high as well as low levels of body surface burned, those in the self-hypnosis group used significantly lower levels of analgesic. These results were strongest for the children and adolescents, possibly because of the greater hypnotic susceptibility of children compared with adults. However, the results are tempered by several methodological flaws: Sample size was small, no measures were obtained for perceived pain or observed distress, and there were no controls for either an expectancy effect or a placebo effect.

Cases involving the use of individual hypnotherapy have also been reported. Gardner and Olness (1981, pp. 231–232, 170–171) used self-hypnosis with great success to help a 4-year-old girl and a 13-year-old boy cope with BDC. There is no question that once a child has learned self-hypnosis he can use it in related situations. In a dramatic example of such transfer, Betcher (1960) reported the case of a 10-year-old girl who used self-hypnosis successfully for BDC and then used it 6 months later when she was unable to have general anesthesia with surgery for severe flexion contractures. Successful use of hypnosis has been described with other cases of severe burns in children (Bernstein, 1963, 1965; LaBaw, 1973; Woodley, 1959) but, as Turner and Chapman (1982b) have pointed out, these studies have generally not been controlled so other factors could be operative in the treatment.

To reduce BDC distress in four children ages 6 to 11, Elliott and Olson (1983) used a treatment package that included attention-distraction procedures, reinforcement of coping skills, emotive imagery, and breathing-induced relaxation. A combined multiple baseline and reversal design included behavioral observations with the Procedural Behavior Rating Scale (PBRS) (Katz et al., 1980). Substantial reductions in distress were reported when the therapist was present in a coaching role, but the benefits did not generalize to noncoaching days. Walker and Healy (1980) also used a treatment package, but theirs included behavior modification, relaxation training, story-telling techniques, play therapy, and parent counseling. The patient was an 8-year-old girl with second- and third-degree burns whose fear of the treatment procedures, primarily the BDC, had generalized to all experiences involving nurses, causing her to scream uncontrollably and lash out physically when they approached. The treatment package interventions were successful in helping the child adjust to the trauma and treatment and to establish a degree of personal control. Kelley, Jarvie, Middlebrook, McNeer, and Drabman (1984) used cartoons as distractors and reinforcers for distress reduction below baseline in a reversal design assessing the impact of distress-attenuating procedures on two girls (CA 4 and CA 6) with second- and third-degree burns. Frequency of distress behaviors was assessed by independent observers with the PBRS (Katz et al., 1980). Both children exhibited significant reductions in distress during intervention as well as the expected return to baseline levels under the reversal condition. Shorkey and Taylor (1973) demonstrated the value for the severely burned child of an unequivocal signal that a BDC that had to be performed at his bedside was imminent. St. Lawrence and Drabman (1983) used a response-interruption device with a 10-month-old burn patient whose self-excoriation of grafted skin had exacerbated her injuries. The procedure proved to be highly effective in halting further self-inflicted tissue damage. Knudson-Cooper (1981) has reported the successful use of relaxation and biofeedback in the treatment of severely burned children.

Comment

Bonica (1980, p. 7) has noted that major advances in the critical care of burns have increased the survival rate of burn victims but that the problem of pain relief for them has received little attention:

> Burns . . . produce continuous pain that is aggravated each time the patient moves the area of the burn; it is an excruciating experience for the patient and those who care for him . . . each time the dressing is changed. The psychologic, emotional, and physiologic stress of burn pain on the patient, the family, and the health care team is immeasurable. Despite its overwhelming clinical importance, no serious research on burn pain has been done and little effort has been spent on devising more effective methods of relieving the pain. This is another serious health care problem in which massive efforts have been made to improve the care of all the other aspects of the disorder but the pain problem has been completely neglected.

A similar criticism could be leveled at the lack of investigative interest in psychological intervention for children with burns in comparison to that in other painful conditions of a less serious nature, such as recurrent abdominal pain and headaches. New directions in psychological intervention that should be considered for pediatric burn patients include the following. A series of cartoon films could be prepared to show sequential modeling within each phase of the burn treatment process. A coping model in the form of a cartoon character would progress through the burn treatment process just ahead of the child; for example, the model would be shown in the emergent phase and then move into the acute phase just ahead of the child. During each sequence the model would display coping strategies, discuss reasons for the procedures, and mention novel ideas such as the fact that the procedure is not easy for the burn treatment team. All of this information would be presented within a reasonably interesting and as cheerful as possible, continued story framework, with the child seeing the film perhaps every 2 or 3 days, if not oftener.

In comparison with other health-related concepts such as illness (Neuhauser, Amsterdam, Hines, & Steward, 1978), the concept of healing is a difficult one for the child to grasp. It is even more difficult for him to view an unsightly burn area as a positive step in the healing process. These ideas could be depicted with great clarity in a cartoon presentation.

Clinical studies (Fordyce, 1976) and experimental investigations (Locke, Shaw, Saari, & Latham, 1981) have demonstrated the efficacy of setting quotas in managing chronic pain problems and improving tolerance for experimental pain. Dolce, Doleys, et al. (1986) reported similar results and also found that with their volunteer undergraduate subjects, offering monetary prizes for quota achievement did not increase pain tolerance levels already reached with quotas alone. These general findings are consistent with other research demonstrating that performance motivation can be enhanced by having the subjects compare ongoing performance with a set standard. When the subjects themselves set the standard, high positive correlations have been obtained between actual tolerance and the quota set (Dolce, Doleys, et al., 1986). This quota procedure could be adapted for use with burn patients in the pediatric setting. To establish a baseline of performance, the child's behavior during BDC could be observed with respect to time, that is, number of seconds before he becomes disruptive. On the basis of this information, the child would then set a quota for the duration of time that he thinks he can go without becoming disruptive, and the BDC is done with attention to this amount of time.

It is possible that the quota procedure is improving self-control rather than effecting a change in pain tolerance, but it is also likely that it would help the child through the procedure with less upset. In support of this idea, Kleck et al. (1976) have provided some evidence for the positive effects of outward calm on reducing inner turmoil. The quota procedure also functions as a distractor and enhances the child's feeling of being in control, which in itself contributes to his self-esteem. If the aforementioned cartoon modeling procedure is used, the quota system lends itself to competition in quotas between child and film model. The model could slowly increase his aspirations about his quota and sometimes drop back. It would be essential to avoid putting undue pressure on the child and to maintain the model at a coping rather than a mastery level.

Migraine Headache

Traditionally, a dichotomous model of headaches has distinguished migraine from the tension or muscle-contraction headache (Ad Hoc Committee on Classification of Headache, 1962). However, some investigators have questioned this dichotomy and have supported a continuous model. On the basis of a factor analytic study of adult headache patients, Ziegler, Hassanein, and Hassanein (1972), for example, have proposed that the two headache types might be on the same etiological continuum and that the differences in symptomatology might be attributed to different degrees of underlying vascular involvement. Other factor analytic studies, such as that of Kroner (1983), have disputed these findings by documenting stable and valid syndrome factors that distinguish the tension and migraine categories. Until the issue is decided by further rigorous evaluation of the continuum model, the dichotomous model will likely prevail. In this discussion we shall treat migraine as distinct from tension headache.

Prevalence estimates of migraine in children, reported in epidemiological studies conducted in Europe (Andrasik, Blake, & McCarran, 1986), vary widely from 2.7% to 18.8% of the pediatric population (Waters, 1971). In the first decade of life, migraine presents in an estimated 2% to 4% of infants and children (Ryan & Ryan, 1978). In studying children with more severe migraine, Bille (1981) found that two children at ages 1 and 2 had recurrent periods of crying, pallor, and vomiting that at age 3 were accompanied by complaints of headaches. The prognosis for spontaneous remission is better for boys than for girls (Bille, 1981) and, in both groups, is better if the onset occurs in childhood rather than in puberty (Neinstein, 1984). In a sophisticated epidemiological study conducted in Sweden (Bille, 1962), evidence of a sex × age interaction was documented. Prior to age 10 there were no sex differences in probability of migraine headaches, but after that point more girls than boys suffered from migraine, and this sex difference was maintained into adulthood. These findings have been supported by recent studies in Sweden (Egermark-Eriksson, 1982) and Finland (Sillanpaa, 1983), but the etiological factors related to the differential incidence that occurs in early adolescence have not been identified. Although there is no direct evidence of a causative relationship between increased migraine headaches in girls and the onset of puberty and menarche (Deubner, 1977), the female hormone estrogen, which is a natural vasodilator, appears to be implicated in migraines in women. Many adolescent girls and women report that migraine attacks coincide with their menstrual periods, a point when estrogen production is high; the estrogen in oral contraceptives precipitates attacks of migraine; and migraines diminish in frequency and intensity with menopause, a time when estrogen production also diminishes.

Experienced investigators have attributed the migraine headache to an interaction between a constitutional predisposition, probably genetically transmitted, which makes the child vulnerable to migraine but is not sufficient in itself to cause it, and an environmental precipitant or trigger. Some support for a heritability factor comes from studies that have documented a high incidence of recurrent headaches in the biological relatives of migraineurs (Bille, 1981; Lance & Anthony, 1966; Ziegler, 1978). However, when the criteria used are rigorous, the prevalence of migraine among relatives drops sharply (Bakal, 1982), and when studies of twins are reviewed, the evidence for a genetic factor becomes less impressive. Bille (1981) has suggested the possibility that transmission of a predisposition to migraines is sex linked, with headache-prone offspring being predominantly female, in other words, a mother–daughter heritability link. Although these approaches to the question of heritability have merit, several methodological problems make it difficult to accept the various findings as firm support for it. One of the criteria for establishing a diagnosis of migraine is the presence of migraine in one or more first-degree relatives and, as Waters (1971) has pointed out, this selection bias artificially inflates the family concordance rate. Then, too, the data are retrospective reports from the migraine patients themselves, and the size of the sample is small. An additional complication is the fact that research on the transmission of other chronic or recurring conditions suggests that observational learning could be operative in the etiology of migraine (Craig, 1978; Hughes & Zimin, 1978; Violon & Giurgea, 1984).

Two other predisposing factors that have been investigated are the "migraine personality" and specific personality attributes, such as depression. Although the stereotype for migraineurs suggests an obsessive, rigid, goal-oriented perfectionistic individual, attempts to demonstrate such a construct have floundered in the face of methodological weaknesses including the use of nonstandardized rating scales and incomplete procedural information on how subjects were matched (Andrasik et al., 1986). In any event, there is at present little evidence to support the existence of a well-defined migraine personality. A similar lack of progress has characterized attempts to demonstrate a causal link between depression and migraine (Andrasik et al., 1986). Andrasik and his colleagues (Andrasik, Kabela, Quinn, Blanchard, & Rosenblum (1985) instead report research suggesting that depression may be a consequence of migraine rather than a precursor to it and that this depression may be age related, with older children showing higher levels of depression than younger ones. Research is needed to determine whether depression precedes or follows the development of chronic headache symptoms of migraine. Data should also be collected on children with other forms of chronic pain to determine whether they exhibit similar depressive reactions. In juvenile rheumatoid arthritis, for example, all the clinical evidence points to depression following the onset of arthritis, as the significance of the disease becomes apparent to the child (Beales, Keen, & Holt, 1983).

Precipitating Factors

The most commonly reported migraine precipitant in children and adolescents is psychological stress from a number of sources, such as school demands, unexpected excitement, or pressure (Leviton, Slack, Masek, Bana, & Graham, 1984). It is interesting that neither children (Andrasik, Kabela, Quinn, Blanchard, & Rosenblum, 1985) nor adults (Andrasik, Blanchard, et al., 1982) with recurring migraine headaches differ in levels of stress from headache-free controls. Apparently it is the heightened mode of response to everyday stressors that precipitates the migraine headaches (Andrasik et al., 1986). Note that in all these studies the analyses of the link between stress and headache have been based on retrospective information. What is needed now are prospective studies with repeated assessment to verify the role of stress as a trigger for pediatric migraine. Other precipitants to migraine include physical stressors such as eyestrain, fatigue, and overexertion. In the case of the young adolescent, the hormonal changes that occur prior to menstruation and during it are clearly implicated, as are the hormones in birth control pills for a wider age range. For a minority of children, certain food substances (Bille, 1962) serve as precipitants, but the link between dietary triggers and migraine remains controversial. For a critical review of this issue see Kohlenberg (1982).

The factors that precipitate migraine are not necessarily those that maintain it (Andrasik et al., 1986). In many instances the adult's response to a child's complaint of headache is in the form of physical and verbal attention that may involve secondary gains such as absence from school or being excused from household responsibilities. These social environmental contingencies may function in concert with physiological factors to reinforce headache pain. It follows that predispositional and precipitating factors may be responsible for the occurrence of migraines but that other elements take over for their maintenance. An intriguing shift in the status of the precipitants of migraine has been described by Andrasik et al. (1986, p. 413):

> Although childhood headaches initially appear to be clearly associated with life stresses, as headache severity and frequency increase, a growing autonomy of headache symptoms from identifiable stressors also increases (Joffe et al., 1983). Bakal (1979, 1982) and colleagues have attempted to explain this phenomenon by suggesting that one consequence of recurrent attacks is a physiological and psychological shift in which the symptoms and anticipation of the pain act as triggers themselves. Thus, those with the most severe and more frequent attacks often awaken with a headache in the morning before an anticipated stressful event (Joffe et al., 1983).

Diagnosis

A thorough diagnostic evaluation includes a detailed history, complete physical and neurological examinations, allergy and histamine tests, and careful psychological assessment. This general diagnostic workup should also include tests to eliminate the possibility of brain tumors or cerebral vascular malformations. Although the probability of missing such diagnoses is minimal in cases of childhood migraine (Tal, Dunn, & Crichton, 1984), it cannot be ignored.

Migraine headaches have been categorized as classic, common, cluster, and complicated (Ad Hoc Committee on Classification of Headache, 1962). The majority of childhood migraines fall into the common category, but nearly all types have been recognized from infancy onward. Although this classification system has been accepted, there are no universally accepted criteria for the diagnosis of childhood migraine. Prensky and Sommer (1979) have devised the following criteria: Recurrent headache separated by symptom-free intervals and any three of the following:

1. Abdominal pain, nausea, or vomiting with the headache
2. Hemicrania
3. A throbbing pulsatile quality of pain
4. Complete relief after a brief period of rest
5. A visual, sensory, or motor aura
6. A history of migraine headache in one or more members of the immediate family

The child's headache symptomatology as well as relevant pain parameters such as duration, frequency, intensity, and medication intake may be assessed by interview or questionnaire. Both methods yield retrospective data subject to inaccuracies that in themselves may provide insights on the case. In addition to the commonly used questionnaires specifically for headache, the use of one of the following three general pain questionnaires should also be considered. These are the Children's Comprehensive Pain Questionnaire (McGrath, P.A., 1986), the Varni/Thompson Pediatric Pain Questionnaire (Varni & Thompson, 1985), and the McGill Pain Questionnaire (Melzack, 1975). Self-monitoring of ongoing headache activity with a headache diary has been used by Richter et al. (1986). In addition to tailoring the diary demands to the specific symptomatology of the child (Epstein & Abel, 1977), the effect of the number of demands on self-monitoring compliance should also be considered. In general, the fewer the demands, the greater the probability of compliance by the child.

To assess the child's headache behavior, information should be obtained from him and others on his observable physical and behavioral responses that are headache-relevant as well as on environmental stressors that relate to the headaches but do so in an indirect way so that the sequence effect may not be obvious to the child. The possibility that secondary and tertiary gains are implicated must also be explored. To aid in identifying the variant of migraine that best describes the child's headaches, psychophysiological assessment is also essential.

This information is highly relevant to treatment procedures. For example, if the onset of migraine is sharply defined as in the prodromal period of classic migraine, it might be advantageous to initiate self-control strategies early in the headache cycle. If, as in common migraine, the prodromal phase is not well defined and, in fact, consists of vague autonomic experiences with no clear signal for onset, then such strategies in the early phases would be difficult to implement and would serve little function. On completion of the diagnostic work-up, the child or adolescent should be reassured that the problem is modifiable and primed on the active role that he will be expected to play if marked improvement is to occur.

Pharmacotherapy

Three types of pharmacological agent recommended in the treatment of migraine in adults have also been used with children.

Prophylactic Medication

Prophylactic agents are used to prevent the occurrence of severe, recurrent attacks of migraine and typically are taken daily for a prescribed period. Of the rather heterogeneous group of anticonvulsants, antidepressants, antihypertensives, and other agents that are available, only propranolol (Inderal), papaverine (Pavabid), and clonidine (Catapres) have been subjected to controlled trials in children and adolescents, and of these three, only propranolol has been labeled by the FDA for the treatment of migraine. Propranolol has been widely used with the pediatric population and has the advantage of minimal side effects (fatigue, hypotension, nausea). It is the drug of choice for severe migraine in adolescents, with a recommended initial dosage of 40 to 80 mg per day, increasing up to 240 mg per day as needed (Neinstein, 1984). Contraindications include children with asthma, allergic rhinitis during the pollen season, and heart decompensation.

Experimental data on propranolol have a certain ambivalence. For 21 of the 28 children in Ludvigsson's (1974) double-blind, placebo-control, crossover design study, it proved significantly more effective in that there were either no headaches or only negligible symptoms when compared with placebo, in which such improvements were rare. In contrast to these results, Forsythe, Gillies, and Sills (1984) were unable to demonstrate a more positive effect with propranolol than placebo with regard to frequency, severity, and duration of headaches and, in fact, reported a trend toward increased headache frequency with propranolol. To date, the best study of the efficacy of propranolol in the management of juvenile migraine was one which involved a double-blind, placebo-controlled, single crossover comparison of propranolol (3 mg/kg/d) and self-hypnosis (Olness et al., 1987). Over a 3-month period, self-hypnosis produced a significant reduction in number of headaches in the children ages 6 to 12, who were participating in the study, whereas propranolol proved no more effective than placebo.

In two double-blind, placebo-controlled studies, by Sillanpaa (1977) with clonidine and Sillanpaa and Koponen (1978) with papaverine, both medications proved effective for the short-term prophylaxis of migraine, and in the latter study papaverine was also effective for long-term treatment. However, clonidine was associated with a much higher rate of side effects than was papaverine. Potentially serious side effects in the form of retroperitoneal fibrosis and cardiac fibrosis may occur with another prophylactic agent, maleate (Sansert), so it is not recommended for use with children or adolescents.

The role of placebo in the migraine drug studies is particularly interesting. In marked contrast to the Ludvigsson (1974) data, in the Sillanpaa studies (Sillanpaa, 1977; Sillanpaa & Koponen, 1978) substantial improvement also occurred under placebo conditions. These differential effects may be a function of method variance. Ludvigsson evaluated outcome from diaries kept by the children and their parents, whereas in the Sillanpaa studies interviews with the children served this purpose. Significant discrepancies between diary measures of headache activity and independent retrospective estimates of the same measures obtained from children and their parents during interviews have been reported by Andrasik and his colleagues (Andrasik, Burke, Attanasio, & Rosenblum, 1985).

Abortive Medication

Abortive drugs act to prevent the expansion of blood vessels and therefore are most effective in the early stages of an attack of migraine. The ergot alkaloids in particular have long been the mainstay of migraine treatment in adults. For children and, to a lesser extent, adolescents, the need for precise timing presents difficulties: At these ages the warning signals are less clearly identifiable and are of briefer duration than is the case with adults. The timing factor requires that the child must have the pills with him at all times, which is not always convenient (Shinnar & D'Souza, 1981). In addition, the timing factor serves to focus the child's attention on the possibility of headache onset at any moment, and carrying the pills at all times strengthens this expectation.

There are no controlled studies with children or adolescents, but experienced clinicians (see, for example, Bille, 1962) have recommended the use of ergot preparations, such as ergotamine and caffeine (Cafergot), and ergotamine (Gynergen) at the onset of a migraine attack. The dose for children has not been established (Benitz & Tatro, 1981), but for adolescents Neinstein (1984) has recommended 2 to 4 mg at onset and 1 mg every 30 minutes to a maximum of four doses. Ergotamine preparations are highly effective in aborting migraine attacks if the timing of the initial dose coincides with onset. Side effects include nausea, vomiting, ischemia, paresthesias, and an intensification of pain, a phenomenon known as rebound headache. Antiprostaglandin agents such as tolfenamic acid appear to be as effective as ergotamine with the additional benefit of fewer side effects. These drugs are currently under investigation (see, for example, Hakkarainen, Vapaatalo, Gothoni, & Parantainen, 1979).

Palliative Treatment

The palliative form of treatment is the most common one, with sedatives, analgesics, and antiemetics being given at the onset of the headache. If the attacks are infrequent and relatively mild, nonnarcotic analgesics sometimes suffice in children as well as adolescents (Neinstein, 1984). In the case of severe and recurrent attacks, however, prophylactic treatment is indicated. No controlled studies have been reported on the early use of these medications, but numerous clinical observations have indicated that a reduction occurs in the duration and severity of migraine headaches but not in their frequency.

Controlled studies on the pharmacotherapy of pediatric migraine are rare, and much of the little research that has been done is singularly lacking in methodological rigor. Because of a lack of systematic research there is no firm knowledge on the important issue of the impact of side effects during key growth periods in children who are on long-term dosage. Research with adults has shown that the continuing usage of analgesics (Kudrow, 1982) and ergotamine (Ala-Hurula, Myllyla, & Hokkanen, 1982) can lead to paradoxical effects and rebound headache. In the absence of careful clinical investigations there is no way of knowing whether these paradoxical effects will occur in children. Because of the side effects of drugs and the unknown long-term effects in children, most medical authorities (Brown, 1977) have cautioned against pharmacological treatment as a long-term solution to migraine. By necessity, this opens the door to other modes of management, notably those of a psychological nature.

Psychological Intervention

In the past, pediatric migraine has been considered to be a benign disorder in the sense that it does not lead to tissue damage. Child migraineurs were given optimum treatment primarily for humane reasons. The tenor of treatment has changed markedly in recent years as a result of reports that migraine can be life-threatening in childhood (Ferguson & Robinson, 1982) and that it may be associated with cognitive impairment (Zeitlin & Oddy, 1984) in adults who experience constant and severe attacks over a long period. Several investigators have reported an association between migraine and strokes (Boisen, 1975; Spaccavento, Solomon, & Mani, 1981), and Amery (1982) has cautioned that in every migraine episode there is brain hypoxia, with consequent potential harm over the long term. Findings such as these emphasize the necessity for early intervention and control of pediatric migraine.

The treatment most commonly used for migraine in children and adolescents begins with reassurance that nothing is seriously wrong (Neinstein, 1984) and that successful treatment is a distinct possibility. The reassurance may have to be repeated in various forms throughout treatment in order to counteract television-mediated misconceptions about the meaning of severe headaches, particularly in respect to brain tumors and amnesia. The initial plan of action for the child involves a discussion aimed at identifying emotional and physical stressors in his environment that may be precipitating factors and then, where possible, eliminating or modifying them. Even where such change is difficult, the precipitating factor tends to lose some impact once the child grasps its association with his migraine. Emphasis is placed on having the child identify early warning cues of an incipient migraine: He may keep a headache diary and record in detail events at home and school at the onset of each attack as well as his feelings concerning his life at those points. To do this, he must first see the migraine as a sequence of temporally related events rather than as a single event. Each event in the sequence has external influences in the form of social interactions as well as internal ones covering the child's thoughts and feelings about the event. Research on mood and migraine in adults (Harrigan, Kues, Ricks, & Smith, 1984) has provided the first empirical evidence that moods may predict the onset of migraines, the best predictors being feelings of constraint (being trapped, hemmed in, and frustrated by inability to achieve a goal in the face of maximum effort) and fatigue (lethargy and exhaustion). If specific moods are frequently linked to the migraine, efforts could be directed at helping the child manage the situation at those times more effectively. Such a link might also make it possible to pinpoint stressors that were not directly identifiable. The diary record would also include what action, if any, is taken by the child when he has a headache. In completing this initial step of clarification for both the child and physician, the child is also likely to gain a feeling of being in control. Olness (1985) has noted that child migraineurs often suffer from feelings of helplessness and lack the opportunities (or initiative) for experiencing mastery and a sense of personal competence. Having to play a vital and active role in their own treatment counteracts such feelings to a certain extent and may have a positive effect on their behavior in other situations.

With the information gathered, it should be possible to develop a plan for the child to follow when he has a migraine and buttress it with instruction in skills that will reverse the symptoms or prevent them from escalating to a migraine. If this psychological approach is introduced to the child in a way that fosters compliance and confidence and then is properly implemented, it will circumvent many of the problems inherent in the medical management of pediatric headache. For example, pharmacological intervention, with the possibility of side effects, the implication that the child is sick, and the resultant tendency to set up a schedule that can provide secondary gains could all be bypassed. In respect to the secondary gains problem, Lake (1981) has reported a stable increase in school attendance by an 11-year-old boy with migraine following attention to migraine-consequent events in the boy's environment and modification of them; and Mehegan and his colleagues (Mehegan, Masek, Harrison, Russo, & Leviton, 1987) have reported the use of operant management of excessive demands for attention and special treatment in a successful multicomponent behavioral treatment program for pediatric migraine. In comparison with the number of studies on other forms of chronic or recurring pain in children, studies on the role of secondary gains in maintaining migraine problems are rare.

Biofeedback

Biofeedback in one of two forms, each combined with relaxation training, is a frequently used intervention. In these instances, the relaxation procedures range from active forms, such as progressive muscle relaxation, to meditation and autogenic therapy (see, for example, Diamond & Franklin, 1975; Houts, 1982; Mehegan et al., 1987). In one form, *thermal biofeedback,* hand (or fingertip) temperature is involved, with the child learning to voluntarily raise his hand temperature. Olness (1985) has reported that children as young as three years become very competent at this self-treatment procedure, and these findings are supported by a cluster of systematic case studies (Feuerstein & Adams, 1977; Houts, 1982; Labbé & Williamson, 1983). In addition, controlled group investigations (Andrasik et al., 1984; Engel & Rapoff, 1987; Labbé & Williamson, 1984) in which thermal biofeedback has been combined with autogenic relaxation training attest to the sometimes astonishing success of this combination in reducing the frequency of migraine headaches in children and adolescents. In the second form, *cephalic vasomotor biofeedback,* the task is to directly decrease the blood flow in the temporal artery as a means of aborting a migraine headache. Andrasik et al. (1986) have aptly termed this procedure "the biofeedback equivalent to ergotamine." The difficulty of acquiring this skill precludes its use with children, but Feuerstein and Adams (1977) have used it successfully with an adolescent patient.

As we have noted previously, there is still uncertainty about the reason for the therapeutic effect of biofeedback in any form or combination. Some investigators (Ciccone & Grzesiak, 1984) disparage the view that biofeedback can effect changes through efforts to control the relevant physiological parameter such as hand temperature and, instead, attribute its success to a more constructive attitude on the patient's part toward his pain problem. In contrast to the prevailing noncognitive, physiologically based explanations, this view stresses the cognitive and behavioral changes that occur with feelings of self-efficacy and being in control, changes that are reinforced by the contingent success of biofeedback. Before we move on to other interventions, it should be noted that Chapman's (1986) excellent, comprehensive, and critical review of biofeedback, while not directed at children, would be of immense help for those interested in pursuing biofeedback research with this age group. A cautionary note from Jay, Renelli, and Mead's (1984) biofeedback research with adults that may be applicable to adolescents and possibly children concerns a drug–biofeedback interaction. Adults undergoing biofeedback therapy who regularly used propranolol or amitriptyline had considerable difficulty attaining the training criterion.

Self-Hypnosis

Gardner and Olness (1981) advocate self-hypnosis singly or in combination with other interventions such as biofeedback (Olness & MacDonald, 1981) for children with migraine. Because self-hypnosis requires that the child practice on a daily basis for 4 to 6 weeks in order to acquire a conditioned response that can be invoked at the first signs of onset of a migraine, compliance can be a problem. However, it is one that is readily avoided with sufficient therapist support and contact. The following case study (Gardner & Olness, 1981, p. 206) of a 10-year-old girl is representative of the efficacy of this intervention for migraine:

> N. was referred by a pediatric neurologist for hypnotherapy . . . [for] intractable migraines that were handicapping her life in many areas. Excessive drug therapy was required and results were not ideal. N. and her family were depressed over her chronic illness. . . . At the first visit, N. was told that she could learn a method of headache control that she could use later to treat herself. The therapist explained that it would be important for her to practice regularly for at least 6 weeks so that she would be sure of her skills. Then the therapist drew diagrams of the nervous system, explained the theory of vascular changes which trigger migraines, and explained the concept of using imaginary switches to control pain. N. was delighted at the idea of having her own method, and she learned rapidly. On the third visit, she was taught the jettison technique for letting go of worries. Within one month, she was off all medications and in complete control of her headaches. When she sensed an aura of migraine, she was able to stop its progression.

Cognitive Coping Strategies

Strategies such as imagery have proved effective with adult migraineurs (Brown, 1984) but have rarely been subjected to systematic investigations in pediatric migraine. In one of the few such studies, Richter et al. (1986) compared cognitive coping, in the form of cognitive restructuring involving the alteration of dysfunctional thought processes, with progressive deep muscle relaxation. There were no differences between these interventions, and both proved superior to a credible placebo intervention in reducing overall headache activity and frequency. Duration and intensity were not affected. Initial headache severity was an important factor in treatment outcome: Children with severe headaches responded better to the treatment interventions than did those with milder headaches. In the placebo condition, an intriguing and unexplained effect occurred in which children with low-severity headaches were markedly responsive to the placebo treatment, but those with high-severity headaches showed significantly less response. The children and adolescents in the two experimental conditions showed continuing improvement over a 16-week follow-up period.

In subjective accounts, children ($n = 7$) with migraine have reported the spontaneous and successful use of imagery (Ross & Ross, 1982a), combined, in most cases, with relaxation:

> I lie down and then I let myself go all over like I'm the laundry bag emptied on the bed, you know? Like all over. Then I start right at the beginning of the game [baseball] against [rival school] and it's not just a shut-out, it's like a real *massacre*, the whole nine innings we do everything great and I hit a homer. (Boy, CA 11)

The most unusual strategy reported by the headache group (Ross & Ross, 1982a) related to the unilaterality of migraines. An 11-year-old girl stated that what would have helped most would have been to move the throbbing pain from the left side of her head, where it always was, to the other side in order to give the left side a rest. Although she was unable to do this, she was persisting in attempting it. The interesting thing about her account is that the same strategy has been reported by a man with severe burns all over his body (Fairley, 1978, p. 62):

> I made myself believe that the pain was only in one half of my body. Every morning I would wake up and mentally drive the pain into, say, my left half. I would then think only of my right side. Next day I would drive it across to the right, and think only of my left. I found out, that way, I could live with the pain—it only seemed half as bad.

Others have reported its use: At a meeting in which D. M. Ross presented a paper, three nurses recounted their successful use of this strategy in childhood with unilateral pains associated with migraine, an abscessed tooth, and appendicitis.

Rebreathing

The possibility that attacks of migraine could be aborted with rebreathing (Dexter, 1982) deserves serious investigation. This procedure consists of rebreathing the patient's own expired air from a paper bag during the period of aura that precedes a migraine attack. The bag is placed over the patient's head and held or secured in such a way that no influx of outside air occurs. For children, it would be essential that the bag not be secured in any way that might cause panic and that an adult be present throughout the 10- to 20-minute period required for this procedure. Rebreathing has been used by six adult patients at the City of London Migraine Clinic, who were able to abort or ease their attacks of migraine. There are no reports of its use with children. Although the mechanism of therapeutic effect has not been established, Dexter (1982, p. 312) has speculated on factors that may be involved:

> The rise in carbon dioxide pressure, or other associated changes . . . seemed to be important. . . . If the carbon dioxide pressure is important this may explain why exercise and excitement with increased ventilation can provoke attacks and why sleep, perhaps due to reduced ventilation, can cut short attacks. Nevertheless, the beneficial effects of rebreathing may be due not to the raised carbon dioxide pressure but to other changes associated with rebreathing. For instance, it has been postulated (Santiago, Remolina, Scolles, & Edelman, 1981) that endorphins minimize the stress of chronic airway obstruction; perhaps rebreathing achieves its therapeutic effect in migraine through the release of endorphins secondary to the respiratory distress it causes.

Comment

Andrasik et al. (1986) have expressed concern that many children with migraine headaches are not being helped to any meaningful degree and have pointed to the need for developing patient $\times$ treatment matches. A contributing factor that should be considered is that of parental resistance to acknowledging the diagnosis of migraine in the child. For some strange reason, occasionally there is stigma associated with such a diagnosis for both the layman and physician: One physician with experience in a college student health center told us that on no account should a student with migraine have this condition noted on his chart because of potential repercussions in relation to his subsequent career aspirations. When these attitudes exist, the child can become the unwitting victim of inadequate treatment.

Intrusive Procedures

Almost all children in Western societies experience a series of intrusive procedures in the form of routine immunizations beginning in infancy and continuing in the preschool years, with assorted and more randomly spaced procedures throughout the school years. Regardless of the degree of pain characteristic of specific procedures, an element of anxiety concerning these events is usually present. Objects that intrude into body openings are often especially threatening in the preschool and early school years. The mouth and anus are basic, early, and important sources of body feelings (Rogers & Head, 1983), so that even painless procedures such as having one's temperature taken orally or rectally or having the most cursory of dental examinations can create significant anxiety in young children. Such a reaction occurs in part because the child feels a loss of autonomy and control, in itself a significant psychological threat, but also because of misconceptions due to immature cognitive levels and the resultant meanings that he imposes on the experience (Ross & Ross, 1982a, 1985; Simeonsson, Buckley, & Monson, 1979). Children often report, for example, that they think the doctor or dentist can tell by the procedures what the child is thinking ("I hate him") and that he will punish the child in some way. Since many of the procedures do involve varying degrees of pain and discomfort, the child's expectations in this situation appear to be confirmed.

It is not uncommon for children to cry, vomit, or have difficulty sleeping when an intrusive procedure is impending, and then become hysterical and so difficult to control during the procedure that they have to be restrained. The ensuing shame and blame add additional negative associations to the whole procedure. Needle procedures are particularly terrifying (see, for example, Fassler, 1985; Lewis, 1978; Menke, 1981; Ross & Ross, 1984b, 1985), and the fears engendered by them often persist into adulthood. Agras, Sylvester, and Oliveau (1969), for example, reported that 14% of the young adults in an epidemiological study of fears reported significant phobias of needle procedures, and Oswalt and Napoliello (1974) found that fear of needles was the major reason for adults' reluctance to donate blood.

Anticipatory Anxiety

The effects of anxiety in situ are further compounded by the anticipatory anxiety that the child brings to the situation. Its sources typically are heterogeneous. Some children may have developed an acute conditioned anxiety reaction from a single traumatic experience in a medical or dental setting, but even those without prior negative experience have cognitions concerning these settings. Information from sibling and peer reports, older children boasting of their bravery during the terrible ordeal, and television programs all contribute to the child's expectations. Parental input in the form of careless comments made within the child's hearing or prior information that often terrifies the child even when supposedly meant well takes its toll, not to speak of the unfortunately quite common instances (Clark, 1987) when intrusive procedures are used as threatened punishment ("If you're not good, I'll get the doctor to give you a shot"). Often, the children's expectations are mediated by inaccurate information. Children of school age, for example, commonly have markedly erroneous ideas concerning their blood. Although they know that their blood is vital to their survival (having seen people on television bleed to death or survive due to a transfusion), they generally do not have the concept of the body continually manufacturing blood so that reasonable amounts lost under normal circumstances are routinely replaced. Consequently, when having a blood test, they are often alarmed about the possibility of losing so much blood that they will die or that the hole from the needle will never close and the blood will all run out. The small hole often visible after venipuncture adds further validity to the latter misconception.

Attempts to cope with the predominantly negative reactions of children to intrusive procedures have focused on three lines of approach: information given the child prior to the procedure, coping skills that he can use both prior to the procedure and during it, and improvements in the procedures themselves.

Prior Information

Prior information for a particular procedure may cover procedural aspects (what will happen), sensory aspects (what it feels like), or the rationale for it (why it is needed). For very young children, such information may be transmitted through doll play (Tucker, 1982), puppets (Lang, 1986), a combination of demonstration and discussion (Adams, 1976; McGrath & de Veber, 1986), fiction and nonfiction picture books (Fassler, 1978; Gibby & Stanford, 1984), and play therapy (Adams, 1976) involving a combination of discussion and desensitization during which the children play with the syringes and related equipment. Lecture-type presentations and films of a factual nature have been used with adolescents as well as children.

The rationale underlying these activities is that prior information will enable the child to absorb the nature of the coming experience, muster his resources, and be better able to cope with the experience than if he were confronted with the unexpected and unknown. The fact is, however, that not all children want to know what is going to happen (Ross & Ross, 1982a). To accommodate the great variation in children's needs, Peterson and Toler (1984) have developed an innovative technique that allows the child to regulate the amount and kind of information that he is given. This technique is in the form of a branching program with choice points at which the child decides what, if anything, he would like to hear next. Preliminary data show an interaction between coping style and amount of information, with sensitizers choosing to hear full details of an impending surgical procedure and repressors managing better with the branching program. Peterson and Toler's (1984) preliminary study represents the first systematic attempt to develop a procedure for arriving at a child × information fit and, as such, represents an important contribution to the literature on preparation for aversive procedures.

Taking a different tack are the management procedures in which positive reinforcements are offered prior to the intrusive procedure to children who have proved unmanageable in the past. Having all the earmarks of bribes, these procedures are nonetheless effective in partially substituting positive anticipation, in the form of reward, for the child's anticipatory anxiety. The coping strategy, thought-stopping (Ross, D. M., 1984), described in Chapter 6, can be used for the child whose anxiety exhausts him and his parents before they ever reach the aversive situation. The child who is emotionally exhausted after hours or days of worry is ill prepared to cope; thought-stopping could enable him to arrive for his appointment in a relatively calm state. McGrath and de Veber (1986) have developed and tested an exemplary program to help leukemic children before and during lumbar punctures. This program is based on the premise that having accurate expectations about the pain source, some control over it, and an altered awareness of the significance of the pain could minimize fear and anxiety.

Coping Skills

Two coping skills are particularly suited to needle procedures of short duration and can be taught in the needle situation. The first one, called *holding on,* consists of holding tightly to one's mother, teddy bear, the arms of the chair, or any other piece of furniture or safe equipment within easy reach. Holding on can function both as a distractor and, if the child holds on tightly enough, as a counterirritant.

The second procedure, *blowing out the pain* (LePage, 1986), has proved highly successful with preschool and young children. Here the child is taught to blow out as hard as he can at the first sign of pain. The effect of this apparently simple procedure is quite complex. It changes the meaning of the aversive stimulus by making the child see the first sharp pain of the needle as a signal for action rather than as a pain per se. At the same time, he is distracted from the thought of pain by the fact that he must be alert to act when he gets the signal. He also feels in control because he is the one who can take the pain and hurl it outside his body. This is a very powerful coping skill that the preschool and young school-age child can learn in a minute or two. It is particularly appropriate for this age group because at this cognitive level children have confidence in magic and there is an element of magic in being able to blow out the pain that heightens the strategy's credibility; they also see things concretely so that it is a big piece of pain that is being blown out.

Improving the Techniques

The concern on the part of pediatric personnel about the effects of needle procedures on children has led to a number of efforts to reduce the pain by improving the techniques. Several investigators have focused on the pain associated with intramuscular (IM) injections. The causes of pain in such injections are the mechanical trauma to the muscle from inserting the needle, distention of the tissue as fluid is forced into the muscle, and increased pain from the fluid if an irritant chemical is being injected. In a study with children (CA 4–5) who were undergoing routine IM immunization injections, Eland (1981) used a 2×2 factorial design to assess the efficacy of spraying a skin coolant, Frigiderm, on the injection site immediately prior to the injection. The use of the coolant spray resulted in a significantly greater reduction in pain than did aerosol air sprayed on the leg for children in the control condition.

Several studies with adults have implications for the reduction of pain from IM injections in children. On the basis of the central inhibitory balance theory (Kerr, 1975) that nonnoxious stimuli delivered before the noxious stimulus (the needle) could decrease pain by reducing the activity of those cells responsible for pain transmission, Wachter-Shikora (1980) demonstrated that mechanostimulation with a nonnoxious vibrator before the IM injection decreased the pain. Kruszewski, Lang, and Johnson (1979) found that discomfort could be minimized by positioning the patient so that the gluteus maximus muscle is relaxed during the injection. The simple procedure for inducing relaxation in this muscle requires only that the femur be extended and internally rotated with the patient in the prone position. Both of these procedures appear to be highly appropriate for children. Locsin (1983) is among those who have used a counterirritant, the pinch-grasp technique, with a consequent decrease in pain. This technique consists of grasping the deltoid muscle by pinching it hard enough to elicit some discomfort prior to inserting the needle: Its success has been attributed, in part, to distraction. We have reservations about its use with the pediatric population, having heard of an 11-year-old girl who reported indignantly that she "didn't mind the needle so much but first she gave me a really mean pinch" (Waechter, 1971).

In a randomized double-blind study of 51 children (CA 8–17), Möller (1985) used a topical anesthetic that contained lidocaine and prilocaine to reduce venipuncture pain. The patients assessed the pain using a three-category graphic rating scale (GRS) ("no pain," "slight pain," "severe pain"); the staff used a three-category verbal rating scale to assess ease of performing the venipuncture ("easier than usual," "as usual," "more difficult than usual") and a four-category scale to rate visible redness and edema of the treated skin. With this injection procedure the patients reported significantly less pain than with placebo, the staff thought that venipuncture was easier to perform with it, and skin reactions were rated as clinically insignificant. A methodological weakness here concerns the small number of choices on the GRS: There should be a minimum of four and preferably five choices. One disadvantage in using this topical anesthetic is its comparatively long application time; it must be applied at least one hour prior to injection. However, additional support for its use with children comes from an earlier study (Hallen & Uppfeldt, 1982) in which it proved effective in reducing pain associated with the insertion of intravenous catheters.

Of the needle developments, one of the most promising is the Syrijet II, referred to by children and staff as the Mizzy Gun, an interesting contradiction of the dangers of using the word *shot*. The Mizzy Gun is a method of performing bone marrow aspirations (BMAs) that was developed by Dyment (1978) and his associates as a way to obtain local anesthesia without using a needle. To do this, they adapted a spring-powered dental device that administers a spray of local anesthesia through a jet-type nozzle. According to children's self-reports and clinic staff observations, this form of anesthesia is significantly less painful and also faster than the infiltration technique. Support for the contribution of speed as a factor in minimizing Mizzy Gun pain comes from a study by Colby, Lanzetta, and Kleck (1977) on undergraduates, in which pain tolerance levels were higher for rapidly ascending shock than for slowly ascending shock. Whatever the reason, children who have undergone BMAs by the traditional method almost without exception prefer the Mizzy Gun (Walsh, 1981).

Modifying the Cognitive and Affective Facets The foregoing improvements in the mechanics of intrusive procedures are limited to the sensory aspects of the pain experience. During the ongoing procedure, attention should also be given to modifying the cognitive and affective facets of the child's pain experience. For the child who momentarily is to have blood taken and may have the common fears of bleeding to death or of having too much blood taken, a simple procedure would be to show him two cartoon-like visual presentations in color: One of these would show the volume of blood in the body in relation to the almost infinitesimal amounts taken with a finger stick or venipuncture as well as the amount lost in common bleeding events such as having a scraped knee, nosebleed, or minor cut; a second would show how the "blood factory" inside the child is constantly manufacturing more blood. In the case of venipuncture, with the likelihood of going in more than once should the child show active resistance, an additional procedure is recommended in which the child is shown in a 2- or 3-minute presentation what is involved in venipuncture. Materials needed are toy syringes and a doll with veins large enough to allow entry by a needle. (As Lang [1986] has noted, there are dolls with detachable scars, plaster casts, veins that show up with pressure, a hole in the throat for a tracheostomy tube, and so on, that are not unduly expensive.) Using these materials, show the child what has to be done and explain how the tourniquet speeds up blood withdrawal and consequently shortens the time the needle is in the arm. Mention that it is normal to jump at having your arm pricked so if someone holds the child's arm they are just helping to keep it still, they are not holding him prisoner. Now show the child how hard it is to put the needle in the doll's vein if the doll is jumping around. Let the child try to do this while you make the doll jump and kick.

For short, foolproof procedures, such as finger sticks or subcutaneous and IM injections, have a clock on the wall with a big second hand, emphasize how short a second is, and tell the child that the procedure will take exactly X number of seconds and no longer. To give implicit support to this statement, have the child choose a Band-Aid from a colorful assortment and hold it during the procedure.

For intrusive procedures such as cardiac catheterizations and endoscopies that are lengthy and uncomfortable, three treatment components are optimal for the child who is amenable to having prior information. The child should be shown a colored cartoon explaining what will happen immediately before it happens. He should have a coach in the form of a friendly adult whose function is to talk the child through the procedure with a combination of reports on progress, praise, and reassurance. When the procedure starts, the coach's remarks should be linked to a graphic presentation in the form of a picture on an overhead screen that should show how much has been done and how much further there is to go. At the conclusion of the procedure, the coach should accompany the child back to his room or parents and give him some small age- and sex-appropriate tangible reward. One of the paradoxes of the pediatric setting is the tendency to give the child balloons or toys following treatments such as routine checkups involving minimal aversive stimulation, only to skip these rewards when he has undergone some really painful treatment. In the latter situation, even verbal pats on the back are frequently withheld.

Other methods of reducing trauma have been investigated. For example, Caire and Erickson (1986) have reported that the use of earphones and tapes of the child's favorite music had high utility in cardiac catheterizations of a wide range of patients, from infants to children in Grade 6. Some of these children brought their own tapes from home, others were supplied. An additional benefit of the earphones was that they masked out conversation between the pediatric personnel as well as other verbal and nonverbal sounds in the setting that had anxiety-arousing potential.

Comment

More use should be made of audiovisual materials for providing information prior to impending pain procedures and during them. Many of the film presentations are extraordinarily dull. There is no reason why these materials could not be attractive and, where appropriate, exciting and funny while at the same time being absolutely accurate. Cartoons offer several important advantages. Children have highly positive associations with cartoons, and the images themselves have a clarity that facilitates transmission of the message. Attention-directing animal characters and events can be used; for example, the crocodile could be shown having a tube down because he had swallowed the treasure map. Cartoons can be used to depict progress through an uncomfortable or painful treatment procedure with a clarity difficult to achieve with a film strip of a live model undergoing the same procedure. The steps to completion of the treatment procedure can be shown in a way that accurately indicates the temporal duration of each step.

Using a hand-controlled pointer projected on the screen the coach can show very clearly where the child is in relation to the goal. The use of cartoons lends itself to the demonstration of coping strategies, such as imagery, that also could provide an opportunity for some very funny, and consequently distracting, sequences. For children facing long-term treatment, a series of cartoons could be prepared with the cartoon character finding more and more ways to cope with the demands.

There is no question that the type of films proposed here are expensive to produce. However, it is also a fact that this kind of project has great appeal to corporations, foundations, and private donors interested in funding activities related to the welfare of sick children. In addition, many universities have graduate-level film programs whose faculty members welcome small projects for their students, thus providing a setup that would permit pediatric personnel to be involved in decision making throughout the production period. Given this kind of funding climate, the only obstacles that we can see are a lack of initiative on the part of pediatric personnel or, more likely, an administration that downgrades the potential that psychological contributions have for the management of pediatric pain.

8

Current Developments and Future Directions

In assessing the state of our basic knowledge and understanding of pain, Wall (1984, p. 1) has commented that

> there are reasons for optimism because there is at present a real increase of knowledge which comes in part from the abandoning of old concepts which were wrong and which held the subject in a strait-jacket.

Although not referring specifically to childhood pain, Wall's comment accurately describes the current state of affairs in this emerging field. In the past decade the conceptualization of childhood pain has undergone radical changes: Some erroneous beliefs have been dispelled, certain established stances have been challenged in productive controversy, and a cluster of well-entrenched but groundless ideas has been significantly weakened (Owens, 1984; Rosenblith & Sims-Knight, 1985). With these advances, some formidable barriers to the study of childhood pain have given way. The result has been to transform what was, as recently as the mid-1970s, merely a fringe topic in the field of pain research into a small but significant area of investigation with a steadily expanding base of clinical and empirical information.

The picture of childhood pain that has emerged is one in which sensitivity to noxious stimulation is intact early in the first year of life, with the infant and young child becoming increasingly efficient in modulating pain reactivity (Barr, 1982; Craig et al., 1984) and the preschool child showing responsivity to the meaning of pain events as well as increasing discrimination and skill in pain description and expressivity. The process of increasing control, refinement, and differentiation continues throughout the middle childhood years until in early adolescence pain expressivity begins to approximate the adult level. The changing face of pain expressivity is paralleled by orderly and predictable Piagetian shifts in the child's understanding of pain (Gaffney, 1983; Gaffney & Dunne, 1986; Ross & Ross, 1987). From the preschool years through early adolescence, the child's concept of pain gradually evolves from the simple and concrete to the significantly more complex, abstract, and sophisticated; from the subjective and egocentric to the more objective and less egocentric; and from the prelogical to the logical. Throughout this period the child demonstrates increasing competence in self-report of pain and acquires a diversity of coping strategies, some of which may involve the maladaptive use of pain for secondary gains. Along the way any tendencies to attribute pain to unrelated transgressions diminish and the focus shifts from an almost exclusive concern with the physiological aspects of pain to an appreciation of its psychological facets. The child's ability to cope independently with pain increases as does his concern for maintaining control, a concern that can make for unpredictable and apparently irrational behavior during painful procedures.

This base of information has had far-reaching and, in some instances, catalytic effects. Some of the resultant advances have stemmed directly from the clinical and empirical data on childhood pain, whereas others can be attributed to the newly perceived link between certain findings in the adult pain field and problems in childhood. Representative advances of the current decade are described in the following sections.

Procedural Refinements

The expanding base of information on childhood pain has compelled clinicians and investigators to reevaluate different facets of pediatric pain management, with the result that refinements have occurred in certain well-established beliefs and related procedures. Consider, for example, the changing views on the issue of preparatory information for impending pain events. In the United States, the consensus on this issue in the 1970s was that an accurate and complete description of the pain event should be provided a day or two prior to the event in the case of preschool children and a week or more ahead for older children (see Azarnoff, 1983, for English and Australian views on this issue). The assumption was that the child needed accurate information as well as time to muster his psychological resources in order to cope with the event. The fallacy in this age-based formula approach was the total disregard for individual differences. In reports from the children themselves (Ross & Ross, 1982a, 1985; Ross, S. A., 1984), marked variability in preferences for both content and timing of information occurred across age levels. A related recent advance is the preparation procedure developed by Peterson and Toler (1984) that allows the child to decide at choice points in the information session the type of information he would like to be given next. This innovative approach in turn suggests a whole new direction in advance information procedures. A logical next step in this sequence would be self-regulated film presentations in which the child has a choice of sensory, procedural, or distractor sequences. The first two would have coping or mastery model choices and the third, content irrelevant to pain. A variation in the prior information procedures would be to allow the child a timing × type of information choice.

Peterson and Toler's (1984) approach exemplifies the increasing awareness in the field of pediatric pain of the need to consider the quality of the intervention × child fit. An impressive example of fit is the Well Doll Clinic Project (Khan, 1985) which was designed to introduce young preschool children to the pediatric setting in a way that would minimize fears and maximize confidence about subsequent encounters with it. In this ongoing project, children are invited to bring a sick doll or toy animal to the hospital for consultation with a pediatrician. They are encouraged to ask questions, make disclosures, and give opinions (Khan, 1985, p. 1):

> At immunization clinics, the doctor or nurse listen to doll's heartbeat and ask what's wrong with the "baby," giving children an opportunity to express fears or concerns they may have. Immunization shots (if required) and a discussion of general health care follows. Children are allowed to assist with shots if they wish. The doll receives a bravery badge.

This cognitively based experience helps the child understand what the doctor does, what a hospital is, what happens there, and why children sometimes have to go there, all within a toy-mediated, reassuring, and non-fear-arousing framework. The immediate benefits center on reduced trauma associated with pediatric visits. For children who have had unpleasant prior experiences in medical settings, the Well Doll Clinic helps them to talk about their fears through the medium of the sick doll in a nonthreatening atmosphere (Widger, 1985, p. 1B):

> Three-year-old Rachel . . . solemnly hands him [the doctor] her doll, Marley, for examination. Marley needs a shot, the doctor says, and invites Rachel to administer it on the doll's thigh. Rachel is willing, and pushes the plunger down. Then they rub the spot to make Marley feel better, and give her a badge for being a good girl.
> The play-acting is important therapy for Rachel. . . . She has already had a hospital experience so traumatic that she would cry if riding in a car passing by outside. Then came the Well Doll Clinic. . . . Every other month, doll parents . . . bring their "babies" in for visits similar to their own check-ups. By bringing her doll in, Rachel was able to work through her own anxieties and eventually became more comfortable with doctor visits.

For those with no prior experience, the Clinic provides an outstanding orientation to the medical setting. In either case, there are likely to be immediate benefits in the form of the attenuation of stress related to pediatric visits and, possibly most important, long-term benefits centering around promotion of a positive attitude toward health care.

Another ingenious example of fit comes from a treatment study (Rozensky & Pasternak, 1985) with 10- to 12-year-old boys who were afflicted with severe migraine headaches. The boys, who were described as overachievers, initially were resistant to any component of the medical, thermal biofeedback, and relaxation training treatment package, a not-unexpected reaction in view of their achievement patterns (see, for example, Leikin, Firestone, & McGrath, 1987). However, when relaxation instructions based on Obi-Wan Kenobi's training of Luke Skywalker in the ways of The Force in the film *Star Wars* were incorporated into the treatment regimen, the boys responded immediately and with great enthusiasm.

A Conceptual Framework

The developmental progression that has been documented in the child's understanding of pain has served an important explanatory function by providing the pediatrician with a conceptual framework that enables him to understand and accept behavior that ordinarily would provoke impatience or anger. For example, the resistant, obstructive distress characteristic of the preschool child who is confronted with a painful treatment procedure becomes reasonable when viewed in the light of the limitations within which the child is attempting to function: He has difficulty in expressing his feelings, doubts, and nebulous anxieties about the procedure and often does not understand the reasons for it. He has a very poor concept of time, so the probable duration of the noxious stimulation is an unknown. He brings few, if any, coping strategies to the situation and has no control over it. Often, the pediatric personnel are seen as deliberately mean. Given these conditions, it is completely rational that a child who is functioning at such a severe psychological disadvantage should resist. In fact, in view of the known odds against him, the preschool child who is really "good" in this situation should give the pediatrician pause (Adams, 1976; Hyson et al., 1982).

New Directions

Throughout this text we have described a diversity of new directions in the study of pediatric pain. These have included refinements in assessment procedures, such as the recognition that the child's placement of categories in measuring instruments constitutes an important element (Eland, 1981; P. A. McGrath et al., 1985), as well as radical changes in pain management, a notable example being the participation strategy for burn treatment advocated by Kavanagh (1983a). In terms of research methodology, a major development with far reaching implications has been the empirical demonstration by Grunau and Craig (1987b) of variations in pain expression following heel lance in the newborn that reflect such perinatal variables as maternal obstetric medication and mode of delivery. This finding negates the assumption underlying research on neonatal pain behavior that healthy neonates represent a homogeneous group, and emphasizes the necessity for specifying sample selection when studying their responses to nociceptive input. It also opens up new possibilities for the investigation of maternal and child factors that might mediate variability in neonatal pain expression, for example, sleep and waking states (Grunau & Craig, 1987a), neonatal size (Grunau, Gilbert, & Craig, 1987), and the possible transmission of endorphins from nonmedicated mothers to children, length of labor, and maternal and child temperament (Grunau & Craig, 1987b). These investigators' neonatal research represents a major contribution in its demonstration of the complexity of factors underlying pain expression in the earliest days of life. Their work also serves as a model of careful investigative procedure for other researchers to follow.

The increasing attention currently being paid to childhood pain has also brought into focus other behaviors and events justifying research attention on the grounds that they might have potential relevance for effective pain management. One of these behaviors (and one that impedes pain management) is *catastrophizing,* defined here as a tendency toward a negative bias in the appraisal of a pain experience. In the pain situation, the child who catastrophizes tends to attend to and magnify the perceived negative aspects of the aversive stimulation, for example, how much it hurts and the dangers in the situation ("All my blood's running out and he can't stop it"), and to create fantasies about it ("The dentist is an evil man, he's got me"). A strong element of helplessness is involved that often triggers sympathy in the onlooker, the unfortunate result being that the child is usually rewarded for his catastrophizing. The sequence also triggers sympathetic arousal, anxiety, and other emotional repercussions in the child: It potentiates pain and distress. Recent research by Brown et al. (1986) has shown that catastrophizing occurs from middle childhood through late adolescence at a rate they describe as "alarming." An innovative and productive feature of this research was the procedure of having the children verbalize their thoughts when confronted with hypothetical pain and other stress situations.

There is no question that the catastrophizing sequence should be interrupted when it occurs in the immediate pain situation, preferably with an unemotional and detached presentation of simple facts that functions neither as reward nor punishment for the child's behavior. The main thrust, though, should be directed at developing training procedures for combatting it. To do this, clinicians and researchers should examine the socialization processes and other factors that function as antecedents to catastrophizing. In terms of effect on pain responsivity, it is possible that for children who catastrophize, procedures preventing or modifying the self-generated influx of negative ideas might be more important in pain relief than learning to use coping strategies. In a recent study of adults with chronic back pain (Turner & Clancy, 1986), decreased catastrophizing was related to significant decreases in pain intensity. Further evidence of a potential link between catastrophizing and heightened response to nociceptive stimulation, as well as of the informational value of going beyond pain ratings to the patient's cognitions concerning the pain experience, comes from an experimental study by Genest, Meichenbaum, and Turk (1977). In this study, adult women were first exposed to a cold pressor task for a maximum of 5 minutes. Next, they were shown a videotape of their task performance and were asked to describe their cognitions, "even if it was brief or random, and even if it seems trivial," during the immersion period. In the low-tolerance group (1 minute or less immersion), two response patterns were present that were absent in the high-tolerance group (endured the full 5-minute trial). One was negative self-referent verbal ideation (for example, "I'm just not good at this sort of thing") and the other was vivid and aversive imagery (for example, seeing their arms "sawed off" at the water line, imagining gangrene spreading up their arms) that became progressively worse during the immersion period.

The role of *humor* in pain attenuation has long been recognized at the anecdotal level, and pediatric personnel have, for some time, been convinced of its potential. Reports from pediatric wards (Clarke, 1965; Smith, 1986), for example, have indicated that on the weekly party night, a festive occasion with very funny cartoons, children needed significantly lower dosages of analgesics or none at all, in marked contrast to their needs on routine nights. The analgesic potential of humor was catapulted into the limelight by Norman Cousins' (1976, p. 1461) report that "ten minutes of genuine belly laughter had an anesthetic effect and would give me at least two hours of pain-free sleep." Nevertheless, a glaring void still exists in respect to scientific evidence either supporting or refuting the role of humor in pain attenuation. There is one clinical report (Wessell, 1975) that has documented the use of humor in a 15-year-old girl who was hospitalized for a prolonged and painful treatment of scoliosis. There is also some empirical support of an admittedly indirect nature from experimental studies of pain with healthy university students (Kleck et al., 1976): Social manipulations that led to a reduction in facial expressions of pain (laughter would have this effect) also led to a reduction in autonomic and self-report indices of pain.

If there is a laughter-analgesic effect relationship, the mediator of such an effect has not been identified. However, there are some possible explanations. The effect could be endorphin mediated if the hearty and almost continuous laughter that occurs with a very funny cartoon qualifies as exercise, since exercise is known to stimulate the release of endorphins. Hearty laughter could also qualify as a strong emotion, which, according to the gate-control theory (Melzack & Wall, 1965), can trigger the gating mechanism that controls the transmission of noxious stimulation. Postlaughter limpness might also be a factor, since relaxation is known to modify some pains. Simmons (1986) has reported that in 1906 a French physician, Israel Waynbaum, compared laughter to taking a "nice, cozy, deep bath of oxygen." Waynbaum's theory of emotional expression, which Zajonc (1985) has restated in terms of contemporary neurophysiological knowledge, is consistent with spontaneous laughter attenuating pain intensity by diminishing the reactive component of pain.

As a treatment method, humor has notable advantages that should justify an intensive investigation of its potential on both the clinical and experimental fronts. It is noninvasive and, with the exception of certain postoperative conditions, is completely safe; it can be administered on a group or individual basis and is inexpensive; it has a strong, positive association with enjoyable events outside the medical setting, such as Saturday cartoons on television. If humor does have the analgesic effect that the anecdotal evidence supports, establishing this status would constitute at least a minor breakthrough on the pain management front.

If we were designing a blueprint for pediatric pain research in the next decade, we would advocate increased clinical and research attention to the *effect of models on pain expression*. The efficacy of film modeling procedures in the preparation of children for impending pain events has already been discussed in Chapter

6. However, of relevance here is the research by Craig and his associates (see, for example, Craig, 1983; Craig & Patrick, 1984; Craig & Prkachin, 1980) on the influence of models on pain expression in healthy young adults in a laboratory setting. Representative of their findings having important implications for the assessment and management of pediatric pain are the following: The degree of pain tolerance exhibited by a model affected the observers' willingness to endure noxious stimulation and influenced their reports of the intensity of pain experienced; subjects exposed to pain-tolerant models showed no increases in autonomic measures of subjective distress as a function of noxious stimulation; and nonverbal expressions of pain were less subject to modeling influences than were verbal reports. With some ingenuity, many of Craig's findings could ethically be subjected to empirical test with older children and adolescents. If the same modeling effects could be demonstrated, they could provide an empirical basis for devising management procedures for the attenuation of clinical pain.

Endorphins and Childhood Pain

Evidence of the etiological role of the endorphins in congenital analgesia has led to speculations that these endogenous opiates may be implicated in pediatric conditions in which pain is a feature but whose causes have never been satisfactorily determined. In the recurrent abdominal pain syndrome (RAP), in which pain is the primary symptom, the possibility that the endogenous opiates may be etiologically implicated has led to a hypothesis (Gaffney & Gaffney, 1987) that RAP may result from a differential gastrointestinal (GI) response to stress mediated by the endogenous opiate system. This empirically based hypothesis rests on the similarities between certain clinical features of RAP and the effects of exogenous opiates on the GI tract, as well as on the fact that the biological action of endogenous opiates in the digestive system resembles that of the exogenous opiates on the GI tract. In addition, the onset of RAP and increases in endorphinergic activity are both associated with stress.

A second example of the endorphins having a possible etiological role in a pediatric condition in which pain is a feature has been provided by Herman (1987). On the basis of preliminary findings, she has speculated that an excess of endorphins may be etiologically implicated in some cases of childhood autism. Such an excess could account for two characteristics of the autistic child, namely, his notable lack of pain responsivity and his failure to bond to his parents and form attachments to others. Underlying the latter characteristic is the hypothesis that in bonding and attachment human infants and young animals receive a surge of euphoria-producing opioid peptides with every loving contact with their parents which, in effect, "addicts" them to their parents. Because autistic children already have high levels of opioid peptides, they do not need the euphoria that affection provides and consequently may never learn attachment.

Implications for Pain in Adulthood

Perhaps the most important effect of the increase in information on childhood pain has been to provide an empirical base and logical reason for looking at the long-standing problem of the chronic pain syndrome (CPS) in adulthood from the vantage point of childhood. Conceptually, the CPS can be viewed as a shift in the status of a pain problem from a noxious and unpleasant part of a person's life to preoccupation with the pain almost to the exclusion of other interests. This shift occurs as a result of an interaction between an initial traumatic event (such as accident or surgery) and a precipitating factor in the individual (e.g., inability to cope with school or work) along with multiple social-environmental influences. Typically, secondary gains, such as social rewards or monetary compensation, compound the problem by serving a dual function as precipitants of the shift and reinforcers of it. It is clear from the clinical, behavioral, and psychiatric literature, as well as from interview data (Ross & Ross, 1982a), that potential precursors of such a shift are present in childhood and adolescence.

Current management of the CPS reflects the treatment-oriented philosophy of the American medical system, primarily in the form of pain clinics. Although these clinics constitute an important advance in the treatment of chronic pain and the CPS, in a sense they are a stopgap. The multifaceted nonmonetary costs of the CPS have been discussed earlier in this text. Of concern here are the financial statistics, which estimate the costs of chronic pain in 1985 to be $60 billion (Aronoff, 1985). Although there is no way of knowing what proportion of that amount is attributable to the CPS, it is reasonable to assume that it would be substantial (Aronoff & Wagner, 1986). In addition, it is a fact that the potential CPS population is increasing: More chronic pain children are surviving and the over-50 population is increasing at a rate greater than that accounted for by general population increases (Cataldo et al., 1980). The concern about CPS-related costs is part of the larger problem of the spiraling costs of general health care (see Table 8-1). These costs have soared to the point where cost containment strategies of some kind are mandatory. Between 1975 and 1985 the cost of being sick tripled, far outstripping the rise in inflation for that period.

The efforts at cost containment have ranged from increased use of paramedics, same-day surgicenters as an alternative to hospitalization, and hospital rate setting, to sweeping cuts in the form of restrictions in access to health care targeted at those on the margin of poverty. The cruel and shortsighted 1981 cuts in funding for Aid to Families with Dependent Children, for example, resulted in a loss of eligibility for 500,000 people (Mundinger, 1985). Despite these and other efforts the nation's health-care expenditures are expected to double every 6 years: from $384 billion in 1984 to $690 billion in 1990 and to $1.9 trillion by the end of the century (Tyson & Merrill, 1984). It is possible that such cost containment attempts are relatively ineffective because in a prevention–treatment dichotomy, the large majority fall into the treatment category. Within this category, the ideal solu-

Table 8-1 Rising National Health-Care Costs

| | Expenditures | |
Year	Billions of dollars	% of GNP
1975	133	8.2
1977	170	8.4
1979	215	8.6
1981	286	9.8
1983	355	10.5
1985	425	10.7
1990	690[a]	11.5[b]

Source: Bureau of Data Management & Strategy, Health Care Financing Administration.
[a]Independent forecasts (Tyson & Merrill, 1984).
[b]Merrill (1987).

tion would be to eliminate certain expenditures without jeopardizing the quality of health care. This would involve evaluating outcomes, assessing techniques, and weeding out ineffective treatments. One procedure that could be virtually eliminated without risk is routine neonatal circumcision, the most common surgical procedure performed on male infants in the United States and one that results in an annual expenditure of $60 million. Although a careful study and considerable debate by the American Academy of Pediatrics (Thompson, King, Knox, & Korones, 1975) has established that there is no medical indication for routine circumcision,[1] the rate for it in the United States (80% to 90% of males) has remained unchanged (Metcalf, Osborn, & Mariani, 1983), probably because most health insurance companies will pay for it. This pattern is consistent with Abelson's (1976, p. 619) comment that

> When the major fraction of medical costs is borne by a third party, demand for care is practically infinite.

Support for this view is provided by Lindeke, Iverson, and Fisch (1986). In England the rate of circumcision plummeted from almost 60% to 0.5% when the National Health Insurance would no longer pay for the operation.

However, no matter how pared down the costs by treatment-related "solutions," this approach represents a holding action that does not address the basic problems. To do so, it is essential that prevention-related strategies be invoked. These represent an approach that has little of the appeal of the cure-related treat-

---

[1]Note, however, that in a more recent and worldwide study of 427,698 infants born in U.S. Army Hospitals during the decade since the American Academy of Pediatrics' report, Wiswell, Enzenauer, Holton, Cornish, and Hankins (1987) have documented a *decrease* in the circumcision frequency rate from 85% in the late 1970s to 70.5% in 1984 and a concomitant 11-fold *increase* in urinary tract infections in uncircumcised as compared to circumcised boys. Wiswell et al. conclude that uncircumcised male infants are at increased risk for infection, but, pending information on long-term effects, they do not advocate routine neonatal circumcision.

ment strategies: There are no immediate returns or dramatic statistical swings; assessment of results is fragmented over a long period of time and definitive data may never be available; and the population involved can be defined only in the broadest terms. Nevertheless, there is a scattering of well-established prevention-based medical procedures, such as immunization programs and cardiovascular-disease-related forms of abstinence. Of particular relevance is the idea of early secondary prevention targeting the CPS in adulthood that has been voiced by Menges (1984, pp. 1259–1260):

> . . . [an] extremely important area . . . is the . . . *prevention* of chronic pain. It appears that in some cases of chronic pain, medicalization has reached staggering proportions. Both professional helpers and social scientists are realizing more and more that their efforts to provide adequate therapy are coming too late for many patients suffering from chronic pain.
>
> At this point several relevant questions may by posed: What signals do we need to look for in the early stages of pain which point towards a developing chronic pain syndrome and what is the most adequate reaction to these signals?

Other crucial questions that should be raised in the service of prevention are: What predisposing factors or developmental precursors should we look for in children and adolescents that suggest that they may be at risk for the CPS or other pain-related maladaptive categories? What action should be taken concerning these factors? It is evident from the clinical, behavioral, and psychiatric literature that such precursors do exist. Consider, for example, certain clusters of children with chronic pain conditions. One such cluster has chronic pain that is characterized by *marginality* (Barker, Wright, & Gonick, 1953). A child in this category has a pain problem that is not visible, so he receives none of the benefits or consideration that a visible disability would elicit. Although he is at a disadvantage psychologically and physiologically, he is expected to function like the healthy child. Under these circumstances the child may begin to move toward a shift in pain status as a coping method and as a means of creating a sanctuary, a pattern that has been observed in some children with juvenile rheumatoid arthritis. Children with chronic pain-related visible disabilities, who have been absent from school for long periods during treatment and lack the coping skills essential for successful school reentry (Katz, Kellerman, Rigler, Williams, & Siegel, 1977), may also seek the shelter that a shift in the status of the pain problem could provide (Kagen-Goodheart, 1977). Children with leukemia are particularly vulnerable because of such problems as extreme pallor, chemotherapy-related baldness, and prednisone-induced obesity (Tucker, 1982). Some of these children reported that their "worst pain ever" was their classmates' derision and taunting about their appearance. One 11-year-old boy said sadly, "I was waiting and waiting to get out [of hospital] and now I sort of think it was nicer there" (Ross & Ross, 1984d).

As a result of parental mishandling of their pain problems, some children with chronic pain (and also some with acute pain) acquire a psychological overlay that they find highly rewarding. Consequently, they strive to maintain the circumstances relevant to it. The following quotation is from a 12-year-old girl who was strongly resistant to the idea that her migraine headaches possibly could be aborted with medication:

> Well, my mom had migraines and so did my grandmother and my mom always said I'd get them, too . . . So whenever I had a headache my mom would ask all about it to see if my migraines had started yet. I finally got my first one when I was eight and it was like being grown up . . . like much better than starting periods. (Girl, CA 12, Ross & Ross, 1982a)

Socialization experiences may also have great impact on the child's tendency to develop a predisposition to the CPS. Some parents use combinations of direct teaching, contingent reinforcement, and modeling to shape their children's behavior in the direction of what Pennebaker (1982) has termed excessive concern with symptoms. Children are sometimes encouraged to use pain for secondary gains in the form of extra privileges and avoidance of disliked activities (Dunn-Geier et al., 1986). Engel (1959) has identified children with early antecedents of what he calls the "pain-prone patient" in adulthood. These children have histories of painful illnesses, trauma, parental aggression, and severe punishment, with prominent illness behavior patterns in their parents or close relatives and with love and affection contingent on their being in pain. A third group of children have parents or families who have a need for them to be ill or in pain (Payne & Norfleet, 1986). In some instances, the mothers obtain tertiary gains out of having a child in pain and exproprate the child's coping ability in the service of these gains, thus facilitating a move toward pre-CPS behavior patterns.

With this sampling of possible predisposing factors and developmental precursors available as a starting point for a focus on early intervention of a preventive kind, the next question concerns the actions that should be taken. At the pediatric level, the optimal prevention strategy involves a two-pronged attack of *primary prevention* for children in general and *early secondary prevention* for chronic pain children in whom early predisposing factors appear to exist but not to a degree that any action has been initiated, as well as for children with experiences or social environmental factors that might put them in the possible risk category. Excluded from these two target groups are cases in which the pain condition and factors in the child, such as developmental level, have resulted in certain well-established pain behaviors for which individualized intervention by skilled pediatric professionals is mandatory. The three-year-old girl with burns (Varni et al., 1980) described earlier would be an example of such a case.

It is our belief that intervention in the school years directed at children in general, including those with physical or environmental characteristics that may put them at risk, could act as a deterrent to the development of the CPS in some cases and, in addition, could influence the general pain-related behaviors of a much larger group by providing a base of knowledge conducive to the development of appropriate pain-related concepts. This intervention strategy would consist of a pain instruction program that would begin within the school setting as part of the general curriculum, at intervals drawing on a range of pediatric professionals in other settings. Health-related programs in the school setting have proliferated in the past decade: These include smoking (Evans, 1982; Pederson, Stennett, & Lefcoe, 1981), diet (Coates, Jeffery, & Slinkard, 1981), back pain (Fine, 1982), relaxation (Setterlind & Uneståhl, 1978), cardiovascular health (Kristein et al., 1977), and active participation in one's own health care (Igoe, 1980; Lewis et al., 1977). Most of these have followed a narrowly defined format involving one instructor, a single topic directly approached, a short-term period of instruction with objective pre- and posttest evaluation, and long-term follow-up within 1 or 2 months of the end of the instruction period. Such programs should be viewed as a preliminary step in the development of a prevention program. This step is useful in establishing that the kind of content and instruction approach appear to be effective. An example relevant to the present discussion is the pain instruction pilot study by Ross and Ross (1985) with children in a mixed Grade 3 and 4 class. Table 8-2 shows the topics that were taught in that 20-lesson program.

Proposed Prevention Program

The kind of prevention program that we envision is a multifaceted, broad-based, long-term program that centers in the school but is implemented across several sectors of the children's lives by professionals from different disciplines. Of a far more comprehensive nature than other school health programs, it would begin at the preschool level and extend into junior high school, covering a wide range of topics from those with a direct and obvious relationship with specific pain subject matter to those with a seemingly tenuous relationship. The goal of the program would be to equip the child and adolescent with a rational perspective of pain; an understanding of the logic of pain treatment procedures; coping skills for attenuation of pain and prepain anxiety, some of which would also have utility in a variety of nonmedical stress situations; simple, safe, medically based and behavioral–cognitive self-management skills, such as Hoku point pressure for headache or stretching for growing pains (Clark, 1987); and a feeling of competence and an ensuing sense of some control in the pain situation.

The school personnel involved would include the class teacher and school nurse. One component of the teacher's role would be to teach the formal pain instruction program with lesson content similar to that in Table 8-2 but appropriate to age and grade level. Another component would require the teacher to be alert to such behaviors as frequent absences with no obvious reason, the effects of the television-mediated specter of pain that inundates many children's concepts of pain (Ross & Ross, 1982a; 1985) and carries over into their conversation, and ex-

Table 8-2   Pain Instruction Program for Third and Fourth Grades

Content (20-lesson program)

Common childhood injuries, spontaneous and iatrogenic pain events
When a pain report is mandatory, how to get help if alone
What to report, pain parameters: localization, duration, intensity, etc.
Simple self-treatment for minor injuries and pains; medication and parent permission
Concepts of emergency, first aid
Value of pain: warning function, diagnostic aid, treatment evaluator, problems of congenital analgesia
Iatrogenic pain settings: hospital, surgicenter, doctor/dentist's offices, school immunization clinic
Painless diagnostic and treatment procedures: x ray, cast removal, vision and hearing tests
Putting needle procedures in perspective: simple explanations for stitches, analgesic procedures, immunization, blood counts
Coping strategies: attention diversion, thought-stopping
Maladaptive pain usage

Teaching Procedures

Direct teaching; discussion; interviews with child concerning specific pain experiences; live and symbolic modeling procedures; demonstration; related fiction/nonfiction picture books; class debate about pain issues such as, advance information re impending pain events and sex differences in sensitivity to pain

cessive reliance on external help in pain relief. The teacher would also seize opportunities that occur spontaneously to encourage generalization of skills and ideas and to teach pain-related skills in the context of other school subjects, for example, coping strategies such as thought-stopping (D. Ross, 1984) when the child is nervous about an impending solo performance, or quota setting to help him through a disliked or difficult task (Dolce, Crocker et al., 1986).

The pediatrician and other pediatric personnel would have to be alert to signs of secondary-gain pain events in children in general and to the needs of children with special problems that might predispose them to maladaptive pain usage. The medical personnel should also note and dispel television-mediated fears and misconceptions, particularly those that hinder pain management. They would have to be prevention oriented, which means extending their inquiries well beyond the immediate and visible problem. The significance of destructive parental and family behavior patterns should be recognized and steps taken to modify them. If such change is unrealistic, attention should be focused on helping the child to counteract these influences. A preventive approach requires concern for the patient in his environment, and there is encouraging evidence (Scott & Neighbor, 1985) that many beginning physicians have this orientation.

Ideally, parents should function as an integral part of the preventive process, with a strong working liaison among school, parents, and pediatrician. They are the primary resource in terms of frequency and duration of contact with the child.

Realistically, they may not participate at all. However, in our preliminary pain instruction projects (Ross & Ross, 1985, 1986), a number of parents were drawn in inevitably, at least to some extent, by the force of the other participants (child and teacher). Some parents, for example, had their maladaptive pain usage behaviors spelled out for them by their children. In any event, the proposed prevention program does not depend on parental input while at the same time it encourages such participation.

Short-Term Results

Some aspects of the program lend themselves to objective measurement: Tests would be used to assess the acquisition of subject-matter content; observational data could be collected on how the child behaves during any medical/dental events that occur routinely in the school setting; and statistical data are always available on absenteeism. However, many of the intended results are not readily quantifiable in the course of the daily school routine: The child should acquire coping skills for use in immediate pain situations and be better able to cope in other stress situations; in medical situations he should experience less fear and have increased feelings of control; his concepts of the hospital and medical procedures should show a broader grasp of these topics; and he should be better able to express his concerns, describe his feelings, and seek information when in these settings. His pain descriptions should become far more precise and informative, and his behavior with the pediatrician should represent a more equitable balance of power: There should be a gradual shift in his interactions with medical/dental personnel from the passive, one-way, edict-and-compliance type of communication that Katz (1984) has censured to more productive interactions in which mutual participation and negotiation predominate.

The basis for these expectations concerning the type of pain instruction program described here are the data collected in the course of a pilot study on pain instruction for a mixed Grade 3 and 4 class (Ross & Ross, 1985), which was followed by a full-scale study on pain instruction in kindergarten through Grade 2 (Ross & Ross, 1986). Empirical data in the form of pre- and posttest comparisons from these two studies support our contention that children can acquire a base of knowledge about pain. Anecdotal support in the form of unsolicited comments from teachers and parents showed unequivocal evidence of acquisition and generalization of lesson content. In the following examples, the children were all from the kindergarten group and their behaviors related to three of the areas of pain lesson content that they had been taught:

1. **On what to tell the pediatrician about a pain problem:** The boy's mother had taken her son to their pediatrician because he had a bad earache. Although clearly in discomfort, he spent some time while in the waiting room telling her all the things that he was going to tell the pediatrician about the earache (when it started,

that it was not continuous, that it felt like needles) to help him know how to treat it. After seeing the boy, the pediatrician told the mother that her son's information had been a significant help in diagnosing the middle-ear problem.

2. **On what to tell an adult if in pain:** A kindergarten teacher noted that prior to the pain instruction program children in her class had offered only minimal descriptions of aches and pains ("I don't feel good"). After the lesson on giving as complete information as possible, almost all the children spontaneously offered explicit accounts ("My stomach hurts all the time like squeezing and it started to hurt right after Show and Tell") and they have continued this practice.

3. **On not using pain as an excuse:** One girl who frequently used pain as an excuse to avoid swimming lessons listened intently to the lesson story and group discussion on why it was not good to use pain as an excuse and why it was better to say how you felt about an activity. Her teachers described her as "looking very downcast and nodding soberly" throughout the lesson. Several days later, when her mother picked her up after school and said they were going to her cousin's house, the child said firmly, "I don't want to go. I don't like going there." The mother looked astonished and asked, "What's the matter? Don't you feel well?" To which the child answered emphatically, "I feel good, I just don't want to go there." Her teachers reported that in the school setting she has not used pain as an excuse since that lesson.

Long-Term Results

One characteristic of prevention programs is that assessment of results is difficult, fragmented, and often inadequate because appropriate measuring instruments are available for only the most objective, gross, and clear-cut indicators of change. Definitive data linking a prevention program to a specific change in a definable statistic are rarely attainable except for specific medical conditions such as the incidence of measles in the pediatric population following an immunization program. In the prevention program that we are advocating, the closest approximation of a program–results link would be to document within a school population the percentage of children who as adults became CPS patients and make comparisons with other nonprogram school populations. While satisfying those who have a need for "statistical" data, the results obtained from such an approach would be exceedingly dubious in view of the large number of uncontrollable unknowns and sources of error inherent in such a comparison.

The long-term outcomes as we see them would be nonmeasurable and often diffused and intangible: Attitudes toward medical experiences, reduction in the stress potential involved, awareness of maladaptive pain usage patterns, independence rather than helplessness when faced with a medical problem—these are the kinds of areas in which positive changes are likely to occur.

Sources of Resistance to Such a Program

The topic of pain instruction appears to have a certain aura or mystique surrounding it that is absent when programs on drugs, death, sex education, and acquired immune deficiency syndrome (AIDS) are proposed. These latter programs, although controversial, have all been introduced into some schools.

Parental resistance has taken the form of concern that children might be frightened by the topic of pain. In the course of obtaining subject permission in our interview and pain instruction studies (Ross & Ross, 1982a; 1985; 1986), a small number of parents raised this point and others volunteered the fact that they actively tried to avoid any discussion of pain, particularly if the child had had some prior serious pain experiences. In the interview setting itself, a substantial number of children provided some confirmation of this parental attitude by stating that they seldom had received advance information on impending pain events. It should be noted that these parents all gave permission for their children's participation and that following the studies, neither we nor the schools received any negative feedback of any sort from any parent.

One issue that as far as we know has been raised only by a small group of psychologists concerns the ethics of teaching a formal program on pain in the schools. This group criticized pain instruction on the grounds that it would teach children pain awareness and that the goal of changing children's behavior in pain situations was an undesirable one. In addition, these psychologists stated that teaching children that maladaptive pain usage was wrong could be psychologically damaging to the children. It is difficult to understand why a program whose intent is to equip the child to cope with the inevitable experience of pain should incur the criticism that it is unethical to do so. We mention this issue only because it seems to relate back to the mystique idea, a surprising link in view of the educational level of its proponents. A number of experts prominent in relevant fields, such as pain, developmental psychology, education, theology, psychiatry, and philosophy have unanimously rejected the criticism that it is unethical to teach a formal program on pain of the type we envision in the schools. Representative of this stance is the statement of the eminent pediatric psychologist Gerald Koocher (1986), who is co-author of a recent text, *Ethics in Psychology,* that will be highly influential in the field:

> Children as young as two or three years old are certainly aware of pain, and cognitions related to it are a normal part of parent-child interaction . . .
>
> Insofar as the concern that you may be trying to change a child's behavior; don't all of us (i.e., parents, teachers, therapists, etc.) attempt to do that daily? . . . A large number (of professionals) across the country are actively involved in research to help children tolerate and cope more effectively with chronic pain and painful medical procedures. The cognitive component in the experience and expression of pain has been well documented. There is a sound theoretical basis for the hypothesis that improving a child's understanding of adaptive and maladaptive usage of pain will lead to improved coping. . .
>
> . . . it is naïve to be critical about "teaching that maladaptive pain usage is wrong" . . . any normal child will encounter dozens of experiences per year when a similar message is given to them by much more influential people than an investigator (e.g., when a knee is scraped and a parent exhorts, "Enough crying already!").

. . . I would be quite surprised if any of the colleagues who raised the "ethical" issues have worked with children suffering from painful illnesses . . . or have ever worked in pediatric settings at all.

Costs

In terms of teacher and class time, as well as expenditures for materials, the costs for this pain instruction program would be low. This is particularly true when the offset effect is included, that is, the fact that the provision of one type of service is likely to lead to a reduction in the use of related services, for example, pain clinic treatment. However, if the cost–benefit ratio (CBR) must be demonstrated to be favorable, that is, if the benefits and consequences of the program must exceed the costs in numerical terms, usually dollars, the pain instruction program that we are advocating would never meet that criterion. Unfortunately, the CBR is now being used to evaluate a number of health-related programs and in some instances has led to the conclusion that treatment of sick children is preferable, from a monetary viewpoint, to prevention of their illness. In a scathing commentary on the blatant disregard for humanitarian principles that the use of CBR implies, particularly with respect to education programs, Cousins (1979, p. 8) has pointed out that

> The term [CBR] descends like a death sentence on any proposal that would apply creative imagination to socially essential programs or long-range goals. If ideas are offered that seek to upgrade the quality of education, or that would improve the nutrition of the nation's children, or that would make life a little less squalid or agonizing for millions of Americans . . . someone is certain to say the idea cannot be justified because of CBR . . . but CBR is a fallacy. It ignores the fact that the main source of a nation's wealth is to be found in the developed mind of its citizenry. Perhaps the most obvious example is education. . . . The notion that this process can be evaluated by numbers is as absurd as an attempt to calibrate infinity.

Much of the emphasis throughout this text has been on prevention rather than treatment. The discussions on establishing a rarefaction ecology in the medical treatment setting fell into this category as did, in a broader sense, the emphasis on teaching the child how to cope with a variety of stressors. The pain instruction program we are advocating is yet a further step on the preventive intervention path. Research and development within a prevention framework is of critical importance in the increasingly uneven battle between humane health care and its spiraling costs. The end result of focusing on management almost to the exclusion of preventive intervention in the allocation of funds has been succinctly described by Rosenfeld (1983, p. 6):

> What if the March of Dimes had elected during the decades of the 1940s and 1950s to devote most of its resources to putting polio victims into iron lungs instead of concentrating on basic viral research and vaccine development? We now know that to have spent *less* money in infantile paralysis research would have been a massive extravagance. Think what we would have been spending all these years on polio care

versus the negligible costs of vaccination and prevention, let alone the untold amount of human anguish that has been prevented.

In the pediatric pain field the continuing emphasis on management rather than prevention represents a symptom rather than a cause. The basic issue, as we see it, is an ideological one: Children are overlooked as a major and important resource. The failure to focus adequate clinical and empirical attention on the area of childhood pain reflects a set of priorities established at the federal and state levels and exerting considerable influence on clinicians and researchers in the field. In rebuttal of the outraged denials of these statements, denials that are usually accompanied by earnest claims that children are our most precious resource, we offer the following facts concerning American children:

Ten percent suffer from chronic pain, yet there are, to our knowledge, fewer than a dozen pain clinics that specialize in children's pain problems (Berde, 1987; Chapman, 1987; Hahn, 1986; P. A. McGrath, 1987c). As of 1983, one in five children live in poverty. This number has risen steadily since 1969, which suggts, at best, indifference. Of the 67 million school children below age 16, 10 million receive no medical care; of all children under age 15, 50% have never been to a dentist. Child-nutrition cuts have also been harsh, with the most severe effects on the children of the working poor. Reductions in program funding between 1982 and 1984 closed out 1 million poor children (Mundinger, 1985). Immunization figures show that 19 million have not been fully immunized against measles or German measles.

Alarming as these statistics are, the most chilling of all are the federal health figures: Between 1960 and 1975, federal health dollars invested in child health declined from 1 of every 2 dollars to 1 of every 10 dollars (Mundinger, 1985).

Comment

The past decade has been marked by encouraging changes and advances in the field of childhood pain. To consolidate these gains and ensure that progress continues at an escalating rate, we need now to focus on two broad kinds of investigation. The first of these is characterized by the high-quality clinical study that emphasizes methodological rigor and forms one element in a systematic attack on facets of the variable under study. The investigator is in complete control of the independent variables, with the child's role restricted to that of a recipient of the investigative action. These requirements are applicable to a wide range of pain topic areas. The approach is exemplified by the careful documentation by Craig and his associates of pain expressivity in infancy; it underlies the skillful pursuit of teams led by Szyfelbein, Herman, and others of the role of the endorphins in severe pediatric pain conditions; it can be applied to a sophisticated investigation of the child's interpretation of pain assessment procedures, as P. A. McGrath has shown; and, finally, it is the base for the persistent and unflagging search for interventions for optimal management of iatrogenic pain that Jay and her associates, Kuttner, and others have conducted.

Throughout this text there is unequivocal evidence that when approached in a cognitively appropriate way, children from preschool through adolescence are competent discussants of pain. The second of the two broad kinds of investigation that we are advocating here involves capitalizing on this incredibly rich source as a way to advance our understanding of childhood pain, improve management procedures for it, clarify the link between it and pain in adulthood, and contribute to theoretical formulations. In the case of preschool and school-age children, this resource has barely been tapped, and with adolescents, it is virtually untouched. It is astonishing that in our consumer-oriented society, with audience reaction in its various forms assigned a major role in determining subsequent events, such a pool of information should be so undervalued. Despite generalizations concerning the advisability of active involvement of children in all facets of health care, in the pain setting attention typically focuses on symptoms and techniques, with little interest or concern in the child's immediate or posttreatment thoughts. A notable exception in this pattern of disinterest has been the formation of the Children's Advisory Board to the Milwaukee Children's Hospital (Lowery, 1985). Composed of 16 children between the ages of 8 and 14, this board advises the hospital on ways to improve patient care from the child's point of view.

Assuming a genuine interest on the part of the pediatric personnel, a major obstacle to the free exchange of ideas and opinions between the child and staff concerns the child's fear of retribution. That hospitalized children often feel that their psychological safety is in jeopardy was apparent in our interview study. As one boy age 11 explained apologetically:

> It's like in school if you complain you're still stuck with the same teacher so things get worse. . . . Well, I'm stuck with Old Iceberg here and if she gets any worse I can't stand it, so I'll tell you about it when they let me out.

Even the youngest hospitalized children are aware of the possible threat implicit in criticism. A child life worker (Gilchrist, 1978) gave the following account of her efforts to obtain a candid report from a 4-year-old boy:

> After several searching inquiries about not telling the nurse, the child looked around carefully, including under his bed, then lifted the covers and said in a conspiratorial way, "Come on in and if *she* [nurse] comes, pretend we're just playing."

Clearly, the child who is asked for opinions and ideas must be assured of complete confidentiality and of immunity from repercussions. Equally important, if this informational source is to be tapped, is the need to accord the child the status of expert: It must be clear to him that because of the subjectivity inherent in the pain experience, he is the expert in the situation and, as such, will be shown the respect that that role entails.

In the past decade, these two kinds of investigation have yielded a diversity of information about the child's view of pain along with a cluster of procedural innovations for pain assessment and intervention. The utility of this information has been drastically limited, however, because much of it is not being used in the clinical setting but, instead, is lying dormant in the literature. This implementation lag is particularly true of interventions having a predominantly psychological rather than a medical base. A case in point is self-hypnosis, a procedure with strong empirical support that is admirably suited for use with pain in children but is not as widely used as its potential would indicate. Although in theory the philosophy of treating the whole child is widely endorsed, in practice, pediatric pain management remains predominantly a matter of medical management of physical problems, often with only cursory interest in the inclusion of psychological interventions in the treatment protocol.

If medical interest in the use of psychological procedures in pediatric pain treatment is to be elicited, changes must occur in dissemination practices. As it is now, the procedural information in the journal literature usually is not given in sufficient detail for it to be readily applied to specific cases in the pediatric setting, if indeed it even reaches that setting. The clinical researcher should be willing to invest some time and energy in ensuring that existing information and new findings relevant to intervention are presented in a form sufficiently detailed to foster their use in the pediatric setting. Research papers should include statements on the rationale, applicability, effectiveness, side effects (if any), developmental level at which the procedure has proven useful, and specific steps for implementing it; they should then be published in journals that reach the pediatric community.

In his introduction to the *Textbook of Pain* (Wall, 1984, p. 1), Wall has cautioned that

> So long as one person remains in pain and we cannot help, our knowledge of pain remains inadequate.

To this caveat we would add:

> So long as one child remains in pain and procedures that could help him are not being used, our management of pediatric pain remains grossly inadequate.

It is incumbent on investigators in this emerging field not only to pursue the study of childhood pain, but also to ensure that their findings, especially those in the area of psychological intervention, see the light of day in the pediatric pain setting.

References

Abelson, P. H. Cost-effective health care. *Science,* 1976, *192,* 619.

Abraham, G. E. Primary dysmenorrhea. *Clinical Obstetrics and Gynecology,* 1978, *21,* 139–145.

Abu-Saad, H. The assessment of pain in children. *Issues in Comprehensive Pediatric Nursing,* 1981, *5,* 327–335.

Abu-Saad, H. Cultural components of pain: The Asian-American child. *Children's Health Care,* 1984a, *13,* 11–14.

Abu-Saad, H. Cultural components of pain: The Arab-American child. *Issues in Comprehensive Pediatric Nursing,* 1984b, *7,* 91–99.

Abu-Saad, H. Cultural group indicators of pain in children. *Maternal-Child Nursing Journal,* 1984c, *13,* 187–196.

Abu-Saad, H., & Holzemer, W. L. Measuring children's self-assessment of pain. *Issues in Comprehensive Pediatric Nursing,* 1981, *5,* 337–349.

Ack, M. New perspectives in comprehensive health care for children. *Journal of Pediatric Psychology,* 1976, *1,* 9–11.

Ack, M. Psychosocial effects of illness, hospitalization, and surgery. *Children's Health Care,* 1983, *11,* 132–136.

Adams, B. N. Birth order: A critical review, *Sociometry,* 1972, *35,* 411–439.

Adams, M. A. A hospital play program: Helping children with serious illness. *American Journal of Orthopsychiatry,* 1976, *46,* 416–424.

Ad Hoc Committee on Classification of Headache. Classification of headache. *Journal of the American Medical Association,* 1962, *179,* 717–718.

Adler, S. N. M. The stigma of handicap and its unlearning: A social perspective on children with muscle disease and their families. *Dissertation Abstracts International,* 1973, *34* (3B), 1266–1267.

Agnew, D. C., & Merskey, H. Words of chronic pain. *Pain,* 1976, *2,* 73–81.

Agras, S., Sylvester, D., & Oliveau, D. The epidemiology of common fears and phobias. *Comprehensive Psychology,* 1969, *10,* 151–156.

Ainsworth, M. Patterns of attachment behavior shown by the infant in interaction with his mother. *Merrill-Palmer Quarterly,* 1964, *10,* 51–58.

Ala-Hurula, V., Myllyla, V., & Hokkanen, E. Ergotamine abuse: Results of ergotamine discontinuation with special reference to the plasma concentration. *Cephalalgia,* 1982, *2,* 189–195.

Alexander, A. B. Systematic relaxation and flow rate in asthmatic children: Relationship to emotional precipitants and anxiety. *Journal of Psychosomatic Research,* 1972, *16,* 405–410.

Allmond, B. W., Buckman, W., & Gofman, H. F. *The family is the patient.* St. Louis: Mosby, 1979.

American Hospital Association. *Patients' Bill of Rights.* Chicago: American Hospital Association, 1972.

American Journal of Maternal/Child Nursing. Pain, 1984, *9,* No. 4, pp. 249–276.

American Pain Society. *Minutes of the new Board of Directors of the American Pain Society.* Nutley, NJ: American Pain Society, 1980.

American Psychological Association. *Principles for the care and use of animals.* Washington, DC: APA, 1968.

American Psychological Association. *American Educational Research Association and National Council on Measurement in Education, Standards for Educational and Psychological Tests.* Washington, DC: APA, 1974.

American Psychological Association. *Ethical principles in the conduct of research with human participants.* Washington, DC: APA, 1982.

Amery, W. K. Brain hypoxia: The turning point in the genesis of the migraine attack. *Cephalalgia,* 1982, *2,* 83–109.

Andolsek, K., & Novik, B. Procedures in family practice: Use of hypnosis with children. *Journal of Family Practice,* 1980, *10,* 503–507.

Andrasik, F., Attanasio, V., Blanchard, E. B., Burke, E., Kabela, E., McCarran, M., Blake, D. D., & Rosenblum, E. L. Behavioral treatment of pediatric migraine headache. Paper presented at the meeting of the Association for Advancement of Behavior Therapy, Philadelphia, 1984.

Andrasik, F., Blake, D. D., & McCarran, M. S. A biobehavioral analysis of pediatric headache. In N. A. Krasnegor, J. D. Arasteh, & M. F. Cataldo (Eds.), *Child health behavior: A behavioral pediatrics perspective.* New York: Wiley Interscience, 1986, pp. 394–434.

Andrasik, F., Blanchard, E. B., Arena, J. G., Saunders, N. L., & Barron, K. D. Psychophysiology of recurrent headache: Methodological issues and new empirical findings. *Behavior Therapy,* 1982, *13,* 407–429.

Andrasik, F., Blanchard, E. B., Arena, J. G., Teders, S. J., Teevan, R. C., & Rodichok, L. D. Psychological functioning in headache sufferers. *Psychosomatic Medicine,* 1982, *44,* 171–182.

Andrasik, F., Burke, E. J., Attanasio, V., & Rosenblum, E. L. Child, parent, and physician reports of a child's headache pain: Relationships prior to and following treatment. *Headache,* 1985, *25,* 421–425.

Andrasik, F., & Holroyd, K. A. A test of specific and nonspecific effects in the biofeedback treatment of tension headache. *Journal of Consulting and Clinical Psychology,* 1980a, *48,* 575–586.

Andrasik, F., & Holroyd, K. A. Reliability and concurrent validity of headache questionnaire data. *Headache,* 1980b, *12,* 44–46.

Andrasik, F., Kabela, E., Quinn, S., Blanchard, E. B., & Rosenblum, E. L. Psychological functioning of children who have recurrent migraine. Unpublished manuscript, State University of New York at Albany, 1985.

Angell, M. The quality of mercy. *New England Journal of Medicine,* 1982, *306,* 98–99.

Ansell, B. M. *Rheumatic disorders in children.* London: Butterworths, 1980.

Apley, J. *The child with abdominal pain,* 2nd ed. London: Blackwell, 1975.

Aradine, C. R., Beyer, J. E., & Tompkins, J. M. Children's pain perceptions before and after analgesia: A study of instrument construct validity and related issues. *Journal of Pediatric Nursing,* in press, 1987.

Arney, W. R., & Bergen, B. J. *Medicine and the management of living.* Chicago: University of Chicago Press, 1984.

Aronoff, G. M. Psychological aspects of nonmalignant chronic pain: A new nosology. In G. M. Aronoff (Ed.), *Evaluation and treatment of chronic pain.* Baltimore: Urban & Schwarzenberg, 1985, pp. 471–484.

Aronoff, G. M., Evans, W. O., & Enders, P. L. A review of follow-up studies of multidisciplinary pain units. In G. M. Aronoff (Ed.), *Evaluation and treatment of chronic pain.* Baltimore: Urban & Schwarzenberg, 1985, pp. 511–521.

Aronoff, G. M., & Wagner, J. M. Pain centers: A community resource. *Mediguide to Pain,* 1986, *7,* 1–4.

Artz, C. P., Moncrief, J. A., & Pruitt, B. A. (Eds.). *Burns: A team approach*. Philadelphia: Saunders, 1979.

Atkinson, R. S., Hamblin, J. J., & Wright, J. E. C. *Handbook of intensive care*. London: Chapman & Hall, 1981.

Averill, J. R. Personal control over aversive stimuli and its relationship to stress. *Psychological Bulletin*, 1973, *80*, 286–303.

Axline, V. M. *Play therapy*. New York: Ballantine, 1969.

Ayer, W. Use of visual imagery in needle-phobic children. *Journal of Dentistry for Children*, 1973, *40*, 41–43.

Azarnoff, P. The care of children in hospitals: An overview. *Journal of Pediatric Psychology*, 1976, *1*, 5–6.

Azarnoff, P. (Ed.). *Preparation of young healthy children for possible hospitalization: The issues*. Monograph No. 1, Santa Monica, CA: Pediatric Projects Inc., 1983.

Azarnoff, P., & Woody, P. D. Preparation of children for hospitalization in acute care hospitals in the United States. *Pediatrics*, 1981, *68*, 361–368.

Bailey, C. A., & Davidson, P. O. The language of pain: Intensity. *Pain*, 1976, *2*, 319–324.

Bailey, W. C. (Ed.). *Pediatric burns*. Miami, FL: Symposia Specialists, 1979.

Bain, J. A. *Thought control in everyday life*. New York: Funk & Wagnalls, 1928.

Bakal, D. A. *Psychology and medicine: Psychobiological dimensions of health and illness*. New York: Springer, 1979.

Bakal, D. A. *The psychobiology of chronic headache*. New York: Springer, 1982.

Bakal, D. A., Demjen, S., & Kaganov, J. A. Cognitive behavioral treatment of chronic headache. *Headache*, 1981, *21*, 81–86.

Bakal, D. A., Demjen, S., & Kaganov, J. A. The continuous nature of headache susceptibility. *Social Science and Medicine*, 1984, *19*, 1305–1311.

Bakal, D. A., & Kaganov, J. A. Muscle contraction and migraine headache: Psychophysiologic comparison. *Headache*, 1977, *17*, 208–215.

Bandura, A. *Principles of behavior modification*. New York: Holt, Rinehart, 1969.

Bandura, A. Self-referent thought: A developmental analysis of self-efficacy. In J. H. Flavell & L. Ross (Eds.), *Social cognitive development: Frontiers and possible futures*. Cambridge, England: Cambridge University Press, 1981, pp. 200–239.

Bandura, A. Self-efficacy mechanism in human agency. *American Psychologist*, 1982, *37*, 122–147.

Banks, M. H., Beresford, S. A., Morrell, D. C., Waller, J. J., & Watkins, C. J. Factors influencing demand for primary medical care in women aged 20–44 years: A preliminary report. *International Journal of Epidemiology*, 1975, *4*, 189–194.

Barber, T. X. Toward a theory of pain: Relief of chronic pain by prefrontal leucotomy, opiates, placebos, and hypnosis. *Psychological Bulletin*, 1959, *56*, 430–460.

Barker, R. G., Wright, B. A., & Gonick, M. A. *Adjustment to physical handicap and illness: A survey of the social psychology of physique and disability*, (Rev.). New York: Social Science Research Council, 1953.

Barnard, C. The colors of pain. *Discover*, 1981, *2*, 62, 64.

Barnes, C. School-age children's recall of the intensive care unit. *A.N.A. Clinical Sessions*. New York: Appleton-Century-Crofts, 1974, pp. 73–91.

Barnes, R. B. The early history of thermography. In S. Uematsu (Ed.), *Medical thermography, theory and clinical applications*. Los Angeles: Brentwood, 1976, pp. 1–14.

Barnett, H. L. *Pediatrics*. New York: Appleton-Century-Crofts, 1977.

Barr, R. G. Pain tolerance and developmental change in pain perception. In M. D. Levine, W. B. Carey, A. C. Crocker, & R. T. Gross (Eds.), *Developmental-behavioral pediatrics*. Philadelphia: Saunders, 1982, pp. 505–512.

Barr, R. G., & Feuerstein, M. Recurrent abdominal pain syndrome: How appropriate are our basic clinical assumptions? In P. J. McGrath & P. Firestone (Eds.), *Pediatric and adolescent behavioral medicine: Issues in treatment*. New York: Springer, 1983, pp. 13–27.

Barr, R. G., Kramer, M. S., Leduc, D. G., Boisjoly, C., McVey, L., & Pless, I. B. Validation of a parental diary of infant cry/fuss behavior by a 24-hour voice-activated infant recording (VAR) system. Unpublished manuscript, Montreal Children's Hospital, 1987.

Bartlett, J. C., Burleson, G., & Santrock, J. W. Emotional mood and memory in young children. *Journal of Experimental Child Psychology*, 1982, *34*, 59–76.

Basmajian, J. V. Control and training of individual motor units. *Science*, 1963, *141*, 440–441.

Bayrakal, S. A group experience with chronically disabled adolescents. *American Journal of Psychiatry*, 1975, *132*, 1291–1294.

Beales, J. G. Pain in children with cancer. In J. J. Bonica & V. Ventfridda (Eds.), *Advances in pain research and therapy*, Vol. 2. New York: Raven Press, 1979, pp. 89–98.

Beales, J. G. Factors influencing the expectation of pain among patients in a children's burns unit. *Burns*, 1983, *9*, 187–192.

Beales, J. G., Holt, P. J., Keen, J. H., & Mellor, V. P. Children with juvenile chronic arthritis: Their beliefs about their illness and therapy. *Annals of the Rheumatic Diseases*, 1983, *42*, 481–486.

Beales, J. G., Keen, J. H., & Holt, P. J. The child's perception of the disease and the experience of pain in juvenile chronic arthritis. *Journal of Rheumatology*, 1983, *10*, 61–65.

Beaver, W. T. Aspirin and acetaminophen as constituents of analgesic combinations, *Archives of Internal Medicine*, 1981, *141*, 293–300.

Beaver, W. T. Measurement of analgesic efficacy in man. In J. J. Bonica, U. Lindblom, & A. Iggo (Eds.), *Advances in pain research and therapy*, Vol. 5. New York: Raven Press, 1983. pp. 411–434.

Beecher, H. K. Relationship of significance of wound to the pain experienced. *Journal of the American Medical Association*, 1956, *161*, 1609–1613.

Beecher, H. K. *Measurement of subjective responses*. New York: Oxford University Press, 1959.

Benitz, W. E. Personal communication, January, 1987.

Benitz, W. E., & Tatro, D. S. *The pediatric drug handbook*. Chicago: Year Book Medical Publishers, 1981.

Bensen, V. B. One hundred cases of post-anesthetic suggestion in the recovery room. *American Journal of Clinical Hypnosis*, 1971, *14*, 9–15.

Berde, C. Personal communication, January, 1987.

Bergmann, T. *Children in the hospital*. New York: International University Press, 1965.

Berkowitz, B. A. The relationship of pharmacokinetics to pharmacological activity; morphine, methadone and naloxone. *Clinical Pharmacokinetics*, 1976, *1*, 219–230.

Bernick, S. M. Relaxation, suggestion, and hypnosis in dentistry: What the pediatrician should know about children's dentistry. *Clinical Pediatrics*, 1972, *11*, 72–75.

Bernstein, N. R. Management of burned children with the aid of hypnosis. *Journal of Child Psychology and Psychiatry*, 1963, *4*, 93–98.

Bernstein, N. R. Significant values of hypnoanesthesia: Three clinical examples. *American Journal of Clinical Hypnosis*, 1965, *7*, 259–260.

Bernstein, N. R. *Emotional care of the facially burned and disfigured*. Boston: Little, Brown, 1976.

Bernstein, N. R., & Robson, M. C. (Eds.). *Comprehensive approaches to the burned person*. New Hyde Park, NY: Medical Examination Publishing Co., 1983.

Bernstein, N. R., Sanger, S., & Fras, I. The functions of the child psychiatrist in the management of severely burned children. *Journal of the American Academy of Child Psychiatry,* 1969, *8,* 620–636.

Betcher, A. M. Hypnosis as an adjunct in anesthesiology. *New York State Journal of Medicine,* 1960, *60,* 816–822.

Beuf, A. H. *Biting off the bracelet.* Philadelphia: University of Pennsylvania Press, 1979.

Beyer, J. E. *The Oucher: A user's manual and technical report.* Evanston, IL: The Hospital Play Equipment Co., 1984.

Beyer, J. E. Cluster studies to examine the reliability and validity of an instrument to measure the intensity of children's pain experiences. Unpublished manuscript, University of Rochester, School of Nursing, 1985.

Beyer, J. E., & Aradine, C. R. Content validity of an instrument to measure young children's perceptions of the intensity of their pain. *Journal of Pediatric Nursing,* 1986, *1,* 386–395.

Beyer, J. E., & Aradine, C. R. Patterns of pain intensity: A methodological investigation of a self-report scale. *Clinical Journal of Pain,* in press, 1987a.

Beyer, J. E., & Aradine, C. R. The convergent and discriminant validity of a self-report measure of pain intensity in children. *Children's Health Care,* in press, 1987b.

Beyer, J. E., & Byers, M. L. Knowledge of pediatric pain: The state of the art. *Children's Health Care,* 1985, *13,* 150–159.

Beyer, J. E., DeGood, D. E., Ashley, L. C., & Russell, G. A. Patterns of postoperative analgesic use with adults and children following cardiac surgery. *Pain,* 1983, *17,* 71–81.

Beyer, J. E., & Knapp, T. R. Methodological issues in the measurement of children's pain. *Children's Health Care,* 1986, *14,* 233–241.

Bibace, R., & Walsh, M. E. Development of children's concepts of illness. *Pediatrics,* 1980, *66,* 912–917.

Bierenbaum, H., & Bergey, S. F. Family therapy training in a pediatric setting, *Journal of Pediatric Psychology,* 1980, *5,* 263–276.

Bille, B. Migraine in school children. *Acta Paediatrica Scandinavica,* 1962, *51,* 1–151.

Bille, B. Migraine in childhood and its prognosis. *Cephalalgia,* 1981, *1,* 71–75.

Bilting, M., Carlsson, C.-A., Menge, B., Pellettieri, L., & Peterson, L.-E. Estimation of time as a measure of pain magnitude. *Journal of Psychosomatic Research,* 1983, *27,* 493–497.

Black, R. G. Management of pain with nerve blocks. *Minnesota Medicine,* 1974, *57,* 189–194.

Black, R. G. The clinical syndrome of chronic pain. In L. K. Y. Ng & J. J. Bonica (Eds), *Pain, discomfort, and humanitarian care.* New York: Elsevier/North-Holland, 1980, pp. 207–231.

Boehncke, H. Pain analysis in childhood. In R. Janzen (Ed.), *Pain analysis.* Bristol, England: John Wright, 1970, pp. 73–81.

Boisen, E. Strokes in migraine: Report on seven strokes associated with severe migraine attacks. *Danish Medical Bulletin,* 1975, *22,* 100–106.

Bok, D. *The President's report 1982–83 to the Board of Overseers.* Cambridge, MA: Harvard University, 1984.

Bokan, J. A., Ries, R. K., & Katon, W. J. Tertiary gain and chronic pain. *Pain,* 1981, *10,* 331–335.

Bond, M. R. *Pain: Its nature, analysis, and treatment.* New York: Churchill Livingstone, 1979.

Bond, M. R. *Pain: Its nature, analysis, and treatment,* 2nd ed. New York: Churchill Livingstone, 1984.

Bonica, J. J. *The management of pain.* Philadelphia: Lea & Febiger, 1953.

Bonica, J. J. Therapeutic acupuncture in the People's Republic of China. *Journal of the American Medical Association,* 1974, *228,* 1544–1551.
Bonica, J. J. Preface. In P. L. LeRoy (Ed.), *Current concepts in the management of chronic pain.* New York: Stratton, 1977, pp. xi–xiii.
Bonica, J. J. The relation of injury to pain. Letter to the Editor. *Pain,* 1979, *7,* 203–207.
Bonica, J. J. Pain research and therapy: Past and current status and future needs. In L. K. Y. Ng & J. J. Bonica (Eds.), *Pain, discomfort, and humanitarian care.* New York: Elsevier/North-Holland, 1980, pp. 1–46.
Bonica, J. J. The importance of education and training in pain diagnosis and therapy: The role of continuing education courses. In R. Rizzi & M. Visentin (Eds.), *Pain Therapy.* Amsterdam: Elsevier Biomedical Press, 1983, pp. 1–10.
Bonica, J. J. Pain research and therapy: Recent advances and future needs. In L. Kruger & J. C. Liebeskind (Eds.), *Neural mechanisms of pain. Advances in Pain Research and Therapy,* Vol. 6. New York: Raven Press, 1984, pp. 1–22.
Bonica, J. J. Importance of the problem. In G. M. Aronoff (Ed.), *Evaluation and treatment of chronic pain.* Baltimore: Urban & Schwarzenberg, 1985a, pp. xxxi–xliv.
Bonica, J. J. Biology, pathophysiology, and treatment of acute pain. In S. Lipton & J. Miles (Eds.), *Persistent pain: Modern methods of treatment,* Vol. 5. London: Grune & Stratton, 1985b, pp. 1–32.
Bower, G. H. Mood and memory. *American Psychologist,* 1981, *36,* 129–148.
Bower, T. G. R. *Development in infancy.* San Francisco: Freeman, 1974.
Boyd, D. B., Merskey, H., & Nielsen, J. S. The pain clinic: An approach to the problem of chronic pain. In W. L. Smith, H. Merskey, & S. C. Gross (Eds.), *Pain: Meaning and management.* New York: SP Medical & Scientific Books, 1980, pp. 159–165.
Bradshaw, C. T. Personal communication, June, 1985.
Brazelton, T. B. Issues for working parents. *American Journal of Orthopsychiatry,* 1986, *56,* 14–25.
Brena, S. F. Ways and attempts to measure pain. In S. F. Brena (Ed.), *Chronic pain: America's hidden epidemic.* New York: Atheneum, 1978, pp. 56–65.
Brena, S. F., & Chapman, S. L. Pain and litigation. In P. D. Wall & R. Melzack (Eds.), *Textbook of pain.* New York: Churchill Livingstone, 1984, pp. 832–839.
Bresler, D. E. *Free yourself from pain.* New York: Simon & Schuster, 1979.
Breslin, P. W. The psychological reactions of children to burn traumata: A review. *Illinois Medical Journal,* 1975, *148,* 519–524; Part II: 595–597, 602.
Brewster, A. B. Chronically ill hospitalized children's concepts of their illness. *Pediatrics,* 1982, *69,* 355–362.
Brody, J. E. Taking the fear out of a child's first hospital stay. *San Francisco Chronicle,* October 20, 1982, p. CC3.
Bronfenbrenner, U. *The ecology of human development.* Cambridge, MA: Harvard University Press, 1979.
Brown, J. K. Migraine and migraine equivalents in children. *Developmental Medicine and Child Neurology,* 1977, *19,* 683–692.
Brown, J. M. Imagery coping strategies in the treatment of migraine. *Pain,* 1984, *18,* 157–167.
Brown, J. M., O'Keefe, J., Sanders, S. H., & Baker, B. Developmental changes in children's cognition to stressful and painful situations. *Journal of Pediatric Psychology,* 1986, *11,* 343–357.
Brown, P. E. Use of acupuncture in major surgery. *Lancet,* 1972, *1,* 1328–1330.
Bruce, S. *Tomorrow is today.* New York: Bobbs-Merrill, 1983.
Bruner, J. S., Jolly, A., & Sylva, K. (Eds.). *Play: Its role in development and evolution.* New York: Basic Books, 1976.

Buckman, W. Personal communication, January, 1973.

Bush, A. F. Personal communication, December, 1982.

Bygdeman, M., Bremme, K., Gillespie, A., & Lundström, V. Effects of the prostaglandins on the uterus. *Acta Obstetricia et Gynecologica Scandinavica*, (Suppl.), 1979, *87*, 33–38.

Cahners, S. S. A strong hospital-school liaison: A necessity for good rehabilitation planning for disfigured children. *Scandinavian Journal of Plastic and Reconstructive Surgery*, 1979, *13*, 173–175.

Caire, J. B., & Erickson, S. Reducing distress in pediatric patients undergoing cardiac catheterization. *Children's Health Care*, 1986, *14*, 146–152.

Cameron, C. O., & Wallace, N. E. Having a bone marrow test: A child's perspective. *Children's Health Care*, 1983, *12*, 41–42.

Campbell, M. C. Personal communication, 1984.

Cannon, W. B. *Bodily changes in pain, hunger, fear and rage*, 2nd ed. New York: Appleton, 1929.

Capperauld, I. Acupuncture, anesthesia and medicine in China today. *Surgery, Gynecology and Obstetrics*, 1972, *135*, 440–445.

Carpenter, D., Engberg, I., & Lundberg, A. Differential supraspinal control of inhibitory and excitatory actions from the FRA to ascending spinal pathways. *Acta Physiologica Scandinavica*, 1965, *63*, 103–110.

Carty, R. M. Children's reaction to the ICU. In M. A. Noble (Ed.), *The ICU environment: Directions for nursing*. Reston, VA: Reston, 1982.

Casey, K. L., & Melzack, R. Neural mechanisms of pain: A conceptual model. In E. L. Way (Ed.), *New concepts in pain and its clinical management*. Philadelphia: Davis, 1967.

Cataldo, M. F., Bessman, C. A., Parker, L. H., Pearson, J. E., & Rogers, M. C. Behavioral assessment for pediatric intensive care units. *Journal of Applied Behavior Analysis*, 1979, *12*, 83–97.

Cataldo, M. F., Jacobs, H. E., & Rogers, M. C. Behavioral/environmental considerations in pediatric inpatient care. In D. C. Russo & J. W. Varni (Eds.), *Behavioral pediatrics: Research and practice*. New York: Plenum Press, 1982, pp. 271–298.

Cataldo, M. F., Russo, D. C., Bird, B. L., & Varni, J. W. Assessment and management of chronic disorders. In J. M. Ferguson & C. B. Taylor (Eds.), *The comprehensive handbook of behavioral medicine*, Vol. 3. New York: Spectrum, 1980, pp. 67–95.

Cautela, J., & Groden, J. *Relaxation: A comprehensive manual for adults, children, and children with special needs*. Champaign, IL: Research Press, 1978.

Cetron, M., & O'Toole, T. *Encounters with the future*. New York: McGraw-Hill, 1982.

Chapman, A. H. *The games children play*. New York: Putnam's, 1971.

Chapman, C. R. Measurement of pain: Problems and issues. In J. J. Bonica & D. Albe-Fessard (Eds.), *Advances in pain research and therapy*, Vol. 1. New York: Raven Press, 1976, pp. 345–354.

Chapman, C. R. The hurtful world: Pathological pain and its control. In E. C. Carterette & M. P. Friedman (Eds.), *Handbook of perception, Vol. VIB: Feeling and hurting*. New York: Academic Press, 1978, pp. 264–301.

Chapman, C. R. New directions in the understanding and management of pain. *Social Science and Medicine*, 1984, *19*, 1261–1277.

Chapman, C. R. Psychological factors in postoperative pain. In G. Smith & B. G. Covino (Eds.), *Acute pain*. London: Butterworths, 1985, pp. 22–41.

Chapman, C. R. Personal communication, February, 1987.

Chapman, C. R., & Bonica, J. J. *Acute pain*. Kalamazoo, MI: Upjohn, 1983. (Current concepts series).

Chapman, C. R., Casey, K. L., Dubner, R., Foley, K. M., Gracely, R. H., & Reading, A. E. Pain measurement: An overview. *Pain*, 1985, *22*, 1–31.

Chapman, S. L. A review and clinical perspective on the use of EMG and thermal biofeedback for chronic headaches. *Pain*. 1986, *27*, 1–43.

Chapman, W. P., & Jones, C. M. Variations in cutaneous and visceral pain sensitivity in normal subjects. *Journal of Clinical Investigation*, 1944, *23*, 81–91.

Cheng, R. S. S., & Pomeranz, B. Electrotherapy of chronic musculoskeletal pain: Comparison of electroacupuncture and acupuncture-like transcutaneous electrical nerve stimulation. *Clinical Journal of Pain*, 1986, *2*, 143–149.

Chesney, M. A., & Tasto, D. L. The development of the menstrual symptom questionnaire. *Behavior Research and Therapy*, 1975a, *13*, 237–244.

Chesney, M. A., & Tasto, D. L. The effectiveness of behavior modification with spasmodic and congestive dysmenorrhea. *Behavior Research and Therapy*, 1975b, *13*, 245–253.

Cholst, I. N., & Carlon, A. T. Oral contraceptives and dysmenorrhea. *Journal of Adolescent Health Care*, 1987, *8*, 121–128.

Christensen, M. F. & Mortensen, O. Long-term prognosis in children with recurrent abdominal pain. *Archives of Disease in Childhood*, 1975, *50*, 110–114.

Christophenson, V. Sociocultural correlates of pain response. Final report, Project No. 1390, Vocational Rehabilitation Administration. Washington, DC: U.S. Dept. of Health, Education, and Welfare, 1966.

Ciccone, D. S., & Grzesiak, R. C. Cognitive dimensions of chronic pain. *Social Science and Medicine*, 1984, *19*, 1339–1345.

Cioppa, F. J., & Thal, A. D. Hypnotherapy in a case of juvenile rheumatoid arthritis. *American Journal of Clinical Hypnosis*, 1975, *18*, 105–110.

Clark, E. B. Personal communication, April, 1987.

Clark, M., Gosnell, M., & Shapiro, D. The new war on pain. *Newsweek*, 1977, *89*, No. 17, 48–58.

Clark, W. C., & Mehl, L. Thermal pain: A sensory decision theory analysis of the effect of age and sex on d', various response criteria, and 50% pain threshold. *Journal of Abnormal Psychology*, 1971, *78*, 202–212.

Clarke, J. P. Personal communication, September, 1965.

Cleland, J. T. The right to live and the right to die. *Resident Physician*, 1968, *14*, 64–66.

Co, L. L., Schmitz, T. H., Havdala, H., Reyes, A., & Westerman, M. P. Acupuncture: An evaluation in the painful crises of sickle cell anaemia. *Pain*, 1979, *7*, 181–185.

Coates, T. J., Jeffery, R. W., & Slinkard, L. A. Heart healthy eating and exercise: Introducing and maintaining changes in health behaviors. *American Journal of Public Health*, 1981, *71*, 15–23.

Cohen, F. L. Postsurgical pain relief: Patients' status and nurses' medication choices. *Pain*, 1980, *9*, 265–274.

Cohen, F., & Lazarus, R. W. Active coping processes, coping disposition and recovery from surgery. *Psychology Reports*, 1979, *45*, 867–873.

Cohen, M. I. Clinical pharmacology and adolescence. *Pediatric Clinics of North America*, 1980, *27*, 45–51.

Cohen, S., & Wills, T. A. Stress, social support, and the buffering hypothesis. *Psychological Bulletin*, 1985, *98*, 310–357.

Colby, C. Z., Lanzetta, J. T., & Kleck, R. E. Effects of the expression of pain on autonomic and pain tolerance responses to subject-controlled pain. *Psychophysiology*, 1977, *14*, 537–540.

Colman, M. D., Dougher, C. A., & Tanner, M. R. Group therapy for physically handicapped toddlers with delayed speech and language development. *Journal of the American Academy of Child Psychiatry*, 1976, *15*, 395–413.

Conners, C. K. Application of biofeedback to treatment of children. *American Academy of Child Psychiatry,* 1979, *18,* 143–153.

Copp, L. A. The spectrum of suffering. *American Journal of Nursing,* 1974, *74,* 491–495.

Corah, N. L. Effect of perceived control on stress reduction in pedodontic patients. *Journal of Dental Research,* 1973, *52,* 1261–1264.

Cousins, N. Anatomy of an illness. *New England Journal of Medicine,* 1976, *295,* 1457–1462.

Cousins, N. The fallacy of cost-benefit ratio (Editorial). *Saturday Review,* 1979, *6,* No. 8, 8.

Cowherd, M. One child's reaction to acute pain. *Nursing Clinics of North America,* 1977, *12,* 639–643.

Craig, K. D. Social modeling influences on pain. In R. A. Sternbach (Ed.), *The psychology of pain.* New York: Raven Press, 1978, pp. 73–109.

Craig, K. D. Ontogenetic and cultural influences on the expression of pain in man. In H. W. Kosterlitz & L. Y. Terenius (Eds.), *Pain and society.* Weinham, Germany: Verlag Chemie, 1980.

Craig, K. D. Modeling and social learning factors in chronic pain. In J. J. Bonica, U. Lindblom, & A. Iggo (Eds.), *Advances in pain research and therapy,* Vol. 5. New York: Raven Press, 1983, pp. 813–827.

Craig, K. D. Psychological aspects of pain in children. In R. Rizzi & M. Visentin (Eds.), *Pain.* Padua, Italy: Piccin/Butterworths, 1984, pp. 263–271.

Craig, K. D. Personal communication, September, 1986.

Craig, K. D., McMahon, R. J., Morrison, J. D., & Zaskow, C. Developmental changes in infant pain expression during immunization injections. *Social Science and Medicine,* 1984, *19,* 1331–1337.

Craig, K. D., & Patrick, C. J. Facial expression during induced pain. *Journal of Personality and Social Psychology,* 1984, *48,* 1080–1091.

Craig, K. D., & Prkachin, K. M. Social influences on public and private components of pain. In I. G. Sarason & C. Spielberger (Eds.), *Stress and anxiety,* Vol. 7. New York: Hemisphere, 1980, pp. 57–72.

Craig, K. D., & Prkachin, K. M. Nonverbal measures of pain. In R. Melzack (Ed.), *Pain measurement and assessment.* New York: Raven Press, 1983, pp. 173–179.

Crocker, E. Play programs in pediatric settings. In E. Gellert (Ed.), *Psychosocial aspects of pediatric care,* New York: Grune & Stratton, 1978, pp. 95–110.

Crocker, E. Reactions of children to health care encounters: Programs that can make a difference. In G. C. Robinson & H. F. Clarke (Eds.), *The hospital care of children.* New York: Oxford University Press, 1980.

Crockett, D. J., Prkachin, K. M., & Craig, K. D. Factors of the language of pain in patient and volunteer groups. *Pain,* 1977, *4,* 175–182.

Crook, J., Rideout, E., & Browne, G. The prevalence of pain complaints in a general population. *Pain,* 1984, *18,* 299–314.

Crook, J., & Tunks, E. Defining the "chronic pain syndrome": An epidemiological method. In H. L. Fields, R. Dubner, & F. Cervero (Eds.), *Advances in pain research and therapy,* Vol. 9. Proceedings of the Fourth World Congress on Pain. New York: Raven Press, 1985, pp. 871–877.

Crue, B. L., Kenton, B., Carregal, E. J. A., & Pinsky, J. J. The continuing crisis in pain research. In W. L. Smith, H. Merskey, & S. C. Gross, (Eds.), *Pain: Meaning and management.* New York: SP Medical & Scientific Books, 1980.

Dahlström, B., Bolme, P., Feychting, H., Noack, G., & Paalzow, L. Morphine kinetics in children. *Clinical Pharmacological Therapy,* 1979, *26,* 354–365.

Dale, J. C. A multidimensional study of infants' responses to painful stimuli. *Pediatric*

Nursing, 1986, *12*, 27–31.

Dalet, R. *How to give yourself relief from pain*. New York: Stein & Day, 1980.

Dalton, K. Premenstrual tension: An overview. In R. C. Friedman (Ed.), *Behavior and the menstrual cycle*. New York: Marcel Dekker, 1982, pp. 217–242.

Dawood, M. Y. Hormones, prostaglandins and dysmenorrhea. In M. Y. Dawood (Ed.), *Dysmenorrhea*. Baltimore: Williams & Wilkins, 1981, pp. 21–52.

DeFee, J. F., Jr., & Himelstein, P. Children's fear in a dental situation as a function of birth order. *Journal of Genetic Psychology*, 1969, *115*, 253–259.

Degenaar, J. J. Some philosophical considerations on pain. *Pain*, 1979, *7*, 281–304.

Dehen, H., Willer, J. C., Prier, S., Boureau, F., & Cambier, J. Congenital insensitivity to pain and the "morphine-like" analgesic system. *Pain*, 1978, *5*, 351–358.

Denholm, C. J., & Ferguson, R. V. Strategies to promote the developmental needs of hospitalized adolescents. *Children's Health Care*, 1987, *15*, 183–187.

Deubner, D. C. An epidemiologic study of migraine and headache in 10–20 year olds. *Headache*, 1977, *17*, 173–180.

Devlin, D., & Magrab, P. R. Bioethical considerations in the care of handicapped newborns. *Journal of Pediatric Psychology*, 1981, *6*, 111–119.

Dexter, S. L. Rebreathing aborts migraine attacks. *British Medical Journal*, 1982, *284*, 312.

Diamond, S., & Franklin, M. Intensive biofeedback therapy in the treatment of headache. Paper presented at the Biofeedback Research Society Annual Meeting, Monterey, CA, 1975.

DiLeo, J. H. *Child development: Analysis and synthesis*. New York: Bruner/Mazel, 1977.

Dodge, J. A. Recurrent abdominal pain in children. *British Medical Journal*, 1976, *1*, 385–387.

Dolce, J. J., Crocker, M. F., Moletteire, C., & Doleys, D. M. Exercise quotas, anticipatory concern and self-efficacy expectancies in chronic pain: A preliminary report. *Pain*, 1986, *24*, 365—372.

Dolce, J. J., Doleys, D. M., Raczynski, J. M., Lossie, J., Poole, L., & Smith, M. The role of self-efficacy expectancies in the prediction of pain tolerance. *Pain*, 1986, *27*, 261–272.

Dubner, R. Peripheral and central mechanisms of pain. In L. K. Y. Ng & J. J. Bonica (Eds.), *Pain, discomfort and humanitarian care*. New York: Elsevier/North-Holland, 1980, pp. 61–82.

Dubuisson, D., & Melzack, R. Classification of clinical pain descriptors by multiple group discriminant analysis. *Experimental Neurology*, 1976, *51*, 480–487.

Dunn-Geier, B. J., McGrath, P. J., Rourke, B. P., Latter, J., & D'Astous, J. Adolescent chronic pain: The ability to cope. *Pain*, 1986, *26*, 23–32.

Dworkin, S. F., & Chen, A. C. N. Pain in clinical and laboratory contexts. *Journal of Dental Research*, 1982, *61*, 772–774.

Dyment, P. G. Safety and efficacy of jet anesthesia for bone marrow aspiration. *Blood*, 1978, *52*, 578–580.

Edwards, P. W., Zeichner, A., Kuczmierczyk, A. R., & Boczkowski, J. Familial pain models: The relationship between family history of pain and current pain experience. *Pain*, 1985, *21*, 379–384.

Egermark-Eriksson, I. Prevalence of headache in Swedish school-children. *Acta Paediatrica Scandinavica*, 1982, *71*, 135–140.

Ekman, R., & Friesen, M. V. The repertoire of nonverbal behavior: Categories, origins, usage and coding. *Semiotica*, 1969, *1*, 49–98.

Eland, J. M. *Children's communication of pain*. Unpublished master's thesis, University of Iowa, Iowa City, 1974.

Eland, J. M. Minimizing pain associated with prekindergarten intramuscular injections. *Issues in Comprehensive Pediatric Nursing,* 1981, *5,* 361–372.

Eland, J. M. Children's pain: Developmentally appropriate efforts to improve identification of source, intensity, and relevant intervening variables. Unpublished manuscript, University of Iowa, Iowa City, 1983.

Eland, J. M. A comparison of the amount of injection pain experienced with the ventrogluteal, vastus lateralis and rectus femorus injection sites. Unpublished report referred to in M. McCaffery, IV morphine for relief of pain in children. *PRN Forum,* 1984, *3,* 1–2.

Eland, J. M., & Anderson, J. E. The experience of pain in children. In A. Jacox (Ed.), *Pain: A source book for nurses and other professionals.* Boston: Little, Brown, 1977, pp. 453–473.

Elkins, P. D., & Roberts, M. C. Reducing medical fears in a general population of children: A comparison of three audiovisual modeling procedures. *Journal of Pediatric Psychology,* 1985, *10,* 65–75.

Ellerton, M.-L., Caty, S., & Ritchie, J. A. Helping young children master intrusive procedures through play. *Children's Health Care,* 1985, *13,* 167–173.

Elliott, C. H., Miller, M. D., Funk, M., & Pruitt, S. D. Implications of children's burn injuries. In D. Routh (Ed.), *Handbook of pediatric psychology.* New York: Guilford, 1987, pp. 426–447.

Elliott, C. H., & Olson, R. A. The management of children's distress in response to painful medical treatment for burn injuries. *Behavior Research and Therapy,* 1983, *21,* 675–683.

Engel, G. L. Psychogenic pain and the pain-prone patient. *American Journal of Medicine,* 1959, *26,* 899–918.

Engel, J. M., & Rapoff, M. A. Biofeedback-assisted relaxation training for adult and pediatric headache disorders. Unpublished manuscript, University of Kansas Medical Center, Kansas City, 1987.

Engelbart, H. J., & Vrancken, M. A. Chronic pain from the perspective of health: A view based on systems theory. *Social Science and Medicine,* 1984, *19,* 1383–1392.

Epstein, L. H., & Abel, G. G. Analysis of biofeedback training effects for tension headache patients. *Behavior Therapy,* 1977, *8,* 37–47.

Erickson, F. Play interviews with four-year-old hospitalized children. *Monographs of the Society for Research in Child Development,* 1958, *3,* 1–77.

Erikson, E. *Childhood and society,* (2nd ed.). New York: Norton, 1963.

Erlen, J. A. The child's choice: An essential component in treatment decisions. *Children's Health Care,* 1987, *15,* 156–160.

Ernst, C., & Angst, J. *Birth order.* New York: Springer-Verlag, 1983.

Evans, C., & Evans, D. E. N. Psychological aspects of anaesthesia. In M. D. Vickers (Ed.), *Medicine for anaesthetists,* 2nd ed. London: Blackwell Scientific Publications, 1982, pp. 580–597.

Evans, M. E., Bhat, R., & Vidyasagar, D. Factors modulating drug therapy and pharmacokinetics. In T. F. Yeh (Ed.), *Drug therapy in the neonate and small infant.* Chicago: Year Book Medical Publishers, 1985, pp. 3–18.

Evans, R. I. Modifying health lifestyles in children and adolescents: Development and evaluation of a social psychological intervention. In A. Baum & J. E. Singer (Eds.), *Handbook of psychology and health.* Hillsdale, NJ: Lawrence Erlbaum Associates, 1982, pp. 231–245.

Fairley, P. *The conquest of pain.* New York: Scribner's, 1978.

Fassler, D. The fear of needles in children. *American Journal of Orthopsychiatry,* 1985, *55,* 371–377.

Fassler, J. *Helping children cope.* New York: Free Press, 1978.

Feldman, W. S., & Varni, J. W. Conceptualizations of health and illness by children with spina bifida. *Children's Health Care,* 1985, *13,* 102–108.

Ferguson, K. S., & Robinson, S. S. Life threatening migraine. *Archives of Neurology,* 1982, *39,* 374–376.

Ferguson, T. Teaching medicine to kids. In T. Ferguson (Ed.), *Medical self-care: Access to medical tools.* New York: Summit Books, 1979.

Fernandez, E. A classification system of cognitive coping strategies for pain. *Pain,* 1986, *26,* 141–151.

Ferrari, M. Chronic illness: Psychosocial effects on siblings: I. Chronically ill boys. *Journal of Child Psychology and Psychiatry and Allied Disciplines,* 1984, *25,* 459–476.

Ferster, C., & Skinner, B. F. *Schedules of reinforcement.* New York: Appleton-Century-Crofts, 1957.

Feuerstein, M., & Adams, H. E. Cephalic vasomotor feedback in the modification of migraine headache. *Biofeedback and Self-Regulation,* 1977, *2,* 241–254.

Feuerstein, M., Barr, R., Francoeur, E., Houle, M., & Rafman, S. Potential biobehavioral mechanisms of recurrent abdominal pain in children. *Pain,* 1982, *13,* 287–298.

Feuerstein, M., & Skjei, E. *Mastering pain.* New York: Bantam Books, 1979.

Field, T., & Goldson, E. Pacifying effects of nonnutritive sucking on term and preterm neonates during heelstick procedures. *Pediatrics,* 1984, *74,* 1012–1015.

Filler, W. W., & Hall, W. C. Dysmenorrhea and its therapy. *American Journal of Obstetrics and Gynecology,* 1970, *106,* 104–109.

Fine, J. Spinal column. *Back to Back,* 1982, *2,* 1–4.

Finer, B. Mental mechanisms in the control of pain. In H. W. Kosterlitz & L. Y. Terenius (Eds.), *Pain and society.* Weinheim, Germany: Verlag Chemie Gmbh., 1980, pp. 223–237.

Fisichelli, V. R., Karelitz, R. M., Fisichelli, R. M., & Cooper, J. The course of induced crying activity in the first year of life. *Pediatric Research,* 1974, *8,* 921.

Fisichelli, V. R., Karelitz, S., & Haber, A. The course of induced crying activity in the neonate. *Journal of Psychology,* 1968, *73,* 183.

Fletcher, B. A., & Johnson, C. The myth of formal operations: Rethinking adolescent cognition in clinical contexts. *Children's Health Care,* 1982, *11,* 17–21.

Fletcher, J. Ethics and euthanasia. *American Journal of Nursing,* 1973, *73,* 670–675.

Florman, A. L. Development and variables of pain in children. *Pain: Current Concepts on Pain and Analgesia,* 1975, *2,* 11–15.

Flower, R. J., Moncada, S., & Vane, J. R. Analgesic-antipyretics and anti-inflammatory agents: Drugs employed in the treatment of gout. In A. G. Gilman, L. S. Goodman, & A. Gilman (Eds.), *The pharmacological basis of therapeutics,* 6th ed. New York: Macmillan, 1980, pp. 494–534.

Foerster, O. *Die leitungsbahnen des schmerzgefühls.* Berlin: Urban & Schwarzenberg, 1927.

Foley, K. M. Adjuvant analgesic drugs in cancer pain management. In G. M. Aronoff (Ed.), *Evaluation and treatment of chronic pain.* Baltimore: Urban & Schwarzenberg, 1985, 425–434.

Folkman, J. Patients yearn for "my doctor." *American Medical News,* May 29, 1981, *24,* 11–12.

Fordyce, W. E. *Behavioral methods for chronic pain and illness.* St. Louis: Mosby, 1976.

Fordyce, W. E. Learning processes in pain. In R. A. Sternbach (Ed.), *The psychology of pain.* New York: Raven Press, 1978, pp. 49–72.

Fordyce, W. E., Fowler, R. S., Lehmann, J. F., & DeLateur, B. J. Some implications of learning in problems of chronic pain. *Journal of Chronic Diseases,* 1968, *21,* 179–190.

Fordyce, W. E., Roberts, A. H., & Sternbach, R. A. The behavioral management of chronic pain: A response to critics. *Pain,* 1985, *22,* 113–125.

Forsythe, W. I., Gillies, D., & Sills, M. A. Propranolol ('Inderal') in the treatment of childhood migraine. *Developmental Medicine & Child Neurology,* 1984, *26,* 737–741.

Foster, M. *Lectures on the history of physiology during the 16th, 17th and 18th centuries.* Translation of R. Descartes, *L'homme.* Cambridge University Press, 1901.

Fox, R. E. Family therapy. In I. B. Weiner (Ed.), *Clinical methods in psychology.* New York: Wiley, 1976.

Framo, J. L. Family theory and therapy. *American Psychologist,* 1979, *34,* 988–992.

Frankl, S., Shiere, F., & Fogels, H. Should the parent remain with the child in the operatory? *Journal of Dentistry for Children,* 1962, *29,* 150–163.

Frankl, V. *Man's search for meaning.* London: Hodder & Stoughton, 1964.

Frederickson, D. S. Welcome to the Conference on Pain, Discomfort, and Humanitarian Care. In L. K. Y. Ng & J. J. Bonica (Eds.), *Pain, discomfort and humanitarian care.* New York: Elsevier/North-Holland, 1980, pp. x–xi.

Freedman, R. R., Lynn, S. J., & Ianni, P. Behavioral assessment of Raynaud's disease. In F. J. Keefe & J. A. Blumenthal (Eds.), *Assessment strategies in behavioral medicine.* New York: Grune & Stratton, 1982, pp. 99–129.

Freeman, L. R. Personal communication, May, 1981.

Freese, A. S. *Pain.* New York: Penguin Books, 1975.

Freud, S. *Beyond the pleasure principle.* (J. Stachey, Trans.), New York: Liveright, 1920.

Friedman, R. Some characteristics of children with "psychogenic" pain: Observations on prognosis and management. *Clinical Pediatrics,* 1972, *7,* 331–333.

Gaal, J. M., Goldsmith, L., & Needs, R. E. The use of hypnosis, as an adjunct to anesthesia, to reduce pre- and post-operative anxiety in children. Paper presented at the Annual Meeting of the American Society of Clinical Hypnosis, Minneapolis, November, 1980.

Gaffney, A. A. *Pain: Perspectives in childhood: A study of the development of non-hospitalized children's verbally mediated ideas about pain between the ages of five and fourteen years,* Vol. 1, Vol. 2. University College, Cork, Ireland: Unpublished doctoral dissertation, 1983.

Gaffney, A. A., & Dunne, E. A. Developmental aspects of children's definitions of pain. *Pain,* 1986, *26,* 105–117.

Gaffney, A. A., & Gaffney, P. R. Recurrent abdominal pain in children and the endogenous opiates: A brief hypothesis. *Pain,* 1987, *30,* 217–220.

Gantt, P. A., & McDonough, P. G. Adolescent dysmenorrhea. *Pediatric Clinics of North America,* 1981, *28,* 389–395.

Gardner, G. G. Childhood, death, and human dignity: Hypnotherapy for David. *International Journal of Clinical and Experimental Hypnosis,* 1976, *24,* 122–139.

Gardner, G. G. Hypnosis with infants and preschool children. *American Journal of Clinical Hypnosis,* 1977, *19,* 158–162.

Gardner, G. G. Teaching self-hypnosis to children. *International Journal of Clinical and Experimental Hypnosis,* 1981, *29,* 300–312.

Gardner, G. G., & Lubman, A. Hypnotherapy for children with cancer: Some current issues. *American Journal of Clinical Hypnosis,* 1983, *25,* 135–142.

Gardner, G. G., & Olness, K. *Hypnosis and hypnotherapy with children.* New York: Grune & Stratton, 1981.

Gardner, W. J., Licklider, J. C., & Weisz, A. Z. Suppression of pain by sound. *Science,* 1960, *132,* 32–33.

Gaston-Johansson, F. Pain assessment: Differences in quality and intensity of the words pain, ache, and hurt. *Pain,* 1984, *20,* 69–76.

Gaudreault, P., Temple, A. R., & Lovejoy, F. H. The relative severity of acute versus chronic salicylate poisoning in children: A clinical comparison. *Pediatrics*, 1982, *70*, 566–569.

Gelfand, S. The relationship of birth order to pain tolerance. *Journal of Clinical Psychology*, 1963, *19*, 406.

Genest, M., Meichenbaum, D., & Turk, D. A cognitive-behavior approach to the management of pain. Paper presented at the 11th Annual Meeting of the Association for the Advancement of Behavior Therapy, Atlanta, December 1977.

Gewanter, H. L., & Baum, J. The use of tolmetin sodium in systemic onset juvenile rheumatoid arthritis. *Arthritis and Rheumatism*, 1981, *24*, 1316–1319.

Gibby, H., & Stanford, G. *You're gonna do what?!* Little Rock, Arkansas: ACH Companies, 1984.

Gilbert, B. O., Johnson, S. B., Spillar, R., McCallum, M., Silverstein, J. H., & Rosenbloom, A. The effects of a peer-modeling film on children learning to self-inject insulin. *Behavior Therapy*, 1982, *13*, 186–193.

Gilchrist, E. B. Personal communication, November, 1978.

Gill, M. M., & Brenman, M. *Hypnosis and related states.* New York: International Universities Press, 1959.

Gilman, A. G., Goodman, L. S., & Gilman, A. (Eds.). *The pharmacological basis of therapeutics*, 6th ed. New York: Macmillan, 1980.

Gilman, A. G., Goodman, L. S., Rall, T. W., & Murad, F. (Eds.). *Goodman and Gilman's The pharmacological basis of therapeutics*, 7th ed. New York: Macmillan, 1985.

Ginott, H. Play group therapy: A theoretical framework. *International Journal of Group Psychotherapy*, 1958, *8*, 160–166.

Ginther, L. J., & Roberts, M. C. A test of mastery versus coping modeling in the reduction of children's dental fears. *Child & Family Behavior Therapy*, 1982, *4*, 41–52.

Glick, R. C., & Nakayama, S. Y. The experience of pain in children: Revisited. In C. Fore & E. C. Poster (Eds.), *Meeting the psychosocial needs of children and families in health care*. Washington, DC: Association for the Care of Children's Health, 1985, pp. 61–66.

Glynn, C. J., Lloyd, J. W., & Folkard, S. The diurnal variation in perception of pain. *Proceedings of the Royal Society of Medicine*, 1976, *69*, 369–372.

Goldscheider, A. *Ueber den schmerz in physiologischer und klinischer hinsicht.* Berlin: Hirschwald, 1894.

Goldstein, A. Opioid peptides (endorphins) in pituitary and brain. *Science*, 1973, *193*, 1081–1086.

Goldstein, A., & Hilgard, E. R. Lack of influence of the morphine antagonist naloxone on hypnotic analgesia. *Proceedings of the National Academy of Sciences*, 1975, *72*, 2041–2043.

Goldstein, A., Lowney, L. I., & Pal, B. K. Stereospecific and nonspecific interactions of the morphine congener levorphanol in subcellular fractions of mouse brain. *Proceedings of the National Academy of Science USA*, 1971, *68*, 1742–1747.

Goldstein, D. P., deCholnoky, C., & Emans, S. J. Chronic pelvic pain in adolescent females. Paper presented at the Annual Meeting of the Society for Adolescent Medicine, San Francisco, October, 1979.

Gordon, D. J. The developmental characteristics of the concept of pain. Unpublished master's thesis, McGill University, Montreal, 1981.

Gorsky, B. H. *Pain: Origin and treatment.* New York: Medical Examination Publishing Co., 1981.

Gracely, R. H. Pain measurement in man. In L. K. Y. Ng & J. J. Bonica (Eds.), *Pain, discomfort and humanitarian care.* New York: Elsevier/North Holland, 1980, pp. 111–137.

Gratch, G. Review of Piagetian infancy research: Object concept development. In W. F.

Overton & J. H. Gallagher (Eds.), *Knowledge and development,* Vol. 1. New York: Plenum Press, 1977.

Graves, D. A., Foster, T. S., Batenhorst, R. L., Bennett, R. L., & Baumann, T. J. Patient-controlled analgesia. *Annals of Internal Medicine,* 1983, *99,* 360–366.

Green, E. C. Normalization: Meeting growth and development needs of children in a pediatric intensive care unit. *Children's Health Care,* 1983, *12,* 43–44.

Grobstein, R. Personal communication, February, 1979.

Gross, S. C., & Gardner, G. G. Child pain: Treatment approaches. In W. L. Smith, H. Merskey, & S. C. Gross (Eds.). *Pain: Meaning and management.* New York: SP Medical & Scientific Books, 1980, pp. 127–142.

Grossi, E., Borghi, C., Cerchiari, E. L., Della Puppa, T., & Francucci, B. Analogue chromatic continuous scale (ACCS): A new method for pain assessment. *Clinical and Experimental Rheumatology,* 1983, *1,* 337–340.

Grossi, E., Borghi, C., & Montanari, M. Measurement of pain: Comparison between visual analog scale and analog chromatic continuous scale. In H. L. Fields, R. Dubner, & F. Cervero (Eds.), *Advances in pain research and therapy,* Vol. 9. Proceedings of the Fourth World Congress on Pain. New York: Raven Press, 1985, pp. 371–376.

Grunau, R. V. E., & Craig, K. D. Pain expression in neonates: Facial action and cry. *Pain,* 1987a, *28,* 395–410.

Grunau, R. V. E., & Craig, K. D. Neonatal pain behavior and perinatal events. Unpublished manuscript, University of British Columbia, Vancouver, 1987b.

Grunau, R. V. E., Gilbert, J. H. V., & Craig, K. D. Pain cry: Fundamental frequency and infant size in healthy neonates. Unpublished manuscript, University of British Columbia, Vancouver, 1987.

Gunsberger, M. Acupuncture in the treatment of sore throat symptomatology. *American Journal of Chinese Medicine,* 1973, *1,* 337–340.

Gurman, A. S., & Kniskern, D. P. Research on marital and family therapy: Progress, perspective, and prospect. In S. L. Garfield & A. E. Bergin (Eds.), *Handbook of psychotherapy and behavior change: An empirical analysis.* New York: Wiley, 1978, pp. 817–901.

Hagbarth, K. E., & Kerr, D. I. B. Central influences on spinal afferent conduction. *Journal of Neurophysiology,* 1954, *17,* 295–307.

Hahn, A. B., Oestreich, S. J. K., & Barkin, R. L. *Mosby's pharmacology in nursing,* 16th ed. St. Louis: Mosby, 1986.

Hahn, Y. S. Behavioral changes that signal pain. *Consultant,* 1983, *23,* 219–220, 225.

Hahn, Y. S. Personal communication, April, 1986.

Hahn, Y. S., & McLone, D. G. Pain in children with spinal cord tumors. *Child's Brain,* 1984, *11,* 36–46.

Haight, W. L., Black, J. E., & DiMatteo, M. R. Young children's understanding of the social roles of physician and patient. *Journal of Pediatric Psychology,* 1985, *10,* 31–43.

Hakkarainen, H., Vapaatalo, H., Gothoni, G., & Parantainen, J. Tolfenamic acid is as effective as ergotamine during migraine attacks. *Lancet,* 1979, *2,* 326–327.

Hallén, B., & Uppfeldt, A. Does lidocaine-prilocaine cream permit painfree insertion of I.V. catheters in children? *Anesthesiology,* 1982, *57,* 240–242.

Halpern, L. M. Psychotropic drugs and the management of chronic pain. In J. J. Bonica (Ed.), *Advances in neurology,* Vol. 4. New York: Raven Press, 1974.

Hannington-Kiff, J. G. *Pain relief.* London: Heineman, 1976.

Harpin, V. A., & Rutter, N. Development of emotional sweating in the newborn infant. *Archives of Diseases in Childhood,* 1982, *57,* 691–695.

Harrigan, J. A., Kues, J. R., Ricks, D. F., & Smith, R. Moods that predict coming migraine headaches. *Pain,* 1984, *20,* 385–396.

Harris, G., & Rollman, G. B. Cognitive techniques for controlling pain: Generality and individual differences. In H. L. Fields, R. Dubner, & F. Cervero (Eds.), *Advances in pain research and therapy,* Vol. 9. Proceedings of the Fourth World Congress on Pain. New York: Raven Press, 1985, pp. 847–851.

Haslam, D. R. Individual differences in pain threshold and level of arousal. *British Journal of Psychology,* 1969, *58,* 139–142.

Hawley, D. D. Postoperative pain in children: Misconceptions, descriptions, and interventions. *Pediatric Nursing,* 1984, *10,* 20–23.

Hazinski, M. F. *Nursing care of the critically ill child.* St. Louis: Mosby, 1984.

Head, H. *Studies in neurology.* London: Kegan Paul, 1920.

Head, H., & Holmes, G. Sensory disturbances from cerebral lesions. *Brain,* 1911, *34,* 102–254.

Hebb, D. O. *The organization of behavior.* New York: Wiley, 1949.

Heczey, M. D. Effects of autogenic temperature training on dysmenorrhea and other menstrual discomforts. Unpublished master's thesis, Hunter College of the City University of New York, 1975.

Heczey, M. D. Effects of biofeedback and autogenic training on dysmenorrhea. In A. J. Dan, E. A. Graham, & C. P. Beecher (Eds.), *The menstrual cycle,* Vol. 1. New York: Springer, 1980, pp. 283–291.

Heel, R. C., Brogden, R. N., Speight, T. M., & Avery, G. S. Buprenorphine: A review of its pharmacological properties and therapeutic efficacy. *Drugs,* 1979, *17,* 81–110.

Heft, M. W., & Parker, S. R. An experimental basis for revising the graphic rating scale for pain. *Pain,* 1984, *19,* 153–161.

Helwick, C. A. A picture of pain. *Health,* 1982, *14,* 17.

Hendler, N. H. *Diagnosis and nonsurgical management of chronic pain.* New York: Raven Press, 1981.

Hendler, N. H. The four stages of pain. In N. H. Hendler, D. M. Long, & T. N. Wise (Eds.), *Diagnosis and treatment of chronic pain.* London: John Wright. PSG, 1982, pp. 1–8.

Herman, B. H. Personal communication, March, 1987.

Hester, N. K. O. The preoperational child's reaction to immunization. *Nursing Research,* 1979, *28,* 250–255.

Hilgard, E. R. Pain as a puzzle for psychology and physiology. *American Psychologist,* 1969, *24,* 103–113.

Hilgard, E. R. The problem of divided consciousness. A neodissociation interpretation. *Annals of the New York Academy of Sciences,* 1977, *296,* 48–59.

Hilgard, E. R., Crawford, H. J., & Wert, A. The Stanford Hypnotic Arm Levitation Test (SHALIT): A six-minute induction and measurement scale. *International Journal of Clinical and Experimental Hypnosis,* 1979, *27,* 111–124.

Hilgard, E. R., & Hilgard, J. R. *Hypnosis in the relief of pain.* Los Altos, CA: Kaufmann, 1975.

Hilgard, J. R., LeBaron, S. Relief of anxiety and pain in children and adolescents with cancer: Qualitative measures and clinical observations. *International Journal of Clinical and Experimental Hypnosis,* 1982, *30,* 417–442.

Hilgard, J. R., & LeBaron, S. *Hypnotherapy and pain in children with cancer.* Los Altos, CA: Kaufmann, 1984.

Hoffman, A., Becker, R., & Gabriel, H. *The hospitalized adolescent: A guide to managing the ill and injured youth.* New York: Free Press, 1976.

Hollien, H. Developmental aspects of neonatal vocalizations. In T. Murry & J. Murry (Eds.), *Infant communication: Cry and early speech.* Houston: College-Hill Press, 1980, pp. 20–55.

Holroyd, K. A., Andrasik, F., & Westbrook, T. Cognitive control of tension headache. *Cognitive Therapy and Research,* 1977, *1,* 121–133.

Houts, A. C. Relaxation and thermal feedback treatment of child migraine headache: A case study. *American Journal of Clinical Biofeedback,* 1982, *5,* 154–157.

Hughes, J., Smith, T. W., Kosterlitz, H. W., Fothergill, L. A., Morgan, B. A., & Morris, H. R. Identification of two related pentapeptides from the brain with potent opiate agonist activity. *Nature London,* 1975, *258,* 577–579.

Hughes, M. C., & Zimin, R. Children with psychogenic abdominal pain and their families. *Clinical Pediatrics,* 1978, *17,* 569–573.

Hull, C. J., & Sibbald, A. Control of postoperative pain by interactive demand analgesia. *British Journal of Anaesthesiology,* 1981, *53,* 385–391.

Hull, C. L. *A behavior system.* New Haven, CT: Yale University Press, 1952.

Huskisson, E. C. Measurement of pain. *Lancet,* 1974, *2,* 1127–1131.

Huskisson, E. C. Visual analogue scales. In R. Melzack (Ed.), *Pain measurement and assessment.* New York: Raven Press, 1983, pp. 33–37.

Huskisson, E. C. Non-narcotic analgesics. In P. D. Wall & R. Melzack (Eds.), *Textbook of pain.* New York: Churchill Livingstone, 1984, pp. 505–513.

Hyson, M. C., Snyder, S. S., & Andujar, E. M. Helping children cope with checkups: How good is the "good patient?" *Children's Health Care,* 1982, *10,* 139–144.

Iacono, C. U., & Roberts, S. J. The dysmenorrhea personality: Actuality or statistical artifact? *Social Sciences and Medicine,* 1983, *17,* 1653–1655.

Iggo, A. Critical remarks on the gate control theory. In R. Janzen, W. D. Keidel, A. Herz, C. Steichele, J. P. Payne, & R. A. D. Burt (Eds.), *Pain.* London: Churchill Livingstone, 1972, pp. 127–128.

Iggo, A. Introduction. In W. R. Lowenstein (Ed.), *Handbook of sensory physiology. Vol. II. Somato-sensory systems.* Berlin: Springer-Verlag, 1973.

Igoe, J. B. Project health PACT in action. *American Journal of Nursing,* 1980, *80,* 2016–2021.

Illich, I. *Medical nemesis—The expropriation of health.* New York: Pantheon, 1976.

Inturrisi, C. E. & Foley, K. M. Narcotic analgesics in the management of pain. In M. Kuhar & G. Pasternak (Eds.), *Analgesics: Neurochemical, behavioral and clinical perspectives.* New York: Raven Press, 1984, pp. 257–288.

Inturrisi, C. E., & Verebely, K. Disposition of methadone in man after a single oral dose. *Clinical Pharmacology Therapy,* 1972, *13,* 923–930.

Irwin, E. C., & McWilliams, B. J. Play therapy for children with cleft palates. *Children Today,* 1974, *3,* 18–22.

Issues in Comprehensive Pediatric Nursing. Children and pain (Special Section), 1984, *5,* 319–380.

Izard, C. E. *Human emotions.* New York: Plenum Press, 1977.

Izard, C. E. The Maximally Discriminative Facial Movement Coding System (MAX). Newark, DE: University of Delaware, Instructional Resources Center, 1979.

Izard, C. E., Dougherty, L. M., & Hembree, E. A. *A system for affect expression identification by holistic judgments (Affex).* Newark, DE: University of Delaware, Instructional Resources Center, 1983.

Izard, C. E., Hembree, E. A., Dougherty, L. M. & Spizzirri, C. C. Changes in facial expressions of 2- to 19-month-old infants following acute pain. *Developmental Psychology,* 1983, *19,* 418–426.

Izard, C. E., Hembree E. A., & Huebner, R. R. Infants' emotion expressions to acute pain: Developmental change and stability of individual differences. *Developmental Psychology,* 1987, *23,* 105–113.

Izard, C. E., Huebner, R. R., Resser, D., McGinness, G. C., & Dougherty, L. M. The infant's ability to produce discrete emotion expressions. *Developmental Psychology,* 1980, *16,* 132–140.

Jackson, D. D. The question of family homeostasis. *Psychiatric Quarterly,* 1957, *31,* 79–90.

Jacox, A. K. The assessment of pain. In W. L. Smith, H. Merskey, & S. C. Gross (Eds.), *Pain: Meaning and management.* New York: SP Medical & Scientific Books, 1980, pp. 75–88.

Jaremko, M. E., Silbert, L., & Mann, T. The differential ability of athletes and nonathletes to cope with two types of pain. A radical behavioral model. *Psychological Record,* 1981, *31,* 265–275.

Jay, G. W., Renelli, D., & Mead, T. The effects of propranolol and amitriptyline on vascular and EMG biofeedback training. *Headache,* 1984, *24,* 59–69.

Jay, S. M. Invasive medical procedures: Psychological intervention and assessment. In D. Routh (Ed.), *Handbook of pediatric psychology.* New York: Guilford, 1987, pp. 401–425.

Jay, S. M., & Elliott, C. H. *Observational Scale of Behavioral Distress—Revised.* Unpublished manuscript, University of Southern California School of Medicine, Los Angeles, 1986.

Jay, S. M., Elliott, C. H., Katz, E. R., & Siegel, S. E. *Treatment of distress in pediatric cancer patients.* National Cancer Institute #CA34871-03, 1984.

Jay, S. M., Ozolins, M., Elliott, C. H., & Caldwell, S. Assessment of children's distress during painful medical procedures. *Health Psychology,* 1983, *2,* 133–147.

Jayson, M. I. V. *Back pain.* New York: Oxford University Press, 1981.

Jeans, M. E. Relief of chronic pain by brief, intense transcutaneous electrical stimulation—a double-blind study. In J. J. Bonica, J. C. Liebeskind, & D. G. Albe-Fessard (Eds.), *Advances in pain research and therapy,* Vol. 3. New York: Raven Press, 1979, pp. 601–606.

Jeans, M. E. Pain in children—a neglected area. In P. Firestone, P. J. McGrath, & W. Feldman (Eds.), *Advances in behavioral medicine with children and youth.* Hillsdale, N.J.: Lawrence Erlbaum Associates, 1983a, pp. 23–37.

Jeans, M. E. The measurement of pain in children. In R. Melzack (Ed.), *Pain measurement and assessment.* New York: Raven, 1983b, pp. 183–189.

Jeans, M. E., & Gordon, D. Developmental characteristics of the concept of pain. Paper presented at the Third World Pain Congress, Edinburgh, Scotland, 1981.

Jeans, M. E., & Johnston, C. C. Pain in children: Assessment and management. In S. Lipton & J. Miles (Eds.), *Persistent pain. Modern methods of treatment,* Vol. 5. London: Grune & Stratton, 1985, pp. 111–127.

Jensen, M. P., Karoly, P., & Braver, S. The measurement of clinical pain intensity: A comparison of six methods. *Pain,* 1986, *27,* 117–126.

Jerrett, M. D. Children and their pain experience. *Children's Health Care,* 1985, *14,* 83–89.

Jessop, C. Personal communication, February, 1987.

Jessup, B. A. Biofeedback. In P. D. Wall & R. Melzack (Eds.), *Textbook on pain.* New York: Churchill Livingstone, 1984, pp. 776–786.

Jewell, E. R. Management of postoperative pain. *Mediguide to Pain,* 1985, *6,* 1–4.

Joffe, R., Bakal, D. A., & Kaganov, J. A self-observation study of headache symptoms in children. *Headache,* 1983, *23,* 20–25.

Johnson, J. E., Kirchhoff, K. T., & Endress, M. P. Altering children's distress behavior during orthopedic cast removal. *Nursing Research,* 1975, *24,* 404–410.

Johnson, M. Assessment of clinical pain. In A. K. Jacox (Ed.), *Pain: A source book for nurses and other health professionals.* Boston: Little, Brown, 1977, pp. 139–166.

Johnston, C. C., & Strada, M. E. Acute pain response in infants: A multidimensional description. *Pain,* 1986, *24,* 373–382.

Jolly, H. *Diseases of children,* 4th ed. London: Blackwell Scientific Publications, 1981.

Jonas, S. *Medical mystery: The training of doctors in the United States.* New York: Norton, 1978.

Kagen-Goodheart, L. Reentry: Living with childhood cancer. *American Journal of Orthopsychiatry,* 1977, *47,* 651–658.

Kane, K., & Taub, A. A history of local electrical analgesia. *Pain,* 1975, *1,* 125–138.

Kao, F. F. Acupuncture therapeutics. New Haven: Eastern Press, 1973.

Kaptchuk, T. J. *The web that has no weaver: Understanding Chinese medicine.* New York: Congdon & Weed, 1983.

Kassowitz, K. Psychodynamic reactions of children to the use of hypodermic needles. *Journal of Diseases of Children,* 1958, *95,* 253–257.

Katz, E. R., Kellerman, J., Rigler, D., Williams, K. O., & Siegel, S. E. School intervention with pediatric cancer patients. *Journal of Pediatric Psychology,* 1977, *2,* 72–76.

Katz, E. R., Kellerman, J., & Siegel, S. E. Behavioral distress in children with cancer undergoing medical procedures: Developmental considerations. *Journal of Consulting and Clinical Psychology,* 1980, *48,* 356–365.

Katz, E. R., Kellerman, J., & Siegel, S. E. Anxiety as an affective focus in the clinical study of acute behavioral distress: A reply to Shacham and Daut. *Journal of Consulting and Clinical Psychology,* 1981, *49,* 470–471.

Katz, E. R., Sharp, B., Kellerman, J., Marston, A. R., Hershman, J. M., & Siegel, S. E. β-Endorphin immunoreactivity and acute behavioral distress in children with leukemia. *Journal of Nervous and Mental Disease,* 1982, *170,* 72–77.

Katz, E. R., Varni, J. W., & Jay, S. M. Behavioral assessment and management of pediatric pain. In M. Hersen, R. M. Eisler, & P. M. Miller (Eds.), *Progress in behavior modification,* Vol. 18. Orlando, Florida: Academic Press, 1984, pp. 163–193.

Katz, J., *The silent world of doctor and patient.* New York: The Free Press, 1984.

Kavaler, L. *A matter of degree: Heat, life, and death.* New York: Harper & Row, 1981.

Kavanagh, C. K. A new approach to dressing change in the severely burned child and its effect on burn-related psychopathology. *Heart and Lung,* 1983a, *12,* 612–619.

Kavanagh, C. K. Psychological intervention with the severely burned child: Report of an experimental comparison of two approaches and their effects on psychological sequelae. *Journal of the American Academy of Child Psychiatry,* 1983b, *22,* 145–156.

Keats, A. S. Postoperative pain: Research and treatment. *Journal of Chronic Disorders,* 1956, *4,* 72–83.

Keefe, F. J., Kopel, S., & Gordon, S. B. *A practical guide to behavioral assessment.* New York: Springer, 1978.

Keele, K. D. The pain chart. *Lancet,* 1948, *2,* 6–8.

Keele, K. D. *Anatomies of pain.* Springfield, IL: Thomas, 1957.

Keeri-Szanto, M., & Heaman, S. Postoperative demand analgesia. *Surgery, Gynecology and Obstetrics,* 1972, *134,* 647–651.

Keith-Spiegel, P., & Koocher, G. P. *Ethics in psychology.* New York: Random House, 1985.

Kelley, M. L., Jarvie, G. J., Middlebrook, J. L., McNeer, M. F., & Drabman, R. S. Decreasing burned children's pain behavior: Impacting the trauma of hydrotherapy. *Journal of Applied Behavior Analysis,* 1984, *17,* 147–158.

Kenny, T. J. The hospitalized child. *Pediatric Clinics of North America,* 1975, *22,* 583–593.

Kerr, F. W. L. Pain: A central inhibitory balance theory. *MAYO Clinic Proceedings,* 1975, *50,* 685–690.

Kerr, F. W., & Wilson, P. R. Pain. *Annual Review of Neuroscience,* 1978, *1,* 83–102.

Kewman, D. G. & Roberts, A. H. Skin temperature biofeedback and migraine headaches, a double blind study. *Biofeedback and Self-Regulation,* 1980, *5,* 327–345.

Khan, M. H. Marlborough Hospital's Well Doll Clinic. Information sheet, 1985. For information: Marlborough Hospital, 57 Union St., Marlborough, MA 01752.

Kibbee, C. J. Personal communication, December, 1984.

King, N. J., & Montgomery, R. B. Biofeedback-induced control of human peripheral temperature: A critical review of the literature. *Psychological Bulletin*, 1980, *88*, 738–752.

Kirya, C., & Werthmann, M. W. Neonatal circumcision and penile dorsal nerve block: A painless procedure. *Journal of Pediatrics*, 1978, *96*, 998–!000.

Kitchell, R. L., & Erickson, H. H. *Animal pain: Perception and alleviation*. Bethesda, MD: American Physiological Society, 1983.

Kleck, R. E., Vaughan, R. C., Cartwright-Smith, J., Vaughan, K. B., Colby, C. Z., & Lanzetta, J. T. Effects of being observed on expressive, subjective, and physiological responses to painful stimuli. *Journal of Personality and Social Psychology*, 1976, *34*, 1211–1218.

Klein, J. R. Update: Adolescent gynecology. *Pediatric Clinics of North America*, 1980, *27*, 141–152.

Klein, J. R., & Litt, I. F. Epidemiology of adolescent dysmenorrhea. *Pediatrics*, 1981, *68*, 661–664.

Klein, J. R., Litt, I. F., Rosenberg, A., & Udall, L. The effect of aspirin on dysmenorrhea in adolescents. *Journal of Pediatrics*, 1981, *98*, 987–990.

Klepac, R. K., Dowling, J., Rokke, P., Dodge, L., & Schafer, L. Interview vs. paper-and-pencil administration of the McGill Pain Questionnaire. *Pain*, 1981, *11*, 241–246.

Klingman, A., Melamed, B. G., Cuthbert, M. I., & Hermecz, D. A. Effects of participant modeling on information acquisition and skill utilization. *Journal of Consulting and Clinical Psychology*, 1984, *52*, 414–422.

Klinzing, D. R., & Klinzing, D. G. Communicating with young children about hospitalization. *Communication Education*, 1977, *26*, 307–313.

Klorman, R., Hilpert, P. L., Michael, R., La Gana, C., & Sveen, O. B. Effects of coping and mastery modeling on experienced and inexperienced pedodontic patients' disruptiveness. *Behavior Therapy*, 1980, *11*, 156–168.

Knudson-Cooper, M. S. Adjustment to visible stigma: The case of the severely burned. *Social Science & Medicine*, 1981, *15B*, 31–44.

Kobasa, S. C. The hardy personality: Toward a social psychology of stress and health. In J. Suls & G. Sanders (Eds.), *Social psychology of health and illness*. Hillsdale, NJ: Erlbaum, 1982.

Kohen, D. P. Relaxation/mental imagery (self-hypnosis) and pelvic examinations in adolescents. *Journal of Developmental and Behavioral Pediatrics*, 1980, *1*, 180–186.

Kohen, D. P., Olness, K. N., Colwell, S. O., & Heimel, A. The use of relaxation-mental imagery (self-hypnosis) in the management of 505 pediatric behavioral encounters. *Developmental and Behavioral Pediatrics*, 1984, *5*, 21–25.

Kohlenberg, R. J. Tyramine sensitivity in dietary migraine: A critical review. *Headache*, 1982, *22*, 30–34.

Kolb, L. Symbolic significance of the complaint of pain. In W. Mosbery (Ed.), *Clinical neurosurgery*, Vol. 8. Baltimore: Williams & Wilkins, 1962, pp. 248–257.

Koocher, G. Personal communication, March, 1986.

Korberly, B. H. Pharmacologic treatment of children's pain. *Pediatric Nursing*, 1985, *11*, 292–294.

Korsch, B. M., Fine, R. N., Grushkin, C. M., & Negrete, V. F. Experiences with children and their families during extended hemodialysis and kidney transplantation. *Pediatric Clinics of North America*, 1971, *18*, 625–637.

Kremer, E. F., Block, A. R., & Atkinson, J. H., Jr. Assessment of pain behavior: Factors that distort self-report. In R. Melzack (Ed.), *Pain measurement and assessment*. New York: Raven Press, 1983, pp. 165–171.

Kremer, E. F., Block, A. R., & Gaylor, M. S. Behavioral approaches to treatment of chronic pain: The inaccuracy of patient self-report measures. *Archives of Physical Medicine and Rehabilitation*, 1981, *62*, 188–191.

Kristein, M. M., Arnold, C. B., & Wynder, E. L. Health economics and preventive care. *Science*, 1977, *195*, 457–462.

Kroner, B. The empirical validity of clinical headache classification. In K. A. Holroyd, B. Schlote, & H. Zenz (Eds.), *Perspectives in research on headache*. Lewiston, NY: C. J. Hogrefe, 1983, pp. 55–65.

Kruger, L., & Liebeskind, J. C. Preface. In L. Kruger & J. C. Liebeskind (Eds.), *Neural mechanisms of pain. Advances in Pain Research and Therapy*, Vol. 6. New York: Raven Press, 1984, pp. vii–viii.

Kruszewski, A. Z., Lang, S. H., & Johnson, J. E. Effect of positioning on discomfort. *Nursing Research*, 1979, *28*, 103–105.

Kudrow, L. Paradoxical effects of frequent analgesic use. In M. Critchley, A. P. Friedman, S. Gorini, & F. Sicuteri (Eds.), *Advances in neurology. Headache: Physiopathological and clinical concepts*, Vol. 33. New York: Raven Press, 1982.

Kueffner, M. Passage through hospitalization of severely burned, isolated school-age children. *Community Nursing Research*, 1976, *7*, 181–197.

Kurylyszyn, N., McGrath, P. J., Cappelli, M., & Humphreys, P. Children's drawings: What can they tell us about intensity of pain? *Clinical Journal of Pain*, 1987, *2*, 155–158.

Kuttner, L. Favorite stories: A hypnotic pain reduction technique for children in acute pain. Paper presented at the American Society for Clinical Hypnosis Conference, San Francisco, November, 1984.

Kuttner, L. *No fears . . . no tears: Children with cancer coping with pain*. (30 min. videotape and manual). Canadian Cancer Society, 955 W. Broadway, Vancouver, B.C., Canada V5Z 3X8, 1986.

Kuttner, L., Bowman, M., & Teasdale, J. M. Psychological treatment of distress, pain and anxiety for young children with cancer. Vancouver, Canada: British Columbia Children's Hospital, unpublished manuscript, 1987.

Kuttner, L., & LePage, T. The development of pictorial self-report scales of pain and anxiety for children. Vancouver, Canada: British Columbia Children's Hospital, unpublished manuscript, 1983.

LaBaw, W. L. Adjunctive trance therapy with severely burned children. *International Journal of Child Psychotherapy*, 1973, *2*, 80–92.

LaBaw, W. L. Autohypnosis in hemophilia. *Haematologia*, 1975, *9*, 103–110.

Labbé, E. E., & Williamson, D. A. Temperature biofeedback in the treatment of children with migraine headaches. *Journal of Pediatric Psychology*, 1983, *8*, 317–326.

Labbé, E. L., & Williamson, D. A. Treatment of childhood migraine using autogenic feedback training. *Journal of Consulting and Clinical Psychology*, 1984, *52*, 968–976.

Lacouture, P. G., Gaudreault, P., & Lovejoy, F. H. Chronic pain of childhood: A pharmacologic approach. *Pediatric Clinics of North America*, 1984, *31*, 1133–1151.

La Greca, A. M., & Ottinger, D. R. Self-monitoring and relaxation training in the treatment of medically ordered exercises in a 12-year-old female. *Journal of Pediatric Psychology*, 1979, *4*, 49–54.

Lake, A. E. Behavioral assessment considerations in the management of headache. *Headache*, 1981, *21*, 170–178.

Lance, J. W., & Anthony, M. Some clinical aspects of migraine. *Archives of Neurology*, 1966, *15*, 356–361.

Lang, L. The puppet hospital. *Health*, 1986, *18*, 18.

Lang, P. J. Imagery in therapy: An information processing analysis of fear. *Behavior Therapy*, 1977, *8*, 862–886.

Lang, P. J. A bio-informational theory of emotional imagery. *Psychophysiology,* 1979, *16,* 495–512.

Larsson, B., & Melin, L. Chronic headaches in adolescents: Treatment in a school setting with relaxation training as compared with information-contact and self-registration. *Pain,* 1986, *25,* 325–336.

Lasoff, E. M., & McEttrick, M. A. Participation versus diversion during dressing change: Can nurses' attitudes change? *Issues in Comprehensive Pediatric Nursing,* 1986, *9,* 391–398.

Latimer, P. B. External contingency management for chronic pain: A critical review of the evidence. *American Journal of Psychiatry,* 1982, *139,* 1308–1312.

Lau, R. R. Origins of health locus of control beliefs. *Journal of Personality and Social Psychology,* 1982, *42,* 322–334.

Lavigne, J. V., Schulein, M. J., & Hahn, Y. S. Psychological aspects of painful medical conditions in children. I. Developmental aspects and assessment. *Pain,* 1986a, *27,* 133–146.

Lavigne, J. V., Schulein, M. J., & Hahn, Y. S. Psychological aspects of painful medical conditions in children. II. Personality factors, family characteristics and treatment. *Pain,* 1986b, *27,* 147–169.

Lavigne, J. V., Schulein, M. J., Hannan, J. A., & Hahn, Y. S. Pain and the pediatric patient: Psychological aspects. In J. L. Echternach (Ed.), *Pain.* New York: Churchill Livingstone, 1987, pp. 267–296.

Lazarus, R. S. Puzzles in the study of daily hassles. *Journal of Behavioral Medicine,* 1984, *7,* 375–389.

Lazarus, R. S., Averill, J. R., & Opton, E. M., Jr. The psychology of coping: Issues of research and assessment. In G. V. Coelho, D. A. Hamburg, & J. E. Adams (Eds.), *Coping and adaptation.* New York: Basic Books, 1974, pp. 249–315.

Lazarus, R. S., & Folkman, S. *Stress, appraisal, and coping.* New York: Springer, 1984.

Leavitt, F., Garron, D. C., McNeill, T. W., & Whisler, W. W. Organic status, psychological disturbance, and pain report characteristics in low-back pain patients on compensation. *Spine,* 1982, *7,* 398–402.

Leavitt, M. Andy was a fighter. *Nursing 79,* 1979, *9,* 62–65.

LeBaron, S., & Zeltzer, L. Assessment of acute pain and anxiety in children and adolescents by self-reports, observer reports, and a behavior checklist. *Journal of Consulting and Clinical Psychology,* 1984, *52,* 729–738.

Lee, R. B. Personal communication, August, 1981.

Leikin, L., Firestone, P., & McGrath, P. J. Physical symptom reporting in Type A and B children. Unpublished manuscript, University of Ottawa, Ontario, 1987.

Lele, P. P., & Weddell, G. Sensory nerves of the cornea and cutaneous sensibility. *Experimental Neurology,* 1959, *1,* 334–359.

Lemchen, M. S. Personal communication, March, 1987.

Lenburg, C. B., Burnside, H., & Davitz, L. J. Inferences of physical pain and psychological distress: 3. In relation to length of time in the nursing education program. *Nursing Research,* 1970, *19,* 399–401.

Leo, K. C. Use of electrical stimulation at acupuncture points for the treatment of reflex sympathetic dystrophy in a child. *Physical Therapy,* 1983, *63,* 957–958.

LePage, T. Personal communication, June, 1986.

LeShan, L. The world of the patient in severe pain of long duration. *Journal of Chronic Diseases,* 1964, *17,* 119–126.

Lethem, J., Slade, P. D., Troup, J. D. G., & Bentley, G. Outline of a fear-avoidance model of exaggerated pain perception. *Behavior Research and Therapy,* 1983, *21,* 401–408.

Levine, J. D., & Gordon, N. C. Pain in prelingual children and its evaluation by pain-induced vocalization. *Pain,* 1982, *14,* 85–93.

Levine, M., & Rappaport, L. A. Recurrent abdominal pain in school children: The loneliness of the long distance physician. *Pediatric Clinics of North America,* 1984, *31,* 969–991.

Levine, R. R. *Pharmacology: Drug actions and reactions,* 3rd ed. Boston: Little, Brown, 1983.

Levinson, J. E., Baum, J., Brewer, E., Jr., Fink, C. W., Hanson, V., & Schaller, J. Comparison of tolmetin sodium and aspirin in the treatment of juvenile rheumatoid arthritis. *Journal of Pediatrics,* 1977, *91,* 799–804.

Leviton, A., Slack, W. V., Masek, B., Bana, D., & Graham, J. R. A computerized behavioral assessment for children with headaches. *Headache,* 1984, *24,* 182–185.

Levy, D. M. The infant's earliest memory of inoculation: A contribution to public health procedures. *Journal of Genetic Psychology,* 1960, *96,* 3–46.

Lewenstein, L. N. Case history. In G. G. Gardiner & K. Olness, *Hypnosis and hypnotherapy with children.* Orlando, FL: Grune & Stratton, 1981, p. 214.

Lewis, C. E. Personal communication, March, 1982.

Lewis, C. E., & Lewis, M. A. The impact of television commercials on health-related beliefs and behaviors of children. *Pediatrics,* 1974, *53,* 431–435.

Lewis, C. E., Lewis, M. A., Lorimer, A., & Palmer, B. B. Child-initiated care: The use of school nursing services by children in an "adult-free" system. *Pediatrics,* 1977, *60,* 499–507.

Lewis, J. W. Pharmacological profile of buprenorphine and its clinical use in cancer pain. In K. M. Foley & C. E. Inturrisi (Eds.), *Advances in pain research and therapy,* Vol. 8. New York: Raven Press, 1986, pp. 267–270.

Lewis, N. The needle is like an animal. *Children Today,* 1978, *7,* 18–21.

Lewis, T., & Law, D. Investigation of certain autonomic responses of children to a specific dental stress. *Journal of American Dental Association,* 1958, *57,* 769–777.

Lewith, G. T., & Machin, D. Acupuncture compared with placebo in post-herpetic pain. *Pain,* 1983, *17,* 361–368.

Li, C., Chung, D., & Doneen, B. Isolation, characterization and opiate activity of β-endorphin from human pituitary glands. *Biochemical and Biophysical Research Communications,* 1976, *72,* 1542–1547.

Libber, S. M., & Stayton, D. J. Childhood burns reconsidered: The child, the family, and the burn injury. *Journal of Trauma,* 1984, *24,* 245–252.

Liebeskind, J. C., & Paul, L. A., Psychological and physiological mechanisms of pain. *Annual Review of Psychology,* 1977, *28,* 41–60.

Liebman, R., Honig, P., & Berger, H. An integrated treatment program for psychogenic pain. *Family Process,* 1976, *15,* 397–405.

Lindeke, L., Iverson, S., & Fisch, R. Neonatal circumcision: A social and medical dilemma. *Maternal-Child Nursing Journal,* 1986, *15,* 31–37.

Lindell, M. H. Humanisation of the hospital. *World Hospitals,* 1982, *18,* 31–33.

Lindsay, S. J. E. The fear of dental treatment: A critical and theoretical analysis. In S. Rachman (Ed.), *Contributions to Medical Psychology,* Vol. 3. Oxford: Pergamon Press, 1984, pp. 193–224.

Linn, S. Puppets and hospitalized children: Talking about feelings. *Journal of the Association for the Care of Children in Hospitals,* 1977, *5,* 5–11.

Linton, S. J. Behavioral remediation of chronic pain: A status report. *Pain,* 1986, *24,* 125–141.

Linton, S. J., Melin, L., & Götestam, K. G. Behavioral analysis of chronic pain and its management. In M. Hersen, R. M. Eisler, & P. M. Miller (Eds.), *Progress in behavior modification*, Vol. 18. Orlando, FL: Academic Press, 1984, pp. 1–42.

Lipsitt, L. P., & Levy, N. Electrotactual threshold in the neonate. *Child Development*, 1959, *30*, 547–554.

Livingstone, W. K. *Pain mechanisms*. New York: Macmillan, 1943.

Lloyd, J. L. Experiences in a pain relief unit 1970–1976. In A. W. Harcus, R. B. Smith, & B. A. Whittle (Eds.), *Pain—New perspectives in measurement and management*. New York: Churchill Livingstone, 1977, pp. 119–127.

Lobsenz, N. M. The hospital that loves children. *Family Circle*, 1982, *95*, pp. 80, 82, 86, 149–150.

Locke, E. A., Shaw, K. N., Saari, L. M., & Latham, G. P. Goal settings and task performance. *Psychological Bulletin*, 1981, *90*, 125–152.

Locsin, R. G. The effect of pinch-grasp technique on the pain of selected patients during intramuscular injection. *ANPHI Papers*, 1983, *18*, 1–6.

Loebach, S. The use of color to facilitate communication of pain in children. Unpublished master's thesis, University of Washington, Seattle, 1979.

Loeser, J. D. Nonpharmacologic approaches to pain relief. In L. K. Y. Ng & J. J. Bonica (Eds.), *Pain, discomfort and humanitarian care*. New York: Elsevier/North-Holland, 1980, pp. 275–292.

Lollar, D. J, Smits, S. J., & Patterson, D. L. Assessment of pediatric pain: An empirical perspective. *Journal of Pediatric Psychology*, 1982, *7*, 267–277.

London, P. *The Children's Hypnotic Susceptibility Scale*. Palo Alto, CA: Consulting Psychologists Press, 1962.

Lonetto, R., *Children's conceptions of death*. New York: Springer, 1980.

Lowe, K., & Lutzker, J. R. Increasing compliance to a medical regimen with a juvenile diabetic. *Behavior Therapy*, 1979, *10*, 57–64.

Lowery, C. Children-for-change-board: The children speak out. Paper presented at the Association for the Care of Children in Hospitals annual meeting, May, 1985.

Ludvigsson, J. Propranolol used in prophylaxis of migraine in children. *Acta Neurologica Scandinavica*, 1974, *50*, 109–115.

Luthe, W. Autogenic training: Method, research, and application in medicine. *American Journal of Psychotherapy*, 1963, *17*, 174–195.

Macdonald, A. *Acupuncture: From ancient art to modern medicine*. London: Unwin, 1984.

Machen, J. B., & Johnson, R. Desensitization, model learning, and the dental behavior of children. *Journal of Dental Research*, 1974, *53*, 83–87.

MacKenzie, R. G. Menstrual disorders in adolescents. In J. T. Y. Shen (Ed.), *The clinical practice of adolescent medicine*. New York: Appleton-Century-Crofts, 1980, pp. 348–361.

MacLeod, S. M., & Radde, I. C. *Textbook of pediatric clinical pharmacology*. Littleton, MA: PSG Publishing, 1985.

MacRae, K. D. The interpretation of pain measurements. In A. W. Harcus, R. B. Smith, & B. A. Whittle (Eds.), *Pain—New perspectives in measurement and management*. Edinburgh: Churchill Livingstone, 1977, pp 21–24.

Madden, E. J. Itch. *Pain*, 1985, *21*, 313–314.

Magrab, P. R. Psychological management and renal dialysis. *Journal of Clinical Child Psychology*, 1975, *4*, 38–40.

Mäkelä, A. L. Naproxen in the treatment of juvenile rheumatoid arthritis: Metabolism, safety and efficacy. *Scandinavian Journal of Rheumatology*, 1977, *6*, 193–205.

Margolis, R. B., Tait, R. C., & Krause, S. J. A rating system for use with patient pain drawings. *Pain*, 1986, *24*, 57–65.

Marks, R., & Sachar, E. Undertreatment of medical inpatients with narcotic analgesics. *Annals of Internal Medicine,* 1973, *78,* 173–181.

Marlow, D. R. *Textbook of pediatric nursing,* 4th ed. Philadelphia: Saunders, 1977.

Martin, W. R. History and development of mixed opioid agonists, partial agonists and antagonists. *British Journal of Clinical Pharmacology,* 1979, *7,* 273S–279S.

Martino, G., Ventafridda, V., Parini, J., & Emanuelli, A. A controlled study on the analgesic activity of indoprofen in patients with cancer pain. In J. J. Bonica & D. Albe-Fessard (Eds.), *Advances in pain research and therapy,* Vol. 1. New York: Raven Press, 1976, pp. 573–578.

Masek, B. J., Russo, D. C., & Varni, J. W. Behavioral approaches to the management of chronic pain in children. *Pediatric Clinics of North America,* 1984, *31,* 1113–1131.

Massey, E. W. Effort headache in runners. *Headache,* 1982, *22,* 99–100.

Masten, A. S. Family therapy as a treatment for children: A critical review of outcome research. *Family Process,* 1979, *18,* 323–335.

Mather, L., & Mackie, J. The incidence of postoperative pain in children. *Pain,* 1983, *15,* 271–282.

Maxwell, G. M. *Principles of paediatric pharmacology.* London: Croom Helm, 1984.

Mayer, D. J., Price, D. D., Barber, J., & Rafii, A. Acupuncture analgesia: Evidence for activation of a pain inhibitory system as a mechanism of action. In J. J. Bonica & D. Albe-Fessard (Eds.), *Advances in Pain Research and Therapy,* Vol. 1. New York: Raven Press, 1976, pp. 751–754.

Mayer, D. J., Price, D. D, & Rafii, A. Antagonism of acupuncture analgesia in man by the narcotic antagonist naloxone. *Brain Research,* 1977, *121,* 368–372.

Mayer, D. J., Wolfle, T. L., Akil, H., Carder, B., & Liebeskind, J. C. Analgesia from electrical stimulation in the brainstem of the rat. *Science,* 1971, *174,* 1351–1354.

McCaffery, M. Brief episodes of pain in children. In A. Bergersen, M. Duffey, M. Lohr, & M. Rose (Eds.), *Current concepts in clinical nursing.* St. Louis: Mosby, 1969, pp. 178–191.

McCaffery, M. Pain relief for the child: Problem areas and selected nonpharmacological methods. *Pediatric Nursing,* 1977, *3,* 11–16.

McCarthy, R. Personal communication, February, 1972.

McCaul, K. D., & Malott, J. M. Distraction and coping with pain. *Psychological Bulletin,* 1984, *95,* 516–533.

McClellan, M. A. The use of the physical examination to promote development of the preschooler. *Children's Health Care,* 1984, *12,* 174–178.

McCollum, A. T. *The chronically ill child.* New Haven, CT: Yale University Press, 1981.

McGrath, P. A. The Children's Comprehensive Pain Questionnaire. Unpublished manuscript. University of Western Ontario, London, 1986.

McGrath, P. A. The management of chronic pain in children. In G. D. Burrows, D. Elton, & G. V. Stanley (Eds.), *The handbook of chronic pain management.* Amsterdam: Elsevier, in press, 1987a.

McGrath, P. A. *Pain in children: The perception, assessment and control of children's pain.* New York: Guilford Press, in press, 1987b.

McGrath, P. A. Personal communication, February, 1987c.

McGrath, P. A. Pediatric pain and behavioral medicine: Pain assessment and the role of an endogenous opiate system in pain relief by psychological intervention. Final report 6606-2244-04. London, Ontario: University of Western Ontario, 1987d.

McGrath, P. A. & de Veber, L. L. The management of acute pain evoked by medical procedures in children with cancer. *Journal of Pain and Symptom Management,* 1986, *1,* 145–150.

McGrath, P. A., de Veber, L. L., & Hearn, M. T. Multidimensional pain assessment in children. In H. L. Fields, R. Dubner, & F. Cervero (Eds.), *Advances in pain research and therapy,* Vol. 9. Proceedings of the Fourth World Congress on Pain. New York: Raven Press, 1985, pp. 387–393.

McGrath, P. J. Migraine headaches in children and adolescents. In P. Firestone, P. J. McGrath, & W. Feldman (Eds.), *Advances in behavioral medicine with children and youth.* Hillsdale, NJ: Lawrence Erlbaum, 1983.

McGrath, P. J., Cunningham, S. J., Goodman, J. T., & Unruh, A. The clinical measurement of pain in children: A review. *Clinical Journal of Pain,* 1986, *2,* 221–227.

McGrath, P. J., Johnson, G., Goodman, J. T., Schillinger, J., Dunn, J., & Chapman, J. A. CHEOPS: A behavioral scale for rating postoperative pain in children. In H. L. Fields, R. Dubner, & F. Cervero (Eds.), *Advances in pain research and therapy,* Vol. 9. Proceedings of the Fourth World Congress on Pain. New York: Raven Press, 1985, pp. 395–402.

McGrath, P. J. & Unruh, A. *Pain in children and adolescents.* New York: Elsevier/North-Holland, in press, 1987.

McGrath, P. J., & Vair, C. Psychological aspects of pain management of the burned child. *Children's Health Care,* 1984, *13,* 15–19.

McNair, D. M., Droppleman, L. F., & Kussman, M. Finger-sweat print tape bands. *Psychophysiology,* 1967, *4,* 75–78.

Mechanic, D. The experience and reporting of common physical complaints. *Health & Social Behavior,* 1980, *21,* 146–155.

Mehegan, J. E., Masek, B. J., Harrison, R. H., Russo, D. C., & Leviton, A. A multicomponent behavioral treatment for pediatric migraine. *Clinical Journal of Pain,* 1987, *2,* 191–196.

Meichenbaum, D. H. Examination of model characteristics in reducing avoidance behavior. *Journal of Personality and Social Psychology,* 1971, *17,* 298–307.

Meichenbaum, D. H. Cognitive factors in biofeedback therapy. *Biofeedback and Self Regulation,* 1976, *1,* 201–216.

Meichenbaum, D. H. *Cognitive-behavior modification: An integrative approach.* New York: Plenum Press, 1977.

Meinhart, N. T., & McCaffery, M. *Pain: A nursing approach to assessment and analysis.* Norwalk, CT: Appleton-Century-Crofts, 1983.

Meissner, W. W., & Nicholi, A. M, Jr. The psychotherapies: Individual, family, and group. In A. M. Nicholi, Jr., (Ed.), *The Harvard guide to modern psychiatry.* Cambridge, MA: Belknap Press, 1978, pp. 357–386.

Melamed, B. G. Behavioral approaches to fear in dental settings. In M. Hersen, R. M. Eisler, & P. M. Miller (Eds.), *Progress in behavior modification,* Vol. 7. New York: Academic Press, 1979, pp. 172–203.

Melamed, B. G., & Siegel, L. J. Reduction of anxiety in children facing hospitalization and surgery by use of filmed modeling. *Journal of Consulting and Clinical Psychology,* 1975, *43,* 511–521.

Melamed, B. G., & Siegel, L. J. *Behavioral medicine: Practical applications in health care.* New York: Springer, 1980.

Melamed, B. G., Yurcheson, R., Fleece, E. L., Hutcherson, S., & Hawes, R. Effects of film modeling on the reduction of anxiety related behaviors in individuals varying in levels of previous experience in the stress situation. *Journal of Consulting and Clinical Psychology,* 1978, *46,* 1357–1367.

Meldman, M. *Diseases of attention and perception.* New York: Pergamon Press, 1970.

Melzack, R. Effects of early experience on behavior: Experimental and conceptual considerations. In P. Hoch & J. Zubin (Eds.), *Psychopathology of perception.* New York: Grune & Stratton, 1965, pp. 271–299.

Melzack, R. *The puzzle of pain.* New York: Basic Books, 1973.

Melzack, R. The McGill Pain Questionnaire: Major properties and scoring methods. *Pain,* 1975, *1,* 277–299.

Melzack, R. (participant). General discussion. In J. J. Bonica (Ed.), *Pain.* Research publications: Association for Research in Nervous and Mental Disease, Vol. 58. New York: Raven Press, 1980, pp. 185–189.

Melzack, R. (Ed.), *Pain measurement and assessment.* New York: Raven, 1983.

Melzack, R. Measurement of the dimensions of pain experience. In B. Bromm (Ed.), *Pain measurement in man.* Amsterdam: Elsevier, 1984a, pp. 327–348.

Melzack, R., Neuropsychological basis of pain measurement. In L. Kruger & J. C. Liebeskind (Eds.), *Neural mechanisms of pain. Advances in Pain Research and Therapy,* Vol. 6. New York: Raven Press, 1984b, pp. 323–339.

Melzack, R., & Casey, K. L. Sensory, motivational and central control determinants of pain: A new conceptual model. In D. Kenshalo (Ed.), *The skin senses.* Springfield, Illinois: Thomas, 1968, pp. 423–443.

Melzack, R., & Dennis, S. G. Neurophysiological foundations of pain. In R. A. Sternbach (Ed.), *The psychology of pain.* New York: Raven Press, 1978, pp. 1–26.

Melzack, R., Guité, S., & Gonshor, A. Relief of dental pain by ice massage of the hand. *Canadian Medical Association Journal,* 1980, *122,* 189–191.

Melzack, R., Katz, J., & Jeans, M. E. The role of compensation in chronic pain: Analysis using a new method of scoring the McGill Pain Questionnaire. *Pain,* 1985, *23,* 101–112.

Melzack, R., & Scott, T. H. The effects of early experience on the responses to pain. *Journal of Comparative Physiology and Psychology,* 1957, *50,* 155–161.

Melzack, R., Stillwell, D. M., & Fox, E. J. Trigger points and acupuncture points for pain: Correlations and implications. *Pain,* 1977, *3,* 3–23.

Melzack, R., & Torgerson, W. S. On the language of pain. *Anesthesiology,* 1971, *34,* 50–59.

Melzack, R., & Wall, P. D. On the nature of cutaneous sensory mechanisms. *Brain,* 1962, *85,* 331–356.

Melzack, R., & Wall, P. D. Pain mechanisms: A new theory. *Science,* 1965, *150,* 971–979.

Melzack, R., & Wall, P. D. *The challenge of pain.* New York: Basic Books, 1983.

Melzack, R., Wall, P. D., & Ty, T. C. Acute pain in an emergency clinic: Latency of onset and descriptor patterns related to different injuries. *Pain,* 1982, *14,* 33–43.

Mendelson, G. Not 'cured by a verdict': Effect of legal settlement on compensation claimants. *Medical Journal of Australia,* 1982, *2,* 132–134.

Mendelson, G. Compensation, pain complaints, and psychological disturbance. *Pain,* 1984, *20,* 169–177.

Menefee, E. E. The internist. *Medical Times,* 1967, *95,* 1177–1179.

Menges, L. J. Pain: Still an intriguing puzzle. *Social Science and Medicine,* 1984, *19,* 1257–1260.

Menke, E. School-aged children's perception of stress in the hospital. *Children's Health Care,* 1981, *9,* 80–86.

Mennie, A. T. The child in pain. In L. Burton (Ed.), *Care of the child facing death.* London: Routledge & Kegan Paul, 1974, pp. 49–59.

Merrill, J. C. Personal communication, April, 1987.

Merskey, H. On the development of pain. *Headache,* 1970, *10,* 116–123.

Merskey, H. Pain, learning and memory. *Journal of Psychosomatic Research,* 1975, *19,* 319–324.

Merksey, H. Pain terms: A list with definitions and notes on usage. Recommended by the International Association for the Study of Pain (IASP) Subcommittee on Taxonomy. *Pain*, 1979, *6*, 249–252.

Metcalf, T. J., Osborn, L. M., & Mariani, E. M. Circumcision: A study of current practices. *Clinical Pediatrics*, 1983, *22*, 575–579.

Micheli, L. J. Overuse injuries in children's sports: The growth factor. *Orthopedic Clinics of North America, 1983, 14,* 337–360.

Michell, J. Measurement scales and statistics: A clash of paradigms. *Psychological Bulletin*, 1986, *100*, 398–407.

Milhorat, T. H. *Pediatric neurosurgery.* Philadelphia: F. A. Davis, 1978.

Miller, A. J., & Kratochwill, T. R. Reduction of frequent stomachache complaints by time out. *Behavior Therapy*, 1979, *10,* 211–218.

Miller, I. W., & Norman, W. H. Learned helplessness in humans: A review and attribution-theory model. *Psychological Bulletin*, 1979, *86,* 93–118.

Miller, J. J., III, Spitz, P. W., Simpson, U., & Williams, G. F. The social function of young adults who had arthritis in childhood. *Journal of Pediatrics*, 1982, *100*, 378–382.

Miller, N. E. Learning of visceral and glandular responses. *Science*, 1969, *163*, 434–445.

Miller, R. R. Evaluation of the analgesic efficacy of ibuprofen. *Pharmacotherapy*, 1981, *1,* 21–27.

Miller, S. W. Personal communication, December, 1980.

Millman, B. S. Acupuncture: Context and critique. *Annual Review of Medicine*, 1977, *28,* 223–234.

Millman, M. *The unkindest cut.* New York: Morrow, 1977.

Minuchin, S., Baker, L., Rosman, B. L., Liebman, R., Milman, L., & Todd, T. C. A conceptual model of psychosomatic illness in children: Family organization and family therapy. *Archives of General Psychiatry*, 1975, *32,* 1031–1038.

Mirvish, I. Hypnotherapy for the child with chronic eczema: A case report. *South African Medical Journal*, 1978, *54*, 410–412.

Miser, A. W., Davis, D. M., Hughes, C. S., Mulne, A. F., & Miser, J. S. Continous subcutaneous infusion of morphine in children with cancer. *American Journal of Diseases in Children*, 1983, *137,* 383–385.

Miser, A. W., Dothage, J. A., Wesley, R. A., & Miser, J. S. The prevalence of pain in a pediatric and young adult cancer population. *Pain*, 1987, *29,* 73–83.

Miser, A. W., McCalla, J., Dothage, J. A., Wesley, M., & Miser, J. S. Pain as a presenting symptom in children and young adults with newly diagnosed malignancy. *Pain*, 1987, *29,* 85–90.

Miser, A. W., Miser, J. S., & Clark, B. S. Continuous intravenous infusion of morphine sulphate for control of severe pain in children with terminal malignancy. *Journal of Pediatrics*, 1980, *96*, 930–932.

Mitchell, S. W., Morehouse, G. R., & Keen, W. W., Jr. *Gunshot wounds and other injuries of nerves.* Philadelphia: Lippincott, 1864.

Mogtader, E. M., & Leff, P. T. "Young healers": Chronically ill adolescents as child life assistants. *Children's Health Care*, 1986, *14*, 174–177.

Mohamed, S. N., Weisz, G. M., & Waring, E. M. The relationship of chronic pain to depression, marital adjustment, and family dynamics. *Pain*, 1978, *5*, 285–292.

Möller, C. A lignocaine-prilocaine cream reduces venipuncture pain. *Upsala Journal of Medical Sciences*, 1985, *90*, 293–298.

Molsberry, D. M. J. Young children's subjective quantification of pain following surgery. Unpublished master's thesis, University of Iowa, 1979.

Mondzac, A. M. In defense of the reintroduction of heroin into American medical practice and H.R. 5290—The Compassionate Pain Relief Act. *New England Journal of Medicine,* 1984, *311,* 532–535.

Monk, M. The nature of pain and responses to pain in adolescent hemophiliacs. Unpublished master's thesis, McGill University, Montreal, 1980.

Morawetz, R. F., Parth, P., & Pöppel, E. Influence of the pain measurement technique on the diurnal variation of pain perception. In B. Bromm (Ed.), *Pain measurement in man.* Amsterdam: Elsevier, 1984, pp. 409–415.

Morbidity and Mortality Weekly Report, Reye Syndrome—United States, 1984–1985, *34,* No. 1, 13–16.

Morgan, A. H., & Hilgard, E. R. Age differences in susceptibility to hypnosis. *International Journal of Clinical and Experimental Hypnosis,* 1973, *21,* 78–85.

Morgan, A. H., & Hilgard, J. R. The Stanford Hypnotic Clinical Scale for Children. *American Journal of Clinical Hypnosis,* 1979, *21,* 148–169.

Morley, J. S. Peptides in nociceptive pathways. In S. Lipton & J. Miles (Eds.), *Persistent pain: Modern methods of treatment,* Vol. 5. London: Grune & Stratton, 1985, pp. 65–91.

Morpurgo, C. V., Nobili, R. M., Leonardi, G., Casati, R., & Cacciabue, F. Rheumatic and orthopaedic pain in children and their environment. In R. Rizzi & M. Visentin (Eds.), *Pain.* Padua, Italy: Piccin/Butterworths, 1984, pp. 358–364.

Morris, F. D., & McFadd, A. The mental health team on a burn unit: A multidisciplinary approach. *Journal of Trauma,* 1978, *18,* 658–663.

Mullen, F. G. The treatment of a case of dysmenorrhea by behavior therapy techniques. *Journal of Nervous and Mental Disorders,* 1968, *147,* 371–376.

Mullen, F. G. Treatment of dysmenorrhea by professional and student behavior therapists. Paper presented at the Fifth Annual Meeting of the Association for the Advancement of Behavior Therapy. Washington, DC, September, 1971.

Mundinger, M. O. Health service funding cuts and the declining health of the poor. *New England Journal of Medicine,* 1985, *313,* 44–47.

Murphy, L. B. Coping, vulnerability, and resilience in childhood. In G. V. Coelho, D. A. Hamburg, & J. E. Adams (Eds.), *Coping and adaptation.* New York: Basic Books, 1974, pp. 69–100.

Murphy, M. E. Letter to the Editor. *Family Circle,* 1982, *95,* No. 13, p. R8.

Murphy, T. M., & Anderson, S. Multidisciplinary approach to managing pain. In C. Benedetti, C. R. Chapman, & G. Moricca (Eds.), *Advances in pain research and therapy,* Vol. 7, *Recent advances in the management of pain.* New York: Raven Press, 1984, pp. 359–371.

Murrin, K. R., & Rosen, M. Pain measurement. In G. Smith & B. G. Covino (Eds.), *Acute pain.* London: Butterworths, 1985, pp. 104–132.

Nafe, J. P. The pressure, pain and temperature senses. In C. A. Murchison (Ed.), *Handbook of general experimental psychology.* Worcester, MA: Clark University Press, 1934.

Nagera, H. Children's reactions to hospitalization and illness. *Child Psychiatry and Human Development,* 1978, *9,* 3–19.

Nathan, P. W. The gate-control theory of pain. A critical review. *Brain,* 1976, *99,* 123–158.

Nathan, P. W. Pain. In W. B. Matthews & G. H. Glaser (Eds.), *Recent advances in clinical neurology.* New York: Churchill Livingstone, 1982, pp. 83–94.

National Commission for the Protection of Human Subjects of Biomedical and Behavioral Research. *Research involving children.* (Publication No. 0577-004). Washington, DC: Department of Health, Education, and Welfare, 1977.

National Health Survey, 1935–36. *The magnitude of the chronic disease problem in the United States.* Washington, DC: Public Health Service, 1938.

Nayman, J. Measurement and control of postoperative pain. *Annals of the Royal College of*

Surgeons, 1979, 61, 419–429.

Neal, H. K. Pain. Bethesda, MD: National Institute of General Medical Sciences, NIH, 1968.

Neal, H. K. The politics of pain. New York: McGraw-Hill, 1978.

Neinstein, L. S. Adolescent health care: A practical guide. Baltimore: Urban & Schwarzenberg, 1984.

Nerlinger, R. E. The technique and recording of thermography. In S. Uematsu (Ed.), Medical thermography, theory and clinical applications. Los Angeles: Brentwood, 1976.

Neuhauser, C., Amsterdam, B., Hines, P., & Steward, M. Children's concepts of healing: Cognitive development and locus of control factors. American Journal of Orthopsychiatry, 1978, 48, 335–341.

Newburger, P. E., & Sallan, S. E. Chronic pain: Principles of management. Journal of Pediatrics, 1981, 98, 180–189.

Newman, R., Painter, J., Seres, J. A therapeutic milieu for chronic pain patients. Journal of Human Stress, 1978, 4, 8–12.

Ng, L. K. Y. Pain and well-being: A challenge for biomedicine. In L. K. Y. Ng & J. J. Bonica (Eds.), Pain, discomfort and humanitarian care. New York: Elsevier/North Holland, 1980, pp. 353–365.

Ng, L. K. Y. (Ed.). New approaches to treatment of chronic pain: A review of multidisciplinary pain clinics and pain centers. National Institute on Drug Abuse Monograph No. 36. Washington, DC: U.S. Government Printing Office, May, 1981.

Ng, L. K. Y. Acupuncture: A neuromodulation technique for pain control. In G. M. Aronoff (Ed.), Evaluation and treatment of chronic pain. Baltimore: Urban & Schwarzenberg, 1985, pp. 539–547.

Ng, L. K. Y., & Bonica, J. J. (Eds.). Pain, discomfort and humanitarian care. Developments in neurology, Vol. 4. New York: Elsevier/North Holland, 1980.

Nicholson, R. H. Medical research with children: Ethics, law, and practice. Oxford, England: Oxford University Press, 1986.

Nissen, K. W., Chow, R. L., & Semmes, J. Effects of restricted opportunity for tactual, kinesthetic, and manipulative experience on the behavior of a chimpanzee. American Journal of Psychology, 1951, 64, 485–507.

Niven, C., & Gijsbers, K. A study of labour pain using the McGill Pain Questionnaire. Social Science and Medicine, 1984, 19, 1347–1351.

Nocella, J., & Kaplan, R. M. Training children to cope with dental treatment. Journal of Pediatric Psychology, 1982, 7, 175–178.

Noordenbos, W. Pain. Amsterdam: Elsevier Press, 1959.

Noordenbos, W. Prologue. In P. D. Wall & R. Melzack (Eds.), Textbook of pain. New York: Churchill Livingstone, 1984, pp. xi–xv.

Notermans, S. L., & Tophoff, M. M. Sex differences in pain tolerance and pain apperception. Psychiatria, Neurologia, Neurochirurgia, 1967, 70, 23–29.

Nover, R. A. Pain and the burned child. Journal of the American Academy of Child Psychiatry, 1973, 12, 499–505.

O'Brien, C. Postoperative pain and analgesics: A comparative study of adults and children. Unpublished master's thesis, McGill University, Montreal, 1984.

Olds, A. R. Psychological considerations in humanizing the physical environment of pediatric outpatient and hospital settings. In E. Gellert (Ed.), Psychosocial aspects of pediatric care. New York: Grune & Stratton, 1978, pp. 111–131.

Olness, K. In-service hypnosis education in a children's hospital. American Journal of Clinical Hypnosis, 1977, 20, 80–83.

Olness, K. In C. Warga, Little swamis. Psychology Today, 1985, 19, 16–17.

Olness, K., & Agle, D. *The enhancement of mastery in the person with hemophilia via relaxation-imagery exercises (self-hypnosis) or biofeedback techniques.* The National Hemophilia Foundation, New York, 1982.

Olness, K., & Gardner, G. G. Some guidelines for uses of hypnotherapy in pediatrics. *Pediatrics,* 1978, *62,* 228–233.

Olness, K., & MacDonald, J. Self-hypnosis and biofeedback in the management of juvenile migraine. *Developmental and Behavioral Pediatrics,* 1981, *2,* 168–170.

Olness, K., MacDonald, J. T., & Uden, D. L. Comparison of self-hypnosis and propranolol in the treatment of juvenile classic migraine. *Pediatrics,* 1987, *79,* 593–597.

Olness, K., Wain, H. J., & Ng, L. K. Y. A pilot study of blood endorphin levels in children using self-hypnosis to control pain. *Developmental and Behavioral Pediatrics,* 1980, *1,* 187–188.

Olson, S. Following aspirin's trail. *Science 85,* 1985, *6,* 20.

O'Neill, J. A. Burns in children. In C. P. Artz, J. A. Moncrief, & B. A. Pruitt (Eds.), *Burns: A team approach.* Philadelphia: Saunders, 1979, pp. 341–350.

Orne, M. T. Hypnotic control of pain: Toward a clarification of the different psychological processes involved. In J. J. Bonica (Ed.), *Pain.* New York: Raven Press, 1980, pp. 155–172.

Orne, M. T., & Dinges, D. F. Hypnosis. In P. J. Wall & R. Melzack (Eds.), *Textbook of pain.* New York: Churchill Livingstone, 1984, pp. 806–816.

Oswalt, R., & Napoliello, M. Motivations of blood donors and nondonors. *Journal of Applied Psychology,* 1974, *59,* 122–124.

Owens, M. E. Pain in infancy: Conceptual and methodological issues. *Pain,* 1984, *20,* 213–230.

Owens, M. E., & Todt, E. H. Pain in infancy: Neonatal reaction to a heel lance. *Pain,* 1984, *20,* 77–86.

Painter, J. R., Seres, J. L., & Newman, R. I. Assessing benefits of the pain center: Why some patients regress. *Pain,* 1980, *8,* 101–113.

Parkin, S. F. The effect of ambient music upon the reactions of children undergoing dental treatment. *Journal of Dentistry for Children,* 1981, *48,* 430–432.

Parlee, M. B. The premenstrual syndrome. *Psychological Bulletin,* 1973, *80,* 454–465.

Passo, M. Aches and limb pain. *Pediatric Clinics of North America,* 1982, *29,* 209–219.

Paulley, J. W., & Haskell, D. J. Treatment of migraine without drugs. *Journal of Psychosomatic Research,* 1975, *19,* 367–374.

Payne, B., & Norfleet, M. A. Chronic pain and the family: A review. *Pain,* 1986, *26,* 1–22.

Pearce, J. D. Case study of play therapy with a 5-year-old boy with Hodgkin's disease. In E. K. Oremland and J. D. Oremland (Eds.), *The effects of hospitalization on children: Models for their care.* Springfield, IL: Thomas, 1973, pp. 211–221.

Pederson, L. L., Stennett, R. G., & Lefcoe, N. M. The effects of a smoking education program on the behavior, knowledge and attitudes of children in grades 4 and 6. *Journal of Drug Education,* 1981, *11,* 141–149.

Peller, L. Models of children's play. *Mental Hygiene,* 1952, *36,* 66–83.

Pennebaker, J. W. *The psychology of physical symptoms.* New York: Springer-Verlag, 1982.

Penticuff, J. H. The effect of filmed peer modeling, cognitive appraisal, and autonomic reactivity in changing children's attitudes about health care procedures and personnel. Case Western Reserve University, doctoral dissertation, 1976. *Dissertation Abstracts,* 1976, *37,* 3089B–3090B.

Peper, E., & Grossman, E. Preliminary observation of thermal biofeedback training in children with migraine. Paper presented at the Biofeedback Research Society Annual Meeting, Colorado Springs, CO, 1974.

Perl, E. R. Is pain a specific sensation? *Journal of Psychiatric Research*, 1971, *8*, 273–287.

Perrin, E. C. & Gerrity, P. C. There's a demon in your belly: Children's understanding of illness. *Pediatrics*, 1981, *67*, 841–849.

Perry, S. W. Undertreatment of pain on a burn unit. *General Hospital Psychiatry*, 1984a, *6*, 308–316.

Perry, S. W. The undermedication for pain. *Psychiatric Annals*, 1984b, *14*, 808–811.

Perry, S., & Heidrich, G. Management of pain during debridement: A survey of U.S. burn units. *Pain*, 1982, *13*, 267–280.

Pert, C., & Snyder, S. Opiate receptor: Demonstration in nervous tissue. *Science*, 1973, *179*, 1011–1014.

Peterschmidt, K. Personal communication, February, 1984.

Peterson, L., & Shigetomi, C. The use of coping techniques to minimize anxiety in hospitalized children. *Behavioral Therapy*, 1981, *12*, 1–14.

Peterson, L., & Ridley-Johnson, R. Pediatric hospital response to survey on prehospital preparation for children. *Journal of Pediatric Psychology*, 1980, *5*, 1–7.

Peterson, L., & Ridley-Johnson, R. Preparation of well children in the classroom: An unexpected contrast between the academic lecture and filmed-modeling methods. *Journal of Pediatric Psychology*, 1984, *9*, 349–361.

Peterson, L., & Toler, S. Self-regulated presurgical preparation for children. Paper presented at the American Psychological Association meeting. Toronto, Canada, 1984.

Peterson, W. J. Personal communication, November, 1983.

Petrie, A. *Individuality in pain and suffering*. Chicago: University of Chicago Press, 1967.

Petrillo, M., & Sanger, S. *Emotional care of hospitalized children*. Philadelphia: Lippincott, 1972.

Piaget, J. *Play, dreams, and imitation in childhood*. London: Heinmann, 1951.

Piaget, J. *The child and reality—problems of genetic psychology*. New York: Grossman, 1973.

Piaget, J., & Inhelder, B. *The psychology of the child*. New York: Basic Books, 1969.

Pickles, V. H. A plain-muscle stimulant in the menstrum. *Nature*. 1957, *180*, 1198.

Pickles, V. R., Hall, W. J., Best, F. A., & Smith, G. N. Prostaglandins in endometrium and menstrual fluid from normal and dysmenorrhoeic subjects. *Journal of Obstetrics and Gynecology of the British Commonwealth*, 1975, *72*, 185–192.

Pilowsky, I., Bassett, D. L., Begg, M. W., & Thomas, P. G. Childhood hospitalization and chronic intractable pain in adults: A controlled retrospective study. *International Journal of Psychiatry in Medicine*, 1982, *12*, 75–84.

Pinsky, J. Chronic intractable benign pain: A syndrome and its treatment with intensive short-term group psychotherapy. *Journal of Human Stress*, 1978, *4*, 17–21.

Pinsky, J. J., & Crue, B. L. Intensive group psychotherapy. In P. D. Wall & R. Melzack (Eds.), *Textbook of pain*. New York: Churchill Livingstone, 1984, pp. 823–831.

Pomeranz, B., Cheng, R., & Law, P. Acupuncture reduces electrophysiological and behavioral responses to noxious stimuli: Pituitary is implicated. *Experimental Neurology*, 1977, *54*, 172–178.

Portenoy, R. K., & Foley, K. M. Chronic use of opioid analgesics in non-malignant pain: Report of 38 cases. *Pain*, 1986, *25*, 171–186.

Porter, J. J. Personal communication, August, 1984.

Porter, J. & Jick, H. Addiction rare in patients treated with narcotics. Letter to the editor. *New England Journal of Medicine*, 1980, *302*, 123.

Pothmann, R., & Goepel, R. Acupuncture therapy of childhood migraine. In R. Rizzi & M. Visentin (Eds.), *Pain*. Padua, Italy: Piccin/Butterworths, 1984a, pp. 335–339.

Pothmann, R., & Goepel, R. Comparison of the *Visual Analog Scale* (VAS) and a *Smiley Analog Scale* (SAS) for the evaluation of pain in children. Paper presented at the IVth

World Congress on Pain of the International Association for the Study of Pain. Seattle, WA, August 1984b.

Pothman, R., Schwammborn, D., Andras, A., Ebell, W., & Jurgens, H. Buprenorphine: Longterm results in therapy of tumor pain in childhood. In R. Rizzi & M. Visentin (Eds.), *Pain*. Padua, Italy: Piccin/Butterworths, 1984, pp. 397–399.

Poznanski, E. O. Children's reactions to pain: A psychiatrist's perspective. *Clinical Pediatrics*, 1976, *15*, 1114–1119.

Prensky, A. L., & Sommer, D. Diagnosis and treatment of migraine in children. *Neurology*, 1979, *29*, 506–510.

Price, D. D., Harkins, S. W., Rafii, A., & Price, C. A simultaneous comparison of fentanyl's analgesic effects on experimental and clinical pain. *Pain*, 1986, *24*, 197–203.

Price, D. D., Rafii, A., Watkins, L. R., & Buckingham, B. A psychophysical analysis of acupuncture analgesia. *Pain*, 1984, *19*, 27–42.

Prudden, B. *Pain erasure: The Bonnie Prudden way.* New York: Evans, 1980.

Pugh, S. T. Pediatric patients: The special situation. *Human Aspects of Anesthesia*, 1985, *7*, 3.

Qualls, P. J., & Sheehan, P. W. Electromyograph biofeedback as a relaxation technique: A critical appraisal and reassessment. *Psychological Bulletin*, 1981, *90*, 21–42.

Quinby, S., & Bernstein, N. Treatment problems with severely burned children—identity problems and adaptation of nurses, Part 1. *American Journal of Psychiatry*, 1971, *128*, 58–63.

Radde, I. C. Topics in adolescent clinical pharmacology. In S. M. MacLeod & I. C. Radde (Eds.), *Textbook of pediatric clinical pharmacology*. Littleton, MA: PSG Publishing, 1985, pp. 341–350.

Radde, I. C., & MacLeod, S. M. Therapeutic and nontherapeutic research in children. In S. M. MacLeod & I. C. Radde (Eds.), *Textbook of pediatric clinical pharmacology*. Littleton, MA: PSG Publishing, 1985, pp. 435–439.

Rae, W. A., & Stieber, D. A. Plant play therapy: Growth through growth. *Journal of Pediatric Psychology*, 1976, *1*, 18–20.

Rafart, A., Espinosa, W., Illa, J., Fabregas, C., & Borrego, A. Different kinds of analgesia in pediatric oncology: Oral medication. In R. Rizzi & M. Visentin (Eds.), *Pain*. Padua, Italy: Piccin/Butterworths, 1984, pp. 401–403.

Ramsden, R. Friedman, B., & Williamson, D. A. Treatment of childhood headache reports with contingency management procedures. *Journal of Clinical Child Psychology*, 1983, *12*, 202–206.

Reading, A. E. The McGill Pain Questionnaire: An appraisal. In R. Melzack (Ed.), *Pain measurement and assessment*. New York: Raven Press, 1983, pp. 55–61.

Reading, A. E., & Newton, J. R. A card sort method of pain assessment. *Journal of Psychosomatic Research*, 1978, *22*, 503–512.

Redd, W. H., Jacobsen, P. B., & Die-Trill, M. Cognitive/attentional distraction in the control of conditioned nausea in pediatric cancer patients receiving chemotherapy. Unpublished manuscript, Memorial Sloan-Kettering Cancer Center, New York, 1986.

Redpath, C. C., & Rogers, C. S. Healthy young children's concepts of hospitals, medical personnel, operations, and illness. *Journal of Pediatric Psychology*, 1984, *9*, 29–40.

Reichmanis, M., & Becker, R. O. Relief of experimentally induced pain by stimulation at acupuncture loci. *Comparative Medicine East and West*, 1977, *5*, 281–288.

Reissland, N. Cognitive maturity and the experience of fear and pain in hospital. *Social Science and Medicine*, 1983, *17*, 1389–1395.

Remen, N. *The human patient.* New York: Anchor Press/Doubleday, 1980.

Renaer, R. Gynecological pain. In P. D. Wall & R. Melzack (Eds.), *Textbook of pain*. Edinburgh: Churchill Livingstone, 1984, pp. 359–375.

Report of the Interagency Committee on New Therapies for Pain and Discomfort: Research needs and opportunities in the control of pain and discomfort. Bethesda, MD: National Institutes of Health, 1978.

Revill, S. I., Robinson, J. O., Rosen, M., & Hogg, M. I. J. The reliability of a linear analogue for evaluating pain. *Anaesthesia*, 1976, *31*, 1191–1198.

Reynolds, D. V. Surgery in the rat during electrical analgesia induced by focal brain stimulation. *Science*, 1969, *164*, 444–445.

Richardson, G. M., McGrath, P. J., Cunningham, S. J., & Humphreys, P. Validity of the headache diary for children. *Headache*, 1983, *23*, 184–187.

Richardson, P. H., & Vincent, C. A. Acupuncture for the treatment of pain: A review of evaluative research. *Pain*, 1986, *24*, 15–40.

Richter, H. G. Emotional disturbances of constant pattern following nonspecific respiratory infections. *Journal of Pediatrics*, 1943, *23*, 315–325.

Richter, I. L., McGrath, P. J., Humphreys, P. J., Goodman, J. T., Firestone, P., & Keene, D. Cognitive and relaxation treatment of paediatric migraine. *Pain*, 1986, *25*, 195–203.

Roberts, A. H. The behavioral treatment of pain. In J. M. Ferguson & C. B. Taylor (Eds.), *The comprehensive handbook of behavioral medicine*, Vol. 2. New York: SP Medical and Scientific Books, 1981, pp. 171–189.

Roberts, M. C., Wurtele, S. K., Boone, R. R., Ginther, L. J., & Elkins, P. D. Reduction of medical fears by use of modeling: A preventive application in a general population of children. *Journal of Pediatric Psychology*, 1981, *6*, 293–300.

Robertson, W. O. Managing pain in children. Letter to the Editor. *Journal of the American Medical Association*, 1981, *245*, 2429–2430.

Robinson, D. Pain: Uncommon enemy/uncommon cures. *Health*, 1982, *14*, 16.

Robson, M. C. Reconstruction and rehabilitation from admission: A surgeon's role at each phase. In N. R. Bernstein & M. C. Robson (Eds.), *Comprehensive approaches to the burned person*. New Hyde Park, NY: Medical Examination Publishing, 1983, pp. 35–48.

Rogers, A. G. The assessment of pain and pain relief in children with cancer. *Pain*, Supplement 1 (1981), S11.

Rogers, E. J., & Vilkin, B. Diurnal variation in sensory and pain thresholds correlated with mood states. *Journal of Clinical Psychiatry*, 1978, *39*, 431–432, 438.

Rogers, F., & Head, B. *Mister Rogers talks with parents*. New York: Berkley Books, 1983.

Romero, R. Autobiographical scrapbooks: A coping tool for hospitalized school children. *Issues in Comprehensive Pediatric Nursing*, 1986, *9*, 247–258.

Rooke, E. D. Benign exertional headache. *Medical Clinics of North America*, 1968, *52*, 801–808.

Rose, M. H. The effects of hospitalization on coping behaviors of children. Unpublished doctoral dissertation, University of Chicago, 1972.

Rosenbaum, P. Where did you get that scar? *Children's Health Care*, 1984, *12*, 190–191.

Rosenblith, J. F., & Sims-Knight, J. E. *In the beginning: Development in the first two years of life*. Monterey, CA: Brooks/Cole, 1985.

Rosenfeld, A. First word. *Omni*, 1983, *5*, No. 5, 6.

Ross, D. M. Thought-stopping: A coping strategy for impending feared events. *Issues in Comprehensive Pediatric Nursing*, 1984, *7*, 83–89.

Ross, D. M. Brief reports of orthodontic pain by young adults. Unpublished manuscript, University of California Medical Center, San Francisco, 1986.

Ross, D. M. The challenge model. Unpublished manuscript, University of California Medical Center, San Francisco, 1987.

Ross, D. M., & Ross, S. A. A study of the pain experience in children. Final report, Ref.

No. 1 ROI HD 13672-01. Bethesda, Maryland: National Institute of Child Health and Human Development, 1982a.

Ross, D. M., & Ross, S. A. *Hyperactivity: Current issues, research, and theory.* New York: Wiley, 1982b.

Ross, D. M., & Ross, S. A. Childhood pain: The school-aged child's perspective. *PRN Forum,* 1983, *2,* 1–2, 4.

Ross, D. M., & Ross, S. A. The importance of type of question, psychological climate and subject set in interviewing children about pain. *Pain,* 1984a, *19,* 71–79.

Ross, D. M., & Ross, S. A. Childhood pain: The school-aged child's viewpoint, *Pain,* 1984b, *20,* 179–191.

Ross, D. M., & Ross, S. A. Stress reduction procedures for the school-age hospitalized leukemic child. *Pediatric Nursing,* 1984c, *10,* 393–395.

Ross, D. M., & Ross, S. A. Teaching the child with leukemia to cope with teasing. *Issues in Comprehensive Pediatric Nursing,* 1984d, *7,* 59–66.

Ross, D. M., & Ross, S. A. Pain instruction with third and fourth grade children: A pilot study. *Journal of Pediatric Psychology,* 1985, *10,* 55–63.

Ross, D. M., & Ross, S. A. The efficacy of pain instruction for the primary grades. Final report, Ref. No. 5 ROI HD17474-03. Bethesda, Maryland: National Institute of Child Health and Human Development, 1986.

Ross, D. M., & Ross, S. A. School children's concepts of pain. Study in progress, Research Institute, Palo Alto Medical Foundation, Palo Alto, CA, 1987.

Ross, M., & Ross, A. P. Commentary: The parents' experience of health care for the terminally ill child. In M. Jospe, J. Nieberding, & B. D. Cohen (Eds.), *Psychological factors in health care.* Lexington, MA: Heath, 1980, pp. 409–424.

Ross, S. A. Impending hospitalization: Timing of preparation for the school-aged child. *Children's Health Care,* 1984, *12,* 1987–189.

Ross, S. A. The repugnant model. Unpublished manuscript, Research Institute, Palo Alto Medical Foundation, Palo Alto, CA, 1987.

Rothenberg, M. B. The unique role of the child life worker in children's health care settings. *Children's Health Care,* 1982, *10,* 121–124.

Rowat, K. M., & Knafl, K. A. Living with chronic pain: The spouse's perspective. *Pain,* 1985, *23,* 259–271.

Roy, R., Bellissimo, A., & Tunks, E. The chronic pain patient and the environment. In R. Roy & E. Tunks (Eds.), *Chronic Pain.* Baltimore: Williams & Wilkins, 1982, pp. 1–9.

Rozensky, R. H., & Pasternak, J. F. Obi-Wan Kenobi, "The Force," and the art of biofeedback: A headache treatment for overachieving young boys. *Clinical Biofeedback & Health: An International Journal,* 1985, *8,* 9–13.

Ruble, D. N., & Brooks-Gunn, J. A developmental analysis of menstrual distress in adolescence. In R. C. Friedman (Ed.), *Behavior and the menstrual cycle.* New York: Marcel Dekker, 1982, pp. 177–197.

Russell, S. W. Development of a behavioral interaction coding system for pain expressions of children. Doctoral dissertation, University of Utah, Salt Lake City, 1984.

Russell, S. W., Strassberg, D. S., & Speltz, M. A behavioral interaction coding system for children's pain experiences and mothers' caregiving responses. Unpublished manuscript, University of Utah, Salt Lake City, 1986.

Ryan, R. E., Sr., & Ryan, R. E., Jr. *Headache and head pain. Diagnosis and treatment.* St. Louis: Mosby, 1978.

Sanders, S. H. Behavioral assessment and treatment of clinical pain: Appraisal of current status. In M. Hersen, R. M. Eisler, & P. M. Miller (Eds.), *Progress in behavior modifica-*

tion, Vol. 8. New York: Academic Press, 1979.

Sanders, S. H. Toward a practical instrument system for the automatic measurement of "uptime" in chronic pain patients. *Pain*, 1980, *9*, 103–109.

Sank, L. I., & Biglan, A. Operant treatment of a case of recurrent abdominal pain in a 10-year-old boy. *Behavior Therapy*, 1974, *5*, 677–681.

Santiago, T. V., Remolina, C., Scolles, V., III, & Edelman, N. H. Endorphins and the control of breathing. *New England Journal of Medicine*, 1981, *304*, 1190–1195.

Sarbin, T. R. Contributions to role-taking theory: I. Hypnotic behavior. *Psychological Review*, 1950, *57*, 255–270.

Sargent, C. Between death and shame: Dimensions of pain in Bariba culture. *Social Science and Medicine*, 1984, *19*, 1299–1304.

Sarles, R. M. The use of hypnosis with hospitalized children. *Journal of Clinical Child Psychology*, 1975, *4*, 36–38.

Saunders, C. *The management of terminal disease*. London: Hospital Medical Publications, 1967.

Savage, C. W. *The measurement of sensation: A critique of perceptual psychophysics*. Berkeley, CA: University of California Press, 1970.

Savage, J. P., & Leitch, I. O. W. Childhood burns: A sociological survey and inquiry into causation. *Medical Journal of Australia*, 1972, *1*, 1337–1342.

Savedra, M. Coping with pain: Strategies of severely burned children. *Canadian Nurse*, 1977, *73*, 28–29.

Savedra, M. Personal communication, May, 1980.

Savedra, M., Gibbons, P., Tesler, M., Ward, J., & Wegner, C. How do children describe pain? A tentative assessment. *Pain*, 1982, *14*, 95–104.

Savedra, M., Tesler, M., Ward, J., & Wegner, C. How adolescents describe pain. Unpublished manuscript, University of California Medical Center, San Francisco, 1985.

Savedra, M., Tesler, M. D., Ward, J. A., Wegner, C., & Gibbons, P. T. Description of the pain experience: A study of school-age children. *Issues in Comprehensive Pediatric Nursing*, 1981, *5*, 373–380.

Schachter, S. *The psychology of affiliation*. Stanford, CA: Stanford University Press, 1959.

Schechter, N. L. Recurrent pains in children: An overview and an approach. *Pediatric Clinics of North America*, 1984, *31*, 949–967.

Schechter, N. L., Allen, D. A., & Hanson, K. Status of pediatric pain control: A comparison of hospital analgesic usage in children and adults. *Pediatrics*, 1986, *77*, 11–15.

Schluderman, E., & Zubek, J. P. Effect of age on pain sensitivity. *Perceptual and Motor Skills*, 1962, *14*, 295–301.

Schmidt, R. F. The gate-control theory of pain: An unlikely hypothesis. In R. Janzen, W. D. Keidel, A. Herz, C. Steichele, J. P. Payne, & R.A.P. Burt (Eds.), *Pain*. London: Churchill Livingstone, 1972, pp. 124–127.

Schollander, D., & Savage, D. *Deep water*. London: Pelham Books, 1971.

Schomer, J. Family therapy. In B. Wolman, J. Egan, & A. Ross (Eds.), *Handbook of treatment of mental disorders in childhood and adolescence*. Englewood Cliffs, NJ: Prentice-Hall, 1978, pp. 91–101.

Schooler, C. Birth order effects: Not here, not now. *Psychological Bulletin*, 1972, *78*, 161–175.

Schorlemer, V. Reflections: A mother's and son's struggle with acute lymphocytic leukemia. *Children's Health Care*, 1984, *12*, 163–183.

Schowalter, J. E. The utilization of child psychiatry on a pediatric adolescent ward. *Journal of the American Academy of Child Psychiatry*, 1971, *10*, 684–699.

Schroeder, P. Use of Eland's color method in pain assessment of burned children. University of Cincinnati, Unpublished master's thesis, 1979.

Schultz, N. V. How children perceive pain. *Nursing Outlook,* 1971, *19,* 670–673.

Schwartz, A. H. Children's concepts of research hospitalization. *New England Journal of Medicine,* 1972, *287,* 589–592.

Scott, C. S., & Neighbor, W. E. Preventive care attitudes of medical students. *Social Science and Medicine,* 1985, *21,* 299–305.

Scott, D. L. Hypnoanalgesia for major surgery—a psychodynamic process. *American Journal of Clinical Hypnosis,* 1973, *16,* 84–91.

Scott, P. J., Ansell, B. M., & Huskisson, E. C. Measurement of pain in juvenile chronic polyarthritis. *Annals of the Rheumatic Diseases,* 1977, *36,* 186–187.

Scott, P. J., & Huskisson, E. C. Graphic representation of pain. *Pain,* 1976, *2,* 175–184.

Scott, R. "It hurts red": A preliminary study of children's perception of pain. *Perceptual and Motor Skills,* 1978, *47,* 787–791.

Scott, V., & Gijsbers, K. Pain perception in competitive swimmers. *British Medical Journal,* 1981, *283,* 91–93.

Seligman, M.E.P. Chronic fear produced by unpredictable shock. *Journal of Comparative Physiology and Psychology,* 1968, *66,* 402–411.

Seligman, M.E.P. *Helplessness: On depression, development and death.* Freeman: San Francisco, 1975.

Seligman, R., Macmillan, B. G., & Carroll, S. S. The burned child: A neglected area of psychiatry. *American Journal of Psychiatry,* 1971, *128,* 52–57.

Seres, J. L., & Newman, R. I. Prevention of chronic pain and strategies for treatment. *Mediguide to Pain,* 1985, *6,* 1–4.

Setterlind, S. Teaching children to relax. Paper presented at the 9th International Congress of Hypnosis and Psychosomatic Medicine. Glasgow, August 1982.

Setterlind, S., & Uneståhl, L.-E. Introducing relaxation training in Swedish schools. Paper presented at the First European Congress of Hypnosis in Psychotherapy and Psychosomatic Medicine, Malmö, Sweden, 1978.

Shacham, S., & Daut, R. L. Anxiety or pain: What does the scale measure? *Journal of Consulting and Clinical Psychology,* 1981, *49,* 468–469.

Shapiro, A. H. Behavior of Kibbutz and urban children receiving an injection. *Psychophysiology,* 1975, *12,* 79–82.

Shapiro, M. B. Personal Questionnaire. London: Unpublished manual, 1961.

Shaw, E. G., & Routh, D. K. Effect of mother presence on children's reaction to aversive procedures. *Journal of Pediatric Psychology,* 1982, *7,* 33–42.

Sheridan, M. Talk time for hospitalized children. *Social Work,* 1975, *20,* 40–44.

Shinnar, S., & D'Souza, B. J. The diagnosis and management of headaches in childhood. *Pediatric Clinics of North America,* 1981, *29,* 79–94.

Shorkey, C. T., & Taylor, J. E. Management of maladaptive behavior of a severely burned child. *Child Welfare,* 1973, *52,* 543–547.

Siaw, S. N., Stephens, L. R., & Holmes, S. S. Knowledge about medical instruments and reported anxiety in pediatric surgery patients. *Children's Health Care,* 1986, *14,* 134–141.

Siegel, L. J. Preparation of children for hospitalization: A selected review of the research literature. *Journal of Pediatric Psychology,* 1976, *1,* 26–30.

Siegel, L. J. Measuring children's adjustment to hospitalization and to medical procedures. In P. Karoly (Ed.), *Handbook of child health assessment: Biosocial perspectives.* New York: Wiley, 1986.

Siegel, L. J. Dental treatment. In D. Routh (Ed.), *Handbook of Pediatric Psychology.* New York: Guilford Press, 1987, pp. 448–459.

Siegel, L. J. & Peterson, L. Stress reduction in young dental patients through coping skills and sensory information. *Journal of Consulting and Clinical Psychology,* 1980, *48,* 785–787.

Siegel, L. J., & Peterson, L. Maintenance effects of coping skills and sensory information on young children's response to repeated dental procedures. *Behavior Therapy,* 1981, *12,* 530–535.

Sigerist, H. E. *A history of medicine. Vol. 1. Primitive and archaic medicine.* New York: Oxford University Press, 1955.

Sillanpaa, M. Clonidine prophylaxis of childhood migraine and other vascular headache: A double blind study of 57 children. *Headache,* 1977, *17,* 28–31.

Sillanpaa, M. Prevalence of headache in prepuberty. *Headache,* 1983, *23,* 10–14.

Sillanpaa, M., & Koponen, M. Papaverine in the prophylaxis of migraine and other vascular headache in children. *Acta Paediatrica Scandinavica,* 1978, *67,* 209–212.

Simeonsson, R., Buckley, L., & Monson, L. Conceptions of illness causality in hospitalized children. *Journal of Pediatric Psychology,* 1979, *4,* 77–84.

Simmons, J. Smile and your brain smiles with you. *Science 86,* 1986, *7,* 69–70.

Simon, E., Hiller, J., & Edelman, I. Stereospecific binding of the potent narcotic analgesic 3H-etorphine to rat brain homogenate. *Proceedings of the National Academy of Sciences of the USA,* 1973, *70,* 1947–1949.

Sinclair, D. C. Cutaneous sensation and the doctrine of specific nerve energies. *Brain,* 1955, *78,* 584–614.

Slade, P. E., Troup, J.D.G., Lethem, J., & Bentley, G. The fear avoidance model of exaggerated pain perception: Preliminary studies of the coping strategies for pain in a student population. *Behavior Research and Therapy,* 1983, *21,* 409–416.

Slavson, S. R., & Schiffer, M. *Group psychotherapies for children.* New York: International Universities Press, 1974.

Slosberg, M. *The August strangers.* New York: Dial Press, 1977.

Smith, D. P. Using humor to help children with pain. *Children's Health Care,* 1986, *14,* 187–188.

Smith, G. A brief review of postoperative pain. In E. Wilkes (Ed.), *Advances in morphine therapy.* Royal Society of Medicine International Congress and Symposium Series No. 64. London: Royal Society of Medicine, 1984, pp. 11–17.

Smith, M. E. The preschooler and pain. In P. Brandt, P. Chinn, & M. E. Smith (Eds.), *Current practice in pediatric nursing.* St. Louis: Mosby, 1976, pp. 198–209.

Smith, R. N. *Anesthesia for infants and children,* 2nd ed. St. Louis: Mosby, 1980.

Smith, W. L., Merskey, H., & Gross, S. C. (Eds.), *Pain: Meaning and management.* New York: SP Medical & Scientific Books, 1980.

Smoller, B., & Schulman, B. *Pain control: The Bethesda program.* Garden City, NY: Doubleday, 1982.

Snyder, C. C., & Saieh, T. A. Burn injuries in children. In V. C. Kelley (Ed.), *Practice of pediatrics.* Philadelphia: Harper & Row, 1984.

Spaccavento, L. J., Solomon, G. D., & Mani, S. An association between strokes and migraines in young adults. *Headache,* 1981, *21,* 121.

Spanos, N. P., Hodgins, D. C., Stam, H. J., & Gwynn, M. Suffering for science: The effects of implicit social demands on response to experimentally induced pain. *Journal of Personality and Social Psychology,* 1984, *46,* 1162–1172.

Spielberger, C. D., Gorsuch, R., & Lushene, R. *The State-Trait Anxiety Inventory.* Palo Alto, CA: Consulting Psychologists Press, 1970.

Sriwatanakul, K., Kelvie, W., & Lasagna, L. The quantification of pain: An analysis of words used to describe pain and analgesia in clinical trials. *Clinical Pharmacology and Therapeutics,* 1982, *32,* 143–148.

Sriwatanakul, K., Kelvie, W., Lasagna, L., Calimlim, J. F., Weis, O. F., & Mehta, G. Studies with different types of visual analog scales for measurement of pain. *Clinical Pharmacology and Therapeutics*, 1983, *34*, 234–239.

Steele, S. *Health promotion of the child with long-term illness* (3rd ed.). Norwalk, CT: Appleton-Century-Crofts, 1982.

Steinmuller, R. The use and abuse of psychiatry in dealing with pain patients. *Pediatric Quarterly*, 1979, *51*, 184–188.

Stern, G. S., & Berrenberg, J. L. Biofeedback training in frontalis muscle relaxation and enhancement of belief in personal control. *Biofeedback and Self-Regulation*, 1977, *2*, 173–183.

Sternbach, R. A. *Pain: A psychophysiological analysis*. New York: Academic Press, 1968.

Sternbach, R. A. Clinical aspects of pain. In R. A. Sternbach (Ed.), *The psychology of pain*. New York: Raven Press, 1978, pp. 241–264.

Sternbach, R. A. The psychologist's role in the diagnosis and treatment of pain patients. In J. Barber & C. Adrian (Eds.), *Psychological approaches to the management of pain*. New York: Brunner/Mazel, 1982, pp. 3–20.

Sternbach, R. A. Acute versus chronic pain. In P. D. Wall & R. Melzack (Eds.), *Textbook of pain*. New York: Churchill Livingstone, 1984, pp. 173–177.

Sternbach, R. A. Survey of pain in the United States: The Nuprin Pain Report. *The Clinical Journal of Pain*, 1986a, 2, 49–53.

Sternbach, R. A. Pain and 'hassles' in the United States: Findings of the Nuprin Pain Report. *Pain*, 1986b, *27*, 69–80.

Sternbach, R. A., Janowsky, D. S., Huey, L. Y., & Segal, D. S. Effects of altering brain serotonin activity on human chronic pain. In J. J. Bonica & D. Albe-Fessard (Eds.), *Advances in pain research and therapy*, Vol. 1. New York: Raven Press, 1976, pp. 601–606.

Sternbach, R. A., Wolf, S. R., Murphy, R. W., & Akeson, W. H. Traits of pain patients: The low-back 'loser.' *Psychosomatics*, 1973, *14*, 226–229.

Stewart, C. M., & Stewart, L. B. *Pediatric medications*. Rockville, MD: Aspen Systems Corporation, 1984.

Stewart, M. L. Measurement of clinical pain. In A. K. Jacox (Ed.), *Pain: A sourcebook for nurses and other health professionals*. Boston: Little, Brown, 1977, pp. 107–137.

Stimmel, B. *Pain, analgesia, and addiction: The pharmacologic treatment of pain*. New York: Raven Press, 1983.

Stinson, R., & Stinson, P. *The long dying of Baby Andrew*. Boston: Little, Brown, 1983.

St. Lawrence, J. S., & Drabman, R. S. Interruption of self-excoriation in a pediatric burn victim. *Journal of Pediatric Psychology*, 1983, *8*, 155–159.

Stoddard, F. J. Coping with pain: A developmental approach to treatment of burned children. *American Journal of Psychiatry*, 1982, *139*, 736–740.

Stravino, V. D. Nature of pain. *Archives of Physical Medicine and Rehabilitation*, 1970, *51*, 37–44.

Strempel, H. Circadian cycles of epicritic and protopathic pain threshold. *Journal of Interdisciplinary Cycle Research*, 1977, *8*, 276–280.

Stroebel, C. F. *QR, the quieting reflex*. New York: G. P. Putnam's, 1982.

Sturner, R. A., Rothbaum, F., Visintainer, M. & Wolfer, J. The effects of stress on children's human figure drawings. *Journal of Clinical Psychology*, 1980, *36*, 324–331.

Sunderland, J. M. Personal communication, March, 1984.

Swafford, L. I., & Allan, D. Pain relief in the pediatric patient. *Medical Clinics of North America*, 1968, *52*, 131–136.

Swanson, D. W. Chronic pain as a third pathologic emotion. *American Journal of Psychiatry*, 1984, *141*, 210–214.

Swanson, D. W., Maruta, T., & Wolff, V. A. Ancient pain. *Pain*, 1986, *25*, 383–387.

Sykes, W. M. Role of the child psychiatrist on the burn team and the psychiatric problems of the burned child. In W. C. Bailey (Ed.), *Pediatric burns*. Miami, Florida: Symposia Specialists, 1979, pp. 107–114.

Syrjala, K. L., & Chapman, C. R. Measurement of clinical pain: A review and integration of research findings. In C. Benedetti, C. R. Chapman, & G. Moricca (Eds.), *Advances in pain research and therapy*, Vol. 7. New York: Raven Press, 1984, pp. 71–101.

Szasz, T. S. *Pain and pleasure: A study of bodily feelings*. New York: Basic Books, 1975.

Szyfelbein, S. K., & Osgood, P. F. The assessment of analgesia by self-reports of pain in burned children. Paper presented at the International Association for the Study of Pain (IASP) Fourth World Congress on Pain. Seattle, WA, August 31–Sept. 5, 1984.

Szyfelbein, S. K., Osgood, P. F., & Carr, D. B. The assessment of pain and plasma β-endorphin immunoactivity in burned children. *Pain*, 1985, *22*, 173–182.

Tainter, M. L. Pain. *Annals of the New York Academy of Sciences*, 1948, *51*, 3–11.

Tal, Y., Dunn, H. G., & Crichton, J. U. Childhood migraine—A dangerous diagnosis? *Acta Paediatrica Scandinavica*, 1984, *73*, 55–59.

Tan, S-Y. Cognitive and cognitive-behavioral methods for pain control: A selective review. *Pain*, 1982, *12*, 201–228.

Tarler-Benlolo, L. The role of relaxation in biofeedback training: A critical review of the literature. *Psychological Bulletin*, 1978, *85*, 727–755.

Tasto, D. L., & Chesney, M. A. Muscle relaxation treatment for primary dysmenorrhea. *Behavior Therapy*, 1974, *5*, 668–672.

Taub, H. A., Beard, M. C., Eisenberg, L., & McCormack, R. K. Studies of acupuncture for operative dentistry. *Journal of American Dental Association*, 1977, *95*, 555–561.

Taylor, H., & Curran, N. M. *The Nuprin Pain Report*. New York: Louis Harris, 1985.

Taylor, P. L. Post-operative pain in toddler and pre-school age children. *Maternal-Child Nursing Journal*, 1983, *12*, 35–50.

Terenius, L. Stereospecific interaction between narcotic analgesics and a synaptic plasma membrane fraction of rat cerebral cortex. *Acta Pharmacology and Toxicology*, 1973, *32*, 317–320.

Terenius, L. Endorphins and pain. *Frontiers of Hormone Research*, 1981, *8*, 162–177.

Terenius, L., & Wahlstrom, A. Endorphins and clinical pain, an overview. *Advances in Experimental Medicine and Biology*, 1979, *116*, 261–267.

Tesler, M. D., Savedra, M., Gibbons, P. T., Ward, J. A., & Wegner, C. Developing an instrument for eliciting children's description of pain. *Perceptual Motor Skills*, 1983, *56*, 315–321.

Tesler, M. D., Wegner, C., Savedra, M., Gibbons, P. T., & Ward, J. A. Coping strategies of children in pain. *Issues in Comprehensive Pediatric Nursing*, 1981, *5*, 351–359.

Thelen, M. H., Fry, R. A., Fehrenbach, P. A., & Frautschi, N. M. Therapeutic videotape and film modeling: A review. *Psychological Bulletin*, 1979, *86*, 701–720.

Thompson, H. C., King, L. R., Knox, E., & Korones, S. B. Report of the Ad Hoc Task Force on Circumcision. *Pediatrics*, 1975, *56*, 610–611.

Thompson, K. L., & Varni, J. W. A developmental cognitive-biobehavioral approach to pediatric pain assessment. *Pain*, 1986, *25*, 283–296.

Thompson, K. L., Varni, J. W., & Hanson, V. Comprehensive assessment of pain in juvenile rheumatoid arthritis: An empirical model. *Journal of Pediatric Psychology*, in press, 1988.

Thompson, R. H., & Stanford, G. *Child life in hospitals: Theory and practice*. Springfield, IL: Thomas, 1981.

Thompson, S. C. Will it hurt less if I can control it? A complex answer to a simple question. *Psychological Bulletin*, 1981, *90*, 89–101.

Tinterow, M. M. The use of hypnotic anesthesia for major surgical procedures. *American Surgeon*, 1960, *26*, 732–737.

Toomey, T. C., Gover, V. F., & Jones, B. N. Spatial distribution of pain: A descriptive characteristic of chronic pain. *Pain*, 1983, *17*, 289–300.

Travell, J. Myofascial trigger points: Clinical view. In J. J. Bonica & D. Albe-Fessard (Eds.), *Advances in pain research and therapy*, Vol. 1. New York: Raven Press, 1976, pp. 919–926.

Travell, J., & Rinzler, S. H. The myofascial genesis of pain. *Postgraduate Medicine*, 1952, *11*, 425–434.

Travis, E. *The chronically ill child and his family*. New York: Holt, Rinehart, & Winston, 1969.

Treaster, J. B. Ballet: The agony behind the ecstacy. *Family Health*, 1978, *10*, No. 10, 29–31, 45–46.

Trevarthen, C., (Discussant). In G. Woistenholme & M. O'Connor (Eds.), *Brain and mind*. Amsterdam: Excerpta Medica, 1979, p. 325.

Tucker, J. B. *Ellie, a child's fight against leukemia*. New York: Holt, Rinehart, and Winston, 1982.

Turk, D. C. Cognitive-behavioral techniques in the management of pain. In J. P. Foreyt & D. P. Rathjen (Eds.), *Cognitive behavior therapy: Research and application*. New York: Plenum, 1978.

Turk, D. C., Meichenbaum, D., & Genest, M. *Pain and behavioral medicine: A cognitive-behavioral perspective*. New York: Guilford, 1983.

Turk, D. C., Rudy, T. E., & Salovey, P. The McGill Pain Questionnaire reconsidered: Confirming the factor structure and examining appropriate uses. *Pain*, 1985, *21*, 385–397.

Turkat, I. D. An investigation of parental modeling in the etiology of diabetic illness behavior. *Behavior Research and Therapy*, 1982, *20*, 547–552.

Turkat, I. D., Guise, B. J., & Carter, K. M. The effects of vicarious experience on pain termination and work avoidance: A replication. *Behavior Research and Therapy*, 1983, *21*, 491–493.

Turner, J. A., & Chapman, C. R. Psychological interventions for chronic pain: A critical review. I. Relaxation training and biofeedback. *Pain*, 1982a, *12*, 1–21.

Turner, J. A., & Chapman, C. R. Psychological interventions for chronic pain: A critical review. II. Operant conditioning, hypnosis, and cognitive-behavioral therapy. *Pain*, 1982b, *12*, 23–46.

Turner, J. A., & Clancy, S. Strategies for coping with chronic low back pain: Relationship to pain and disability. *Pain*, 1986, *24*, 355–364.

Tursky, B., Jamner, L. D., & Friedman, R. The pain perception profile: A psychophysical approach to the assessment of pain report. *Behavior Therapy*, 1982, *13*, 376–394.

Twycross, R. G. Narcotics. In P. D. Wall & R. Melzack (Eds.), *Textbook of pain*. New York: Churchill Livingstone, 1984, pp. 514–525.

Tyler, F. B. Individual psychosocial competence: A personality configuration. *Educational and Psychological Measurement*, 1978, *38*, 309–323.

Tyson, K. W., & Merrill, J. C. Health care institutions: Survival in a changing environment. *Journal of Medical Education*, 1984, *4*, 773–782.

Uematsu, S. Telethermography for the assessment of chronic pain. In R. Rizzi & M. Visentin (Eds.), *Pain therapy*. Amsterdam: Elsevier Biomedical Press, 1983, pp. 107–114.

Uhde, T. W., Siever, L. J., Post, R. M., Jimerson, D. C., Boulenger, J.-P, & Buchsbaum, M. S. The relationship of plasma-free MHPG to anxiety and psychophysical pain in normal volunteers. *Psychopharmacology Bulletin*, 1982, *18*, 129–132.

Ulrich, R. S. View through a window may influence recovery from surgery. *Science*, 1984,

224, 420–421.

University of California Medical Center, San Francisco. Videotapes, Child Study Unit, 1975.

Unruh, A., McGrath, P. J. Cunningham, S. J., & Humphreys, P. Children's drawings of their pain. *Pain*, 1983, *17*, 385–392.

U.S. Department of Health and Human Services. *Protection of human subjects* (Code of Federal Regulations 45 CFR 46). Washington, DC: DHHS March 8, 1983.

Vair, C. The perceptions of coping strategies of seven- to twelve-year-old hospitalized children in response to acute pain. Unpublished master's thesis, University of Toronto, Ontario, 1981.

VanderMeulen, P. R. The parent as a member of the health care team?! *Children's Health Care*, 1985, *14*, 12–13.

Varni, J. W. Self-regulation techniques in the management of chronic arthritic pain in hemophilia. *Behavior Therapy*, 1981, *12*, 185–194.

Varni, J. W. *Clinical behavioral pediatrics: An interdisciplinary biobehavioral approach.* New York: Pergamon Press, 1983.

Varni, J. W. Personal communication, August, 1987.

Varni, J. W., Bessman, C. A., Russo, D. C., & Cataldo, M. F. Behavioral management of chronic pain in children: Case study. *Archives of Physical Medicine and Rehabilitation*, 1980, *61*, 375–379.

Varni, J. W., Gilbert, A., & Dietrich, S. L. Behavioral medicine in pain and analgesia management for the hemophilic child with factor VIII inhibitor. *Pain*, 1981, *11*, 121–126.

Varni, J. W., & Thompson, K. L. The Varni/Thompson Pediatric Pain Questionnaire. Unpublished manuscript, University of Southern California, Los Angeles, 1985.

Varni, J. W., Thompson, K. L. & Hanson, V. The Varni/Thompson Pediatric Pain Questionnaire: I. Chronic musculoskeletal pain in juvenile rheumatoid arthritis. *Pain*, 1987, *28*, 27–38.

Varni, J. W., Wilcox, K. T., Hanson, V., & Brik, R. Chronic musculoskeletal pain and functional status in juvenile rheumatoid arthritis: An empirical model. *Pain*, in press, 1988.

Venham, L. The effect of mother's presence on child's responses to dental treatment. *Journal of Dentistry for Children*, 1979, *46*, 219–225.

Ventafridda, V., Rogers, A., & Valera, L. Pain in the child with cancer. In R. Rizzi & M. Visentin (Eds.), *Pain*. Padua, Italy: Piccin/Butterworths, 1984, pp. 377–382.

Vere, D. The 1983 International Symposium on Pain Control: Summary of the day. In E. Wilkes (Ed.), *Advances in morphine therapy*. Royal Society of Medicine International Congress and Symposium Series No. 64. London: Royal Society of Medicine, 1984, pp. 97–99.

Vernon, D. T. A. Use of modeling to modify children's responses to a natural, potentially stressful situation. *Journal of Applied Psychology*, 1973, *58*, 351–356.

Vernon, D. T. A. Modeling and birth order in responses to painful stimuli. *Journal of Personality and Social Psychology*, 1974, *29*, 794–799.

Vesell, E. S. On the significance of host factors that affect drug disposition. *Clinical Pharmacology and Therapeutics*, 1982, *31*, 1–7.

Villamira, M. A. & Occhiuto, M. G. Psychological aspects of pain in children, particularly relating to their family and school environment. In R. Rizzi & M. Visentin (Eds.), *Pain*. Padua, Italy: Piccin/Butterworths, 1984, pp. 285–289.

Villoldo, A., & Dychtwald, K. (Eds.). *Millennium: Glimpses into the 21st century.* Los Angeles: Tarcher, 1981.

Vincent, C. A., & Richardson, P. H. The evaluation of therapeutic acupuncture: Concepts and methods. *Pain*, 1986, *24*, 1–13.

Violon, A., & Giurgea, D. Familial models for chronic pain. *Pain,* 1984, *18,* 199–203.
Visintainer, M. A., & Wolfer, J. A. Psychological preparation for surgical pediatric patients: The effect on children's and parents' stress responses. *Pediatrics,* 1975, *56,* 187–202.
Vollman, R. F. *The menstrual cycle.* Toronto: Saunders, 1977.
Volpe, J. *Neurology of the newborn.* Philadelphia: Saunders, 1981.
von Frey, M. Beiträge zur physiologie des schmerzsinns. *Ber Sachs. Ges-amte, Wiss. Math-Phys.* 1894, Clone 46, 185.
Wachter-Shikora, N. L. The effects of mechanostimulation on the first and second pain produced by intramuscular injection. Unpublished doctoral dissertation, Catholic University of America, Washington, DC, 1980.
Waechter, E. H. Personal communication, January, 1971.
Wagner, M. M. Pain and nursing care associated with burns. In A. K. Jacox (Ed.), *Pain: A source book for nurses and other health professionals.* Boston: Little, Brown, 1977, pp. 391–403.
Wagner, M. M. The pain of burns. In P. D. Wall & R. Melzack (Eds.), *Textbook of pain.* New York: Churchill Livingstone, 1984, pp. 304–306.
Wakeman, R. J., & Kaplan, J. Z. An experimental study of hypnosis in painful burns. *American Journal of Clinical Hypnosis,* 1978, *21,* 3–12.
Walker, L. J. S., & Healy, M. Psychological treatment of a burned child. *Journal of Pediatric Psychology,* 1980, *5,* 395–404.
Wall, P. D. The gate control theory of pain mechanisms. A re-examination and re-statement. *Brain,* 1978, *101,* 1–18.
Wall, P. D. On the relation of injury to pain: The John J. Bonica lecture. *Pain,* 1979a, *6,* 253–264.
Wall, P. D. Three phases of evil: The relation of injury to pain. In G. Woistenholme & M. O'Connor (Eds.), *Brain and mind.* Amsterdam: Excerpta Medica, 1979b, pp. 293–304.
Wall, P. D. General discussion. In J. J. Bonica (Ed.), *Pain.* New York: Raven Press, 1980, pp. 379–80.
Wall, P. D. Introduction. In P. D. Wall & R. Melzack (Eds.), *Textbook of pain.* New York: Churchill Livingstone, 1984, pp. 1–16.
Wall, P. D., & Sweet, W. H. Temporary abolition of pain in man. *Science,* 1967, *155,* 108–109.
Wallace, N. E., & Cama, R. Humanizing the physical environment of an inpatient pediatric division: Two creative expressive components. *Children's Health Care,* 1983, *11,* 165.
Wallenstein, S. L. The measurement of pain. *PRN Forum,* 1982, *1,* No. 4, 1–2, 5–6, 8.
Walsh, J. Personal communication, April, 1981.
Walsh, T. D. Letter to the Editor. *Pain,* 1984, *19,* 96–97.
Warden, G. D. Kravitz, M., & Schnebly, A. The outpatient management of moderate and major thermal injuries. *Journal of Burn Care,* 1981, *2,* 159–167.
Wasz-Höeckert, O., Lind, J., Vuorenkoski, V., Partanen, T. J., Valanné, E. *The infant cry.* Philadelphia: Lippincott, 1968.
Waters, W. E. Migraine: Intelligence, social class, and familial prevalence. *British Medical Journal,* 1971, *2,* 77–81.
Watzlawick, P., Weakland, J., & Fisch, R. *Change: Principles of problem formation and problem solution.* New York: Norton, 1974.
Webster, S. K. Problems for diagnosis of spasmodic and congestive dysmenorrhea. In A. J. Dan, E. A. Graham, & C. P. Beecher (Eds.), *The menstrual cycle,* Vol. 1. New York: Springer, 1980, pp. 292–304.
Weddell, G. Somesthesis and the chemical senses. *Annual Review of Psychology,* 1955, *6,*

119–136.

Weeks, D. J. Communication to the Editor. *Journal of Psychosomatic Research,* 1983, *27,* 333.

Weighill, V. E. Compensation neurosis: A review of the literature. *Journal of Psychosomatic Research,* 1983, *27,* 97–104.

Weisenberg, M. Pain and pain control. *Psychological Bulletin,* 1977a, *84,* 1008–1044.

Weisenberg, M. Cultural and racial reactions to pain. In M. Weisenberg (Ed.), *The control of pain.* New York: Psychological Dimensions, 1977b.

Weisenberg, M. Cognitive aspects of pain. In P. D. Wall & R. Melzack (Eds.), *Textbook of pain.* Edinburgh: Churchill Livingstone, 1984, pp. 162–172.

Weisenberg, M., Aviram, O., Wolf, Y., & Raphaeli, N. Relevant and irrelevant anxiety in the reaction to pain. *Pain,* 1984, *20,* 371–383.

Weisenberg, M., & Tursky, B. *Pain: New perspectives in therapy and research.* New York: Plenum Press, 1976.

Weitzenhoffer, A. M., & Hilgard, E. R. *Stanford Hypnotic Susceptibility Scale, Forms A and B.* Palo Alto, CA: Consulting Psychologists Press, 1959.

Welch, C. A. Psychiatric medicine and the burn patient. In T. C. Manschreck (Ed.), *Psychiatric medicine update.* New York: Elsevier North Holland, 1981, pp. 179–193.

Werder, D. S. An exploratory study of childhood migraine using thermal biofeedback as a treatment alternative. *Biofeedback Self-Regulation,* 1978, *3,* 242–243.

Wessell, M. L., Sr. Use of humor by an immobilized adolescent girl during hospitalization. *Maternal-Child Nursing Journal,* 1975, *4,* 35–48.

Wester, W. C., II, & Smith, A. H., Jr. *Clinical hypnosis.* Philadelphia: Lippincott, 1984.

Whalen, C. K. Personal communication, January, 1987.

Whalen, C. K., & Henker, B. Psychostimulants and children: A review and analysis. *Psychological Bulletin,* 1976, *83,* 1113–1130.

Whalen, C. K., & Henker, B. (Eds.), *Hyperactive children: The social ecology of identification and treatment.* New York: Academic Press, 1980.

Whalen, C. K., Henker, B., & Dotemoto, S. Methylphenidate and hyperactivity: Effects on teacher behaviors. *Science,* 1980, *208,* 1280–1282.

White, J. C., & Sweet, W. H. *Pain and the neurosurgeon: A forty-year experience.* Springfield, IL: Thomas, 1969.

White, R. Strategies of adaptation: An attempt at systematic description. In G. Coelho, D. Hamburg, & J. Adams (Eds.), *Coping and adaptation.* New York: Basic Books, 1974.

Widger, M. Clinic for sick dolls helps kids lose fear of hospitals. *Middlesex News,* 1985, *14,* No. 312, 1B.

Widholm, O., & Kantero, R. L. III. Menstrual pattern of adolescent girls according to chronological and gynecological ages. *Acta Obstetricia et Gynecologica Scandinavica* (Suppl.), 1971, *14,* 19–29.

Wiggins, J. S. *Personality and prediction: Principles of personality assessment.* Reading, MA: Addison-Wesley, 1973.

Wikler, D. Pain and the senses. (Commentary). In G. Woistenholme & M. O'Connor (Eds.), *Brain and mind.* Amsterdam: Excerpta Medica, 1979, pp. 315–321.

Wilkinson, V. A. Multidisciplinary approach to pain in juvenile arthritis. In R. Rizzi & M. Visentin (Eds.), *Pain.* Padua, Italy: Piccin/Butterworths, 1984, pp. 353–357.

Willems, E. P. Ecological psychology. In D. Stokols (Ed.), *Perspectives on environment and behavior: Theory, research, and applications.* New York: Plenum Press, 1977.

Williams, D. E., Thompson, J. K., Haber, J. D., & Raczynski, J. M. MMPI and headache: A special focus on differential diagnosis, prediction of treatment outcome, and patient-treatment matching. *Pain,* 1986, *24,* 143–158.

Williams, D. T., & Singh, M. Hypnosis as a facilitating therapeutic adjunct in child psychiatry. *Journal of the American Academy of Child Psychiatry,* 1976, *15,* 326–342.

Williamson, P. S., & Williamson, M. L. Physiologic stress reduction by a local anesthetic during newborn circumcision. *Pediatrics,* 1983, *71,* 36–40.

Willis, R. J., & Cousins, M. J. Pain relief in acute care. In S. Lipton & J. Miles (Eds.), *Persistent pain: Modern methods of treatment,* Vol. 5. London: Grune & Stratton, 1985, pp. 33–63.

Winnicott, D. W. *The family and individual development.* London: Tavistock Publications, 1965.

Wisely, D. W., Masur, F. T., & Morgan, S. B., Psychological aspects of severe burn injuries in children. *Health Psychology,* 1983, *2,* 45–72.

Wiswell, T. E., Enzenauer, R. W., Holton, M. E., Cornish, J. D., & Hankins, C. T. Declining frequency of circumcision: Implication for changes in the absolute incidence and male to female sex ratio of urinary tract infections in early infancy. *Pediatrics,* 1987, *79,* 338–342.

Witkin, H. A. The perception of the upright. *Scientific American,* 1959, *200,* 50–56.

Wolberg, L. R., Aronson, M. L., & Wolberg, A. R. (Eds.). *Group Therapy 1977: An overview.* New York: Stratton Intercontinental Medical Book Corp., 1977.

Wolfer, J. A., & Visintainer, M. A. Prehospital psychological preparation for tonsillectomy patients: Effects on children's and parents' adjustment. *Pediatrics,* 1979, *64,* 646–655.

Wolff, B. B. Behavioral measurement of human pain. In R. Sternbach (Ed.), *The psychology of pain.* New York: Raven Press, 1978, pp. 129–168.

Wolff, B. B. Measurement of human pain. In J. J. Bonica (Ed.), *Pain.* New York: Raven Press, 1980, pp. 174–184. General discussion, pp. 185–189.

Wolff, B. B. Methods of testing pain mechanisms in normal man. In P. D. Wall & R. Melzack (Eds.), *Textbook of pain.* Edinburgh: Churchill Livingstone, 1984, pp. 186–194.

Wolff, B. B., & Langley, S. Cultural factors and the response to pain: A review. *American Anthropologist,* 1968, *70,* 494–501.

Wolff, P. H. The natural history of crying and other vocalizations in early infancy. In B. Foss (Ed.), *Determinants of infant behavior,* Vol. 4. London: Methuen, 1969, pp. 81–115.

Wolpe, J., & Lazarus, A. A. *Behavior therapy techniques.* Oxford: Pergamon Press, 1966.

Woodley, J. Psychological management with hypnosis for a severely burned girl. *Medical Journal of Australia,* 1959, *2,* 153–154.

Woodrow, K. M., Friedman, G. D., Siegelaub, A. B., & Collen, M. F. Pain tolerance: Differences according to age, sex, and race. *Psychosomatic Medicine,* 1972, *34,* 548–556.

Woolf, C. F. Transcutaneous and implanted nerve stimulation. In P. D. Wall & R. Melzack (Eds.), *Textbook of pain.* Edinburgh: Churchill Livingstone, 1984, pp. 679–690.

Wortis, H., Stein, M. H., & Joliffe, N. Fibre dissociation in peripheral neuropathy. *Archives of Internal Medicine,* 1942, *69,* 222–237.

Wright, B. *Physical disability: A psychological approach.* New York: Harper & Row, 1960.

Wright, G. Z., & Alpern, G. D. Variables influencing children's cooperative behavior at the first dental visit. *Journal of Dentistry for Children,* 1971, *38,* 124–128.

Yaffe, S. J. Comparative efficacy of aspirin and acetaminophen in the reduction of fever in children. *Archives of Internal Medicine,* 1981, *141,* 286–292.

Yalom, I. D. *The theory and practice of group psychotherapy,* (2nd ed.). New York: Basic Books, 1975.

Ylikorkala, O. C., & Dawood, M. Y. New concepts in dysmenorrhea. *American Journal of Obstetrics and Gynecology,* 1978, *130,* 833–847.

Youssef, A. E. The uterine isthmus and its sphincter mechanism. I. The uterine isthmus under normal conditions. *American Journal of Obstetrics and Gynecology,* 1958a, *75,* 1305–1319.

Youssef, A. E. The uterine isthmus and its sphincter mechanism. II. The uterine isthmus under abnormal conditions. *American Journal of Obstetrics and Gynecology,* 1958b, *75,* 1320–1332.

Zachary, R. A., Friedlander, S., Huang, L. N., Silverstein, S., & Leggott, P. Effects of stress-relevant and -irrelevant filmed modeling on children's responses to dental treatment. *Journal of Pediatric Psychology,* 1985, *10,* 383–401.

Zajonc, R. B. Emotion and facial efference: A theory reclaimed. *Science,* 1985, *228,* 15–21.

Zborowski, M. Cultural components in response to pain. *Journal of Social Issues,* 1952, *8,* 16–30.

Zeitlin, C., & Oddy, M. Cognitive impairment in patients with severe migraine. *British Journal of Clinical Psychology,* 1984, *23,* 27–35.

Zeltzer, L., Dash, J., & Holland, J. P. Hypnotically induced pain control in sickle cell anemia. *Pediatrics,* 1979, *64,* 533–536.

Zeltzer, L., Kellerman, J., Ellenberg, L., Dash, J., & Rigler, D. Psychological effects of illness in adolescence. II. Impact of illness in adolescents—crucial issues and coping styles. *Journal of Pediatrics,* 1980, *97,* 132–138.

Zeltzer, L., & LeBaron, S. Hypnosis and nonhypnotic techniques for reduction of pain and anxiety during painful procedures in children and adolescents with cancer. *Journal of Pediatrics,* 1982, *101,* 1032–1035.

Ziegler, D. K. The epidemiology and genetics of migraine. *Research and Clinical Studies in Headache,* 1978, *5,* 21–33.

Ziegler, D. K., Hassanein, R., & Hassanein, K. Headache syndromes suggested by factor analysis of symptom variables in a headache prone population. *Journal of Chronic Diseases,* 1972, *25,* 353–363.

Zimmerman, J. L., & Elliott, C. H. The relationship of stress to anioneurotic edema: Implications for improved management. *Child and Family Behavior Therapy,* 1984, *6,* 57–62.

Author Index

Abel, G. G., 277
Abelson, P. H., 301
Abraham, G. E., 257
Abu-Saad, H., 36, 44, 46, 47, 50, 51, 53, 99, 115, 137, 143, 157
Ack, M., 32, 104, 168
Adams, B. N., 89
Adams, H. E., 281, 282
Adams, M. A., 222, 223, 224, 248, 286, 296
Adler, S. N. M., 226
Agle, D., 235
Agnew, D. C., 116
Agras, S., 285
Ainsworth, M., 98, 100
Akeson, W. H., 28
Akil, H., 25
Ala-Hurula, V., 279
Alexander, A. B., 32
Allan, D., 194
Allen, D. A., 29, 194, 195
Allmond, B. W., 228
Alpern, G. D., 32
Amery, W. K., 280
Amsterdam, B., 272
Anderson, J. E., 28, 32, 35, 40, 78, 115, 117, 131, 146, 157, 159, 196
Anderson, S., 26
Andolsek, K., 235
Andras, A., 191
Andrasik, F., 127, 159, 204, 205, 274, 275, 276, 278, 281, 284
Andujar, E. M., 173, 296
Angell, M., 195
Angst, J., 89
Ansell, B. M., 61, 115, 117, 137, 138, 182, 184, 193
Anthony, M., 274
Apley, J., 32, 58, 59, 83, 84, 85, 221
Aradine, C. R., 140
Arena, J. G., 159
Arney, W. R., 18
Arnold, C. B., 110, 304
Aronoff, G. M., 22, 300

Aronson, M. L., 226
Artz, C. P., 260
Ashley, L. C., 29, 193, 195
Atkinson, H. H., 21
Atkinson, R. S., 104
Attanasio, V., 278
Averill, J. R., 52, 94, 231
Avery, G. S., 191
Aviram, O., 95
Axline, V. M., 224
Ayer, W., 245
Azarnoff, P., 32, 87, 294

Bailey, C. A., 116, 249
Bailey, W. C., 32
Bain, J. A., 246
Bakal, D. A., 4, 27, 274, 276
Baker, B., 54, 238, 297
Baker, L., 228
Bana, D., 275
Bandura, A., 76, 83, 84, 85, 96, 107, 127, 207, 217, 220, 238, 239, 241, 249
Banks, M. H., 4
Barber, J., 201
Barber, T. X., 13
Barker, R. G., 302
Barkin, R. L., 176, 177
Barnard, C., 163
Barnes, C., 104
Barnes, R. B., 162
Barnett, H. L., 28
Barr, R. G., 29, 31, 32, 59, 88, 99, 127, 293
Barron, K. D., 159
Bartlett, J. C., 119
Basmajian, J. V., 17
Bassett, D. L., 83
Batenhorst, R. L., 193, 195
Baum, J., 183, 184
Baumann, T. J., 193, 195
Bayrakal, S., 226
Beales, J. G., 26, 32, 62, 63, 64, 92, 174, 239, 266, 267, 275

Beard, M. C., 199
Beaver, W. T., 136, 190
Becker, R., 173
Becker, R. O., 200
Beecher, H. K., 13, 19, 76, 92, 200, 231
Begg, M. W., 83
Bellissimo, A., 21
Benitz, W. E., 180, 191, 279
Bennett, R. L., 193, 195
Bensen, V. B., 235
Bentley, G., 23
Berde, C., 310
Beresford, S. A., 4
Bergen, B. J., 18
Berger, H., 228
Bergey, S. F., 229
Bergmann, T., 46
Berkowitz, B. A., 189
Bernick, S. M., 235, 238
Bernstein, N., 32
Bernstein, N. R., 235, 259, 260, 264, 265, 271
Berrenberg, J. L., 206
Bessman, C. A., 89, 213, 215, 216, 270, 303
Best, F. A., 253
Betcher, A. M., 271
Beuf, H. A., 32, 35, 78, 102
Beyer, J. E., 29, 32, 113, 136, 140, 193, 195
Bhat, R., 177
Bibace, R., 35, 36, 41, 42, 43, 44, 45, 46, 141
Bierenbaum, H., 229
Biglan, A., 32, 212
Bille, B., 274, 275, 279
Bilting, M., 101, 120, 146
Bird, B. L., 23, 300
Black, J. E., 46
Black, R. G., 17
Blake, D. D., 274, 275, 276, 284
Blanchard, E. B., 159, 275
Block, A. R., 21, 137
Boczkowski, J., 85, 221
Boehncke, H., 32
Boisen, E., 280
Boisjoly, C., 127
Bok, D., 103, 109
Bokan, J. A., 82
Bolme, P., 194
Bond, M. R., 2, 116, 175

Bonica, J. J., 1, 3, 4, 6, 8, 13, 16, 18, 19, 20, 22, 23, 24, 25, 26, 47, 112, 167, 193, 195, 197, 272
Boone, R. R., 219
Borghi, C., 164
Borrego, A., 188
Boulenger, J.-P., 95
Boureau, F., 25
Bower, G. H., 119
Bower, T. G. R., 38
Bowman, M., 232, 235
Boyd, D. B., 22, 26
Bradshaw, C. T., 98, 99, 231
Braver, S., 142
Brazelton, T. B., 110
Bremme, K., 253
Brena, S. F., 111
Brenman, M., 236
Bresler, D. E., 1, 3, 21, 47, 201
Breslin, P. W., 259, 265
Brewer, E., Jr., 183
Brewster, A. B., 46
Brik, R., 80
Brody, J. E., 110
Brogden, R. N., 191
Bronfenbrenner, U., 78, 98, 100
Brooks-Gunn, J., 252, 253
Brown, J. K., 279, 283
Brown, J. M., 54, 55, 238, 241, 297
Brown, P. E., 87
Browne, G., 3, 238
Bruce, S., 35, 65, 74, 101, 248
Bruner, J. S., 222
Buchsbaum, M. S., 95
Buckingham, B., 200
Buckley, L., 285
Buckman, W., 227, 228
Burke, E. J., 278
Burleson, G., 119
Burnside, H., 156, 157
Bush, A. F., 144
Byers, M. L., 32
Bygdeman, M., 253

Cacciabue, F., 63
Cahners, S. S., 263
Caire, J. B., 290
Caldwell, S., 155, 194
Calimlim, J. F., 137
Cama, R., 107, 108
Cambier, J., 25

Cameron, C. O., 65
Campbell, M. C., 84
Cannon, W. B., 19, 157
Cappelli, M., 130
Capperauld, I., 87
Carder, B., 25
Carlon, A. T., 257
Carlsson, C.-A., 101, 120, 146
Carpenter, D., 25
Carr, D. B., 114, 115, 134, 136, 142,
    143, 144, 148, 161, 162
Carregal, E. J. A., 4
Carroll, S. S., 265
Carter, K. M., 25, 86
Cartwright-Smith, J., 159, 273, 298
Carty, R. M., 89, 104
Casati, R., 63
Casey, K. L., 15, 159
Cataldo, M. F., 23, 89, 104, 213, 215,
    216, 270, 300, 303
Caty, S., 222
Cautela, J., 207
Cerchiari, E. L., 164
Cetron, M., 6
Chapman, A. H., 81, 83
Chapman, C. R., 1, 6, 16, 19, 20, 21,
    23, 35, 76, 79, 111, 112, 134, 135,
    136, 137, 141, 148, 149, 159, 164, 174,
    178, 204, 217, 271, 282, 310
Chapman, J.-A., 152, 155
Chapman, S. L., 32
Chapman, W. P., 88
Chen, A. C. N., 96
Cheng, R., 199, 200, 201
Chesney, M. A., 255, 258
Cholst, I. N., 257
Chow, R. L., 28
Christensen, M. F., 84
Christophenson, V., 87
Chung, D., 25
Ciccone, D. S., 19, 282
Cioppa, F. J., 235
Clancy, S., 297
Clark, B. S., 188, 189
Clark, E. B., 285, 304
Clark, M., 3
Clark, W. C., 88
Clarke, J. P., 298
Cleland, J. T., 18
Co, L. L., 199
Coates, T. J., 304

Cohen, F., 220, 240
Cohen, F. L., 193
Cohen, M. I., 179, 195
Cohen, S., 52, 98, 99
Colby, C. Z., 159, 273, 289, 298
Collen, M. F., 89
Colman, M. D., 226
Colwell, S. O., 237
Conners, C. K., 206
Cooper, J., 29
Copp, L. A., 241
Corah, N. L., 231
Cornish, J. D., 301
Cousins, M. J., 167
Cousins, N., 298, 309
Cowherd, M., 78, 171
Craig, K. D., 29, 30, 32, 42, 75, 76,
    83, 84, 85, 86, 88, 99, 149, 150, 151,
    155, 157, 158, 221, 275, 293, 296,
    299, 310
Crawford, H. J., 233
Crichton, J. U., 276
Crocker, E., 108, 169, 172
Crocker, M. F., 243, 305
Crockett, D. J., 99
Crook, J., 3, 4, 21, 85
Crue, B. L., 4, 15, 21
Cunningham, S. J., 126, 127, 141
Curran, N. M., 4
Cuthbert, M. I., 219

Dåhlstrom, B., 194
Dale, J. C., 29, 160
Dalet, R., 201
Dalton, K., 255
Dash, J., 32, 65
D'Astous, J., 64, 299, 303
Daut, R. L., 155
Davidson, P. O., 249
Davis, D. M., 188
Davitz, L. J., 157
Dawood, M. Y., 252, 253
deCholnoky, C., 252
DeFee, J. F., Jr., 32
Degenaar, J. J., 2, 3
DeGood, D. E., 29, 193, 195
Dehen, H., 25
DeLateur, B. J., 17
Della Puppa, T., 164
Demjen, S., 27
Denholm, C. J., 173

Dennis, S. G., 15
Deubner, D. C., 274
de Veber, L. L., 32, 134, 137, 138, 139, 141, 148, 156, 238, 239, 286, 287, 296
Devlin, D., 18
Dexter, S. L., 284
Diamond, S., 281
Dietrich, S. L., 157, 245
Die-Trill, M., 243
DiLeo, H. H., 127
DiMatteo, M. R., 46
Dinges, D. F., 234, 235
Dodge, J. A., 32
Dodge, L., 124
Dolce, J. J., 243, 272, 273, 305
Doleys, D. M., 243, 272, 273, 305
Doneen, B., 25
Dotemoto, S., 78
Dothage, J. A., 64, 194
Dougher, C. A., 226
Dougherty, L. M., 29, 151, 152, 158
Dowling, J., 124
Drabman, R. S., 271
Droppleman, L. F., 161
D'Souza, B. J., 279
Dubner, R., 11, 16, 159
Dubuisson, D., 42
Dunn, H. G., 276
Dunn, J., 152, 155
Dunne, E. A., 41
Dunn-Geier, B. J., 64, 79, 229, 293, 303
Dworkin, S. F., 96
Dychtwald, K., 6
Dyment, P. G., 207, 288

Ebell, W., 191
Edelman, I., 25
Edelman, N. H., 284
Edwards, P. W., 85, 221
Egermark-Eriksson, I., 274
Eisenberg, L., 199
Ekman, R., 71
Eland, J. M., 28, 32, 35, 40, 50, 78, 111, 115, 117, 131, 143, 144, 145, 146, 148, 157, 159, 187, 194, 196, 287, 296
Elkins, P. D., 218, 220
Ellenberg, L., 65
Ellerton, M.-L., 222

Elliott, C. H., 153, 155, 160, 161, 194, 207, 243, 244, 262, 266, 271
Emans, S. J., 252
Emmanuelli, A., 180
Enders, P. L., 22
Endress, M. P., 32, 135
Engberg, I., 25
Engel, G. L., 22, 303
Engel, J. M., 281
Engelbart, H. J., 23
Enzenauer, R. W., 301
Epstein, L. H., 277
Erickson, F., 222
Erickson, H. H., 4, 10
Erickson, S., 290
Erikson, E., 173, 222
Erlen, J. A., 172
Ernst, C., 89
Espinosa, W., 188
Evans, C., 107, 172
Evans, D. E. N., 107, 172
Evans, M. E., 177
Evans, R. I., 304
Evans, W. O., 22

Fabregas, C., 188
Fairley, P., 8, 9, 283
Fassler, D., 285
Fassler, J., 32, 286
Fehrenbach, P. A., 71, 217, 219
Feldman, W. S., 35
Ferguson, K. S., 280
Ferguson, R. V., 173
Ferguson, T., 32
Fernandez, E., 54, 167, 175, 176
Ferrari, M., 63
Ferster, C., 211
Feuerstein, M., 10, 31, 59, 281, 282
Feychting, H., 194
Field, T., 160
Filler, W. W., 257
Fine, J., 304
Finer, B., 235
Fink, C. W., 183
Firestone, P., 277, 283, 295
Fisch, R., 227
Fisch, Robert, 301
Fisichelli, R. M., 29
Fisichelli, V. R., 29
Fleece, E. L., 159, 161
Fletcher, B. A., 39

Fletcher, J., 18
Florman, A. L., 75, 218
Flower, R. J., 181
Foerster, O., 14
Fogels, H., 98
Foley, K. M., 159, 188, 193, 195
Folkard, S., 52, 90
Folkman, J., 109
Folkman, S., 52
Fordyce, W. E., 9, 17, 21, 22, 24, 63, 214, 263, 272
Forsythe, W. I., 278
Foster, M., 10, 76
Foster, T. S., 193, 195
Fothergill, L. A., 25
Fowler, R. S., 17
Fox, E. J., 199
Fox, R. E., 229
Framo, J. L., 227
Francoeur, E., 31
Francucci, B., 164
Frankl, S., 98
Frankl, V., 101
Franklin, M., 207
Fras, I., 264
Frautschi, N. M., 71, 217, 219
Frederickson, D. S., 4
Freedman, R. R., 163
Freeman, L. R., 197
Freese, A. S., 6
Freud, S., 222
Friedlander, S., 219
Friedman, B., 213
Friedman, G. D., 89
Friedman, R., 11, 32
Friesen, M. V., 71
Fry, R. A., 71, 217, 219
Funk, M., 262

Gaal, J. M., 238
Gabriel, H., 173
Gaffney, A. A., 36, 40, 41, 42, 43, 44, 45, 49, 51, 53, 54, 91, 99, 141, 238, 293, 299
Gaffney, P. R., 299
Gantt, P. A., 252, 253
Gardner, G. G., 29, 32, 207, 232, 233, 234, 235, 236, 237, 238, 252, 253, 271, 282
Gardner, W. J., 95
Garron, D. C., 27

Gaston-Johansson, F., 118
Gaudreault, P., 181, 192, 193
Gaylor, M. S., 137
Gelfand, S., 89
Genest, M., 3, 297
Gerrity, P. C., 46
Gewanter, H. L., 184
Gibbons, P. T., 44, 46, 51, 99, 143
Gibby, H., 286
Gijsbers, K., 66, 70, 119
Gilbert, A., 157, 245
Gilbert, B. O., 219, 220
Gilbert, J. H. V., 296
Gilchrist, E. B., 311
Gill, M. M., 236
Gillespie, A., 253
Gillies, D., 278
Gilman, A., 183, 186
Gilman, A. G., 180, 183, 186, 192
Ginott, H., 222, 224
Ginther, L. J., 218, 219, 220
Giurgea, D., 23, 84, 85, 275
Glick, R. C., 36, 41, 48, 51, 54
Glynn, C. J., 90, 91
Goepel, R., 139, 198
Gofman, H. F., 228
Goldscheider, A., 11
Goldsmith, L., 238
Goldson, E., 160
Goldstein, A., 25, 161
Goldstein, D. P., 252
Gonick, M. A., 302
Gonshor, A., 202
Goodman, J. T., 141, 152, 155, 207, 277, 283
Goodman, L. S., 180, 183, 186, 192
Gordon, D. J., 36, 52, 53, 54, 73, 130, 143
Gordon, N. C., 159
Gordon, S. B., 127
Gorsky, B. H., 1, 201
Gorsuch, R., 94
Gosnell, M., 3
Gôtestam, K. G., 19, 111
Gothoni, G., 279
Gover, V. F., 132, 133
Graceley, R. H., 135, 159
Graham, J. R., 275
Gratch, G., 38
Graves, D. A., 193, 195
Green, E. C., 105

Grobstein, R., 99
Groden, J., 207
Gross, S. C., 1, 29, 32
Grossi, E., 164
Grossman, E., 204
Grunau, R. V. E., 29, 151, 158, 296
Grushkin, C. M., 226
Grzesiak, R. C., 19, 282
Guise, B. J., 86
Guité, S., 202
Gunsberger, M., 198
Gurman, A. S., 229
Gwynn, M., 241

Haber, A., 29
Haber, J. D., 73
Hagbarth, K. E., 25
Hahn, A. B., 176, 177
Hahn, Y. S., 29, 30, 32, 35, 38, 39, 42, 99, 119, 130, 310
Haight, W. L., 46, 101
Hakkarainen, H., 279
Hall, W. C., 257
Hall, W. J., 253
Hallén, B., 288
Halpern, L. M., 17
Hamblin, J. J., 104
Hankins, C. T., 301
Hannan, J. A., 32
Hannington-Kiff, J. G., 27
Hanson, K., 194, 195
Hanson, V., 61, 80, 123, 183
Harkins, S. W., 186
Harpin, V. A., 161
Harrigan, J. A., 280
Harris, G., 240
Harrison, R. H., 281
Haskell, D. J., 3
Haslam, D. R., 88, 194
Hassanein, K., 273
Hassanein, R., 273
Havdala, H., 199
Hawes, R., 159, 161
Hawley, D. D., 39, 119
Hazinski, M. F., 29, 88
Head, B., 94, 110, 285
Head, H., 10, 24
Healy, M., 265, 271
Heaman, S., 193
Hearn, M. T., 32, 134, 135, 137, 138,

139, 141, 148, 156, 296
Hebb, D. O., 29
Heczey, M. D., 257
Heel, R. C., 191
Heft, M. W., 138
Heidrich, G., 157, 194, 264
Heimel, A., 237
Helwick, C. A., 163
Hembree, E. A., 29, 151, 152
Hendler, N. H., 23, 111
Henker, B., 73, 78, 79
Herman, B. H., 299, 310
Hermecz, D. A., 219
Hershman, J. M., 163
Hester, N. K. O., 140
Hilgard, E. R., 17, 35, 161, 233, 235, 236, 237
Hilgard, J. R., 17, 35, 54, 65, 232, 233, 234, 235, 236, 237, 238, 239
Hiller, J., 25, 64
Hilpert, P. L., 218
Himelstein, P., 32
Hines, P., 272
Hodgins, D. C., 241
Hoffman, A., 173
Hogg, M. I. J., 136
Hokkanen, E., 279
Holland, J. P., 32
Hollien, H., 151
Holmes, G., 24
Holmes, S. S., 106, 169
Holroyd, K. A., 127, 204, 205
Holt, P. J., 62, 63, 64, 92, 275
Holton, M. E., 301
Holzemer, W. L., 115, 137
Honig, P., 228
Houle, M., 31
Houts, A. C., 281
Huang, L. N., 219
Huebner, R. R., 151, 158
Huey, L. Y., 192
Hughes, C. S., 188
Hughes, J., 25
Hughes, M. C., 84, 275
Hull, C. L., 27
Humphreys, P. J., 126, 127, 130, 207, 277, 283
Huskisson, E. C., 61, 115, 117, 135, 136, 137, 138, 175, 181
Hutcherson, S., 159, 161
Hyson, M. C., 173, 296

Iacono, C. U., 258
Ianni, P., 163
Iggo, A., 11, 26
Igoe, J. B., 304
Illa, J., 188
Inhelder, B., 88, 108, 130, 141, 205
Inturrisi, C. E., 188, 189
Irwin, E. C., 226
Iverson, S., 301
Izard, C. E., 27, 29, 151, 152, 158

Jackson, D. D., 227
Jacobs, H. E., 104
Jacobsen, P. B., 243
Jacox, A. K., 35, 116, 156, 159
Jamner, L. D., 11
Janowsky, D. S., 192
Jaremko, M. E., 70, 81, 85, 92
Jarvie, G. J., 271
Jay, G. W., 282
Jay, S. M., 153, 155, 160, 161, 194,
    239, 243, 244, 311
Jayson, M. I. V., 200
Jeans, M. E., 28, 32, 52, 53, 54, 73,
    75, 111, 112, 124, 130, 143, 175, 199
Jeffery, R. W., 304
Jensen, M. P., 142
Jerrett, M. D., 36, 50, 51, 99
Jessop, C., 257
Jessup, B. A., 204, 205
Jewell, E. R., 187
Jick, H., 195
Joffe, R., 27, 276
Johnson, C., 39
Johnson, G., 152, 155
Johnson, J. E., 32, 135, 288
Johnson, M., 20
Johnson, R., 218
Johnson, S. B., 219, 220
Johnston, C. C., 39, 75, 151, 157, 160,
    175
Joliffe, N., 14
Jolly, A., 106, 222
Jolly, H., 121
Jonas, S., 109, 110
Jones, B. N., 132, 133
Jones, C. M., 88
Jurgens, H., 191

Kabela, E., 275
Kaganov, J., 27, 276

Kagen-Goodheart, L., 302
Kane, K., 16
Kantero, R. L., 254
Kao, F. F., 197
Kaplan, J. Z., 270
Kaplan, R. M., 207, 243
Kaptchuk, T. J., 197, 198
Karelitz, R. M., 29
Karelitz, S., 29
Karoly, P., 142
Kassowitz, K., 39
Katon, W. J., 82
Katz, E. R., 95, 153, 155, 160, 161, 162,
    243, 244, 271, 302
Katz, Jay, 28, 306
Katz, Joel, 28
Kavaler, L., 163
Kavanagh, C. K., 95, 251, 266, 267,
    268, 269, 270
Keats, A. S., 18
Keefe, F. J., 127
Keele, K. D., 8, 131
Keen, J. H., 62, 63, 64, 92, 275
Keen, W. W., Jr., 9
Keene, D., 207, 277, 283
Keeri-Szanto, M., 193
Keith-Spiegel, P., 30
Kellerman, J., 65, 95, 153, 155, 162,
    271, 302
Kelley, M. L., 271
Kelvie, W., 137, 138, 144
Kenny, T. J., 169
Kenton, B., 4
Kerr, D. I. B., 25
Kerr, F. W., 11, 16, 24, 26
Kewman, D. G., 204, 205
Khan, M. H., 294, 295
Kibbee, C. J., 261
King, L. R., 301
King, N. J., 204
Kirchhoff, K. T., 32, 135
Kirya, C., 29
Kitchell, R. L., 4, 10
Kleck, R. E., 98, 101, 159, 273, 289,
    298
Klein, J. R., 182, 252, 253, 256, 257
Klepac, R. K., 124
Klingman, A., 219
Klinzing, D. G., 218
Klinzing, D. R., 218
Klorman, R., 218

Knafl, K. A., 23
Knapp, T. R., 113
Kniskern, D. P., 229
Knox, E., 301
Knudson-Cooper, M. S., 272
Kobasa, S. C., 55
Kohen, D. P., 237, 238, 258
Kohlenberg, R. J., 276
Kolb, L., 13
Koocher, G. P., 30, 308
Kopel, S., 127
Koponen, M., 278
Korberly, B. H., 181, 182, 183, 190
Korones, S. B., 301
Korsch, B. M., 226
Kosterlitz, H. W., 25
Kramer, M. S., 127, 137
Kratochwill, T. R., 213, 217
Krause, S. J., 131, 132
Kravitz, M., 259
Kremer, E. F., 21, 137
Kristein, M. M., 110, 304
Kroner, B., 273
Kruger, L., 16
Kruszewski, A. Z., 288
Kuczmierczyk, A. R., 85
Kudrow, L., 279
Kueffner, M., 267
Kues, J. R., 280
Kurylszyn, N., 130
Kussman, M., 161
Kuttner, L., 139, 232, 235, 236, 242, 311

LaBaw, W. L., 232, 235, 271
L'Abbé, E. E., 281
Lacouture, P. G., 192
LaGana, C., 218
La Greca, A. M., 32, 207
Lake, A. E., 281
Lance, J. W., 274
Lang, L., 286, 289
Lang, P. J., 245
Lang, S. H., 288
Langley, S., 89
Lanzetta, J. T., 159, 273, 289, 298
Larsson, B., 208
Lasagna, L., 137, 138, 144
Lasoff, E. M., 270
Latham, G. P., 272
Latimer, P. B., 22

Latter, J., 64, 229, 303
Lau, R. R., 85
Lavigne, J. V., 32
Law, D., 98
Law, P., 199, 201
Lazarus, A. A, 246
Lazarus, R. S., 52
Lazarus, R. W., 220, 240
Leavitt, F., 27
Leavitt, M., 32, 78, 266
LeBaron, S., 30, 35, 54, 64, 65, 153,
     156, 232, 233, 234, 235, 236, 237,
     238, 239
Leduc, D. G., 127
Lee, R. B., 197
Lefcoe, N. M., 304
Leff, P. T., 174
Leggott, P., 219
Lehmann, J. F., 17
Leikin, L., 295
Leitch, I. O. W., 259
Lele, P. P., 10
Lemchen, M. S., 95, 243
Lenburg, C. B., 156, 157
Leo, K. C., 198
Leonardi, G., 63
LePage, T., 139, 287
LeShan, L., 20
Lethem, J., 23, 59
Levine, J. D., 159
Levine, M., 59
Levine, R. R., 175, 181, 187, 190, 193
Levinson, J. E., 183
Leviton, A., 275, 281
Levy, D. M., 39
Levy, N., 88
Lewenstein, L. N., 235
Lewis, C. E., 48, 110, 304
Lewis, J. W., 191
Lewis, M. A., 110, 304
Lewis, N., 35, 78, 101, 285
Lewis, T., 98
Lewith, G. T., 199
Li, C., 25
Libber, S. M., 259
Licklider, J. C., 95
Liebeskind, J. C., 4, 9, 12, 16, 25, 26,
     116, 199, 200, 250
Liebman, R., 228
Lind, J., 151, 158
Lindeke, L., 301

Lindell, M. H., 109
Lindsay, S. J. E., 231
Linn, S., 164, 223
Linton, S. J., 19, 20, 22, 111
Lipsitt, L. P., 88
Litt, I. F., 182, 252, 256
Livingstone, W. K., 11
Lloyd, J. L., 114
Lloyd, J. W., 90
Lobsenz, N. M., 106
Locke, E. A., 272
Locsin, R. G., 288
Loebach, S., 143
Loeser, J. D., 200
Lollar, D. J., 37, 50, 113, 146, 147, 148
London, P., 233
Lonetto, R., 35, 46
Lorimer, A., 110, 304
Lossie, J., 272, 273
Lovejoy, F. H., 181, 192, 193
Lowe, K., 213
Lowery, C., 311
Lowney, L. I., 25
Lubman, A., 235
Ludvigsson, J., 278
Lundberg, A., 25
Lundström, V., 253
Lushene, R., 94
Luthe, W., 257
Lutzker, J. R., 213
Lynn, S. J., 163

Macdonald, A., 197
MacDonald, J. T., 238, 278, 282
Machen, J. B., 218
Machin, D., 199
MacKenzie, R. G., 257
Mackie, J., 194, 195
MacLeod, S. M., 176, 178
Macmillan, B. G., 265
MacRae, K. D., 115
Magrab, P. R., 18, 225
Mäkelä, A. L., 183
Malott, J. M., 241, 242, 249
Mani, S., 280
Mann, T., 70
Margolis, R. B., 131, 132
Mariani, E. M., 301
Marks, R., 193, 195
Marlow, D. R., 28
Marston, A. R., 163

Martin, W. R., 180
Martino, G., 180
Maruta, T., 22
Masek, B. J., 63, 275, 281
Massey, E. W., 69
Masten, A. S., 228
Masur, F. T., 259
Mather, L., 194, 195
Maxwell, G. M., 178, 182, 188, 193
Mayer, D. J., 25, 199, 201
McCaffery, M., 3, 19, 32, 38, 40, 78, 115, 157
McCalla, J., 194
McCallum, M., 219, 220
McCarran, M. S., 274, 275, 276, 284
McCarthy, R., 117
McCaul, K. D., 241, 242, 249
McClellan, M. A., 94
McCollum, A. T., 174
McCormack, R. K., 199
McDonough, P. G., 252, 253
McEttrick, M. A., 270
McFadd, A., 264
McGinness, G. C., 151, 158
McGrath, P. A., 32, 117, 120, 123, 127, 134, 137, 138, 139, 141, 148, 156, 238, 239, 277, 286, 287, 296, 310
McGrath, P. J., 32, 64, 126, 127, 128, 141, 152, 155, 207, 229, 270, 277, 283, 295, 303
McLone, D. G., 29, 30, 35, 38, 39, 119, 130
McMahon, R. J., 29, 150, 151, 155, 158, 293
McNair, D. M., 161
McNeer, M. F., 271
McNeill, T. W., 27
McVey, L., 127
McWilliams, B. J., 226
Mead, T., 282
Mechanic, D., 83
Mehegan, J. E., 281
Mehl, L., 88
Mehta, G., 137
Meichenbaum, D. H., 3, 96, 97, 205, 218, 240, 258, 297
Meinhart, N. T., 3, 19, 115, 157
Meissner, W. W., 226
Melamed, B. G., 32, 159, 161, 218, 219, 220
Meldman, M., 96

Melin, L., 19, 111, 208
Mellor, V. P., 62, 64
Melzack, R., 1, 3, 10, 11, 12 13, 14, 15,
    17, 25, 26, 27, 28, 29, 31, 42, 58, 59,
    60, 61, 67, 69, 77, 78, 95, 115, 119,
    124, 125, 126, 174, 199, 202, 203,
    249, 277, 298
Mendelson, G., 27
Menefee, E. E., 18
Menge, B., 101, 120, 146
Menges, L. J., 4, 7, 302
Menke, E., 285
Mennie, A. T., 32
Merrill, J. C., 300, 301
Merskey, H., 1, 2, 22, 29, 116
Metcalf, T. J., 301
Michael, R., 218
Micheli, L. J., 68
Michell, J., 111
Middlebrook, J. L., 271
Milhorat, T. H., 111
Miller, A. J., 213, 217
Miller, I. W., 93
Miller, J. J., III, x, 61, 63
Miller, M. D., 262
Miller, N. E., 17
Miller, R. R., 183
Miller, S. W., 230
Millman, B. S., 197, 200
Millman, M., 109
Milman, L., 228
Minuchin, S., 63, 228
Mirvish, I., 235
Miser, A. W., 64, 188, 189, 194
Miser, J. S., 64, 188, 189, 194
Mitchell, S. W., 9
Mogtader, E. M., 174
Mohamed, S. N., 84
Moletteire, C., 243, 305
Möller, C., 288
Molsberry, D. M. J., 40, 140, 141, 142
Moncada, S., 181
Moncrief, J. A., 260
Mondzac, A. M., 18
Monk, M., 124
Monson, L., 285
Montanari, M., 164
Montgomery, R. B., 204
Morawetz, R. F., 90
Morehouse, G. R., 9
Morgan, A. H., 232, 233

Morgan, B. A., 25
Morgan, S. B., 259
Morley, J. S., 25
Morpurgo, C. V., 63
Morrell, D. C., 4
Morris, F. D., 264
Morris, H. R., 25
Morrison, J. D., 29, 150, 151, 155,
    158, 293
Mortensen, O., 84
Mullen, F. G., 258
Mulne, A. F., 188
Mundinger, M. O., 300, 310
Murad, F., 180, 192
Murphy, L. B., 52
Murphy, M. E., 98, 109
Murphy, R. W., 28
Murphy, T. M., 26
Murrin, K. R., 142
Myllyla, V., 279

Nafe, J. P., 11
Nagera, H., 223
Nakayama, S. Y., 36, 41, 48, 51, 54
Napoliello, M., 285
Nathan, P. W., 15, 26, 200
Nayman, J., 144
Neal, H. K., 18, 32, 78, 93, 231
Needs, R. E., 238
Negrete, V. F., 226
Neighbor, W. E., 305
Neinstein, L. S., 252, 253, 256, 274,
    278, 279, 280
Nerlinger, R. E., 162
Neuhauser, C., 272
Newburger, P. E., 194
Newman, R. I., 20, 22, 23
Newton, J. R., 164, 165
Ng, L. K. Y., 4, 16, 19, 26, 161
Nicholi, A. M., Jr., 226
Nicholson, R. H., 30
Nielsen, J. S., 22
Nissen, K. W., 28
Niven, C., 119
Noack, G., 194
Nobili, R. M., 63
Nocella, J., 207, 243
Noordenbos, W., 4, 11, 12, 14, 15, 16,
    56
Norfleet, M. A., 20, 23, 303
Norman, W. H., 93

Notermans, S. L., 89
Nover, R. A., 32, 264
Novik, B., 235

O'Brien, C., 193, 194
Occhiuto, M. G., 130
Oddy, M., 280
Oestreich, S. J. K., 176, 177
O'Keefe, J., 54, 238, 297
Olds, A. R., 105
Oliveau, D., 285
Olness, K., 161, 204, 207, 232, 233,
    234, 235, 236, 237, 238, 271, 278,
    281, 282
Olson, R. A., 207, 266, 271
Olson, S., 4
O'Neill, J. A., 260
Opton, E. M., Jr., 52
Orne, M. T., 232, 234, 235
Osborn, L. M., 301
Osgood, P. F., 114, 115, 134, 136, 142,
    143, 144, 148, 161, 162, 190
Oswalt, R., 285
O'Toole, T., 6
Ottinger, D. R., 32, 207
Owens, M. E., 28, 29, 30, 32, 88,
    151, 159, 160, 293
Ozolins, M., 155, 194

Paalzow, L., 194
Painter, J. R., 22, 23
Pal, B. K., 25
Palmer, B. B., 110, 304
Parantainen, J., 279
Parini, J., 180
Parker, L. H., 89
Parker, S. R., 138
Parkin, S. F., 207
Parlee, M. B., 255
Partanen, T. J., 151, 158
Parth, P., 90
Passo, M., 32
Pasternak, J. F., 295
Patrick, C. J., 299
Patterson, D. L., 50, 113, 146, 147, 148
Paul, L. A., 4, 9, 12, 16, 26, 116, 199,
    200, 250
Paulley, J. W., 3
Payne, B., 20, 23, 303
Pearson, J. E., 89
Pederson, L. L., 304

Peller, L., 223
Pellettieri, L., 101, 120, 146
Pennebaker, J., 39, 96, 303
Penticuff, J. H., 218, 219
Peper, E., 204
Perl, E. R., 11
Perrin, E. C., 46
Perry, S. W., 157, 193, 194, 195, 196,
    197, 264
Pert, C., 25
Peterschmidt, K., 39, 98, 99, 119, 248
Peterson, Lizette, 87, 160, 218, 219,
    220, 239, 243, 286, 294
Peterson, L.-E., 101, 120, 148
Petrie, A., 29, 89
Petrillo, M., 223
Piaget, J., 38, 46, 62, 88, 108, 130, 141,
    205, 222, 223
Pickles, V. H., 253
Pilowsky, I., 83
Pinsky, J. J., 4, 21, 23
Pless, I. B., 127
Pomeranz, B., 199, 200, 201
Poole, L., 272, 273
Pöppel, E., 90
Portenoy, R. K., 195
Porter, J., 195
Porter, J. J., 84
Post, R. M., 95
Pothmann, R., 139, 191, 198
Poznanski, E. O., 29, 32
Prensky, A. L., 276
Price, C., 186
Price, D. D., 186, 199, 200, 201
Prier, S., 25
Prkachin, K. M., 86, 99, 149, 155, 299
Prudden, B., 202, 203
Pruitt, B. A., 260
Pruitt, S. D., 262
Pugh, S. T., 173

Qualls, P. J., 204, 205
Quinby, S., 32
Quinn, S., 275

Raczynski, J. M., 73, 272, 273
Radde, I. C., 176, 178, 179, 181
Rae, W. A., 223
Rafart, A., 188
Rafii, A., 186, 199, 200, 201
Rafman, S., 31

Rall, T. W., 180, 192
Ramsden, R., 213
Raphaeli, N., 95
Rapoff, M. A., 281
Rappaport, L. A., 59
Reading, A. E., 126, 159, 164, 165
Redd, W. H., 243
Redpath, C. C., 35
Reichmanis, M., 200
Reissland, N., 37, 53, 54
Remen, N., 35, 46, 79, 248
Remolina, C., 284
Renaer, R., 252, 253
Renelli, D., 282
Resser, D., 151, 158
Revill, S. I., 136
Reyes, A., 199
Reynolds, D. V., 25
Richardson, G. M., 126
Richardson, P. H., 198, 199, 200
Richter, H. G., 46
Richter, I. L., 207, 277, 283
Ricks, D. F., 280
Rideout, E., 3
Ridley-Johnson, R., 87, 218, 219, 220
Ries, R. K., 82
Rigler, D., 65, 302
Rinzler, S. H., 199
Ritchie, J. A., 222
Roberts, A. H., 19, 22, 204, 205
Roberts, M. C., 218, 219, 220
Roberts, S. J., 258
Robertson, W. O., 29
Robinson, D., 198
Robinson, J. O., 136
Robinson, S. S., 280
Robson, M. C., 260
Rogers, A. G., 130, 137, 139
Rogers, C. S., 35
Rogers, E. J., 90
Rogers, F., 94, 110, 285
Rogers, M. C., 89, 104
Rokke, P., 124
Rollman, G. B., 240
Romero, R., 108
Rooke, E. D., 69
Rose, M. H., 52
Rosen, M., 136, 142
Rosenbaum, P., 35, 74, 248
Rosenberg, A., 182, 256
Rosenblith, J. F., 28, 29, 88, 89, 293

Rosenbloom, A., 219, 220
Rosenblum, E. L., 275, 278
Rosenfeld, A., 309
Rosman, D. L., 228
Ross, A. P., 35, 66, 110
Ross, D. M., 35, 37, 39, 40, 41, 42,
  44, 45, 46, 50, 51, 53, 54, 55, 56,
  59, 61, 64, 66, 67, 68, 70, 71, 72,
  73, 76, 78, 85, 94, 95, 110, 115,
  118, 120, 121, 134, 136, 142, 146,
  157, 169, 170, 195, 220, 221, 239,
  246, 248, 249, 293, 294, 300, 304,
  305, 306, 308
Ross, M., 35, 66, 110
Ross, S. A., 35, 37, 39, 40, 41, 42,
  44, 45, 46, 50, 51, 53, 54, 55, 56,
  59, 61, 64, 66, 67, 68, 70, 71, 72,
  73, 76, 78, 85, 95, 110, 115, 118,
  120, 121, 134, 136, 142, 146, 157,
  169, 170, 195, 220, 221, 239, 240,
  248, 249, 293, 294, 300, 304, 305,
  306, 308
Rothbaum, F., 130
Rothenberg, M. B., 103
Rourke, B. P., 64, 229, 313
Routh, D. K., 98, 100, 149
Rowat, K. M., 23
Roy, R., 21, 23
Rozensky, R. H., 295
Ruble, D. N., 252, 253
Rudy, T. E., 126
Russell, G. A., 29, 193, 195
Russell, S. W., 156, 158
Russo, D. C., 23, 63, 213, 215, 216,
  270, 281, 300, 303
Rutter, N., 161
Ryan, R. E., Jr., 274
Ryan, R. E., Sr., 274

Saari, L. M., 272
Sachar, E., 193, 195
Saieh, T. A., 259
Sallan, S. E., 194
Salovey, P., 126
Sanders, S. H., 54, 111, 157, 159, 238,
  297
Sanger, S., 223, 264
Sank, L. I., 32, 212
Santiago, T. V., 284
Santrock, J. W., 119
Sarbin, T. R., 236

Sargent, C., 87, 92
Sarles, R. M., 235
Saunders, C., 17
Saunders, N. L., 159
Savage, C. W., 111
Savage, D., 69
Savage, J. P., 259
Savedra, M., 37, 44, 46, 47, 50, 51,
    53, 55, 99, 143, 238
Schachter, S., 89, 98
Schafer, L., 124
Schaller, J., 183
Schechter, N. L., 28, 29, 32, 194
Schiffer, M., 225
Schillinger, J., 152, 155
Schluderman, E., 88
Schmidt, R. F., 26
Schmitz, T. H., 199
Schnebly, A., 259
Schollander, D., 69
Schomer, J., 228
Schooler, C., 89
Schorlemer, V., 65, 66, 101
Schowalter, J. E., 226
Schroeder, P., 143
Schulein, M. J., 32
Schulman, B., 1, 3, 4, 16, 19, 20, 23
Schultz, N. V., 32, 37
Schwammborn, D., 191
Schwartz, A. H., 31
Scolles, V., III, 284
Scott, C. S., 305
Scott, D. L., 17
Scott, P. J., 61, 115, 117, 136, 137, 138
Scott, R., 37, 121, 143, 145, 146
Scott, T. H., 28, 29
Scott, V., 66, 70
Segal, D. S., 192
Seligman, M. E. P., 85, 93, 171, 173,
    239, 247, 249, 267, 268
Seligman, R., 265
Semmes, J., 28
Seres, J. L., 20, 22, 23
Setterlind, S., 32, 204, 208, 304
Shacham, S., 155
Shapiro, A. H., 75, 138, 159, 160, 161,
    165
Shapiro, D., 3
Shapiro, M. B., 164
Sharp, B., 163
Shaw, E. G., 98, 100, 272

Shaw, K. N., 149
Sheehan, P. W., 204, 205
Sheridan, M., 171
Shiere, F., 98
Shigetomi, C., 160, 239
Shinnar, S., 279
Shorkey, C. T., 169, 271
Siaw, S. N., 106, 169
Siegel, L. J., 32, 161, 218, 219, 238,
    239, 243
Siegel, S. E., 95, 153, 155, 160, 161,
    162, 243, 244, 271, 302
Siegelaub, A. B., 89
Siever, L. J., 95
Sigerist, H. E., 8
Silbert, L., 70
Sillanpaa, M., 274, 278
Sills, M. A., 278
Silverstein, J. H., 219, 220
Silverstein, S., 219
Simeonsson, R., 285
Simmons, J., 298
Simon, E., 25
Simpson, U., 61
Sims-Knight, J. E., 28, 29, 88, 293
Sinclair, D. C., 11
Singh, M., 235
Skinner, B. F., 211
Skjei, E., 10
Slack, W. V., 275
Slade, P. D., 23
Slavson, S. R., 225
Slinkard, L. A., 304
Slosberg, M., 100
Smith, A. H., Jr., 235
Smith, D. P., 298
Smith, G., 9
Smith, G. N., 253
Smith, M., 272, 273
Smith, M. E., 32
Smith, R., 280
Smith, R. N., 29
Smith, T. W., 25
Smith, W. L., 1, 4
Smits, S. J., 50, 113, 146, 147, 148
Smoller, B., 1, 3, 4, 16, 19, 20, 23
Snyder, C. C., 259
Snyder, S., 25
Snyder, S. S., 173, 196
Solomon, G. D., 280
Sommer, D., 276

Spaccavento, L. J., 280
Spanos, N. P., 241
Speight, T. M., 191
Speltz, M., 156
Spielberger, C. D., 94
Spillar, R., 219, 220
Spitz, P. W., 61
Spizzirri, C. C., 29, 152
Sriwatanakul, K., 137, 138, 144
Stam, H. J., 241
Stanford, G., 103, 222, 286
Stayton, D. J., 259
Steele, S., 223
Stein, M. H., 14
Steinmuller, R., 9
Stennett, R. G., 304
Stephens, L. R., 106, 169
Stern, G. S., 206
Sternbach, R. A., 4, 5, 9, 19, 22, 28, 29, 47, 58, 77, 90, 192
Steward, M., 272
Stewart, C. M., 176, 183
Stewart, L. B., 176, 183
Stewart, M. L., 142
Stieber, D. A., 223
Stillwell, D. M., 199
Stimmel, B., 8, 19, 191, 192
Stinson, P., 110
Stinson, R., 110
St. Lawrence, J. S., 271
Stoddard, F. J., 78, 98, 239
Strada, M. E., 75, 151, 157, 160
Strassberg, D. S., 156
Stravino, V. D., 17
Strempel, H., 90
Stroebel, C. F., 204, 209
Sturner, R. A., 130
Sunderland, J. M., 121
Sveen, O. B., 218
Swafford, L. I., 29, 194
Swanson, D. W., 22, 23
Sweet, W. H., 15, 17
Sykes, W. M., 264
Sylva, K., 222
Sylvester, D., 285
Syrjala, K. L., 35, 112, 134, 135, 136, 137, 141, 148, 149, 150, 164, 178
Szasz, T. S., 32
Szyfelbein, S. K., 114, 115, 134, 136, 142, 143, 144, 148, 161, 162, 190, 310

Tainter, M. L., 8, 9
Tait, R. C., 131, 132
Tal, Y., 276
Tan, S.-Y., 16, 26, 248, 249
Tanner, M. R., 226
Tarler-Benlolo, L., 204
Tasto, D. L., 255, 258
Tatro, D. S., 180, 279
Taub, A., 16
Taub, H. A., 199
Taylor, H., 4
Taylor, J. E., 169, 271
Taylor, P. L., 30, 88
Teasdale, J. M., 232, 235
Teders, S. F., 275
Teevan, R. C., 275
Temple, A. R., 181
Terenius, L., 15, 25, 161
Tesler, M. D., 44, 46, 51, 99, 143
Thal, A. D., 235
Thelen, M. H., 71, 97, 104, 217, 219
Thomas, P. G., 83
Thompson, H. C., 301
Thompson, J. K., 73
Thompson, K. L., 32, 61, 80, 121, 123, 148, 277
Thompson, R. H., 103, 222
Thompson, S. C., 66, 93, 205, 231
Tinterow, M. M., 17
Todd, T. C., 228
Todt, E. H., 30, 160
Toler, S., 286, 294
Tompkins, J. M., 140
Toomey, T. C., 132, 133
Tophoff, M. M., 89
Torgerson, W. S., 249
Travell, J., 199, 202
Travis, E., 32, 39, 46, 119, 174
Treaster, J. B., 71
Trevarthen, C., 30
Troup, J. D. G., 23
Tucker, J. B., 35, 222, 286, 302
Tunks, E., 21
Turk, D. C., 3, 26, 94, 126, 297
Turkat, I. D., 84, 86
Turner, J. A., 20, 204, 217, 271, 297
Tursky, B., 11
Twycross, R. G., 184, 185, 189, 190
Ty, T. C., 26, 60
Tyler, F. B., 55
Tyson, K. W., 300, 301

Udall, L., 182, 256
Uden, D. L., 238, 278
Uematsu, S., 163
Uhde, T. W., 95
Ulrich, R. S., 105
Uneståhl, L.-E., 32, 208, 304
Unruh, A., 32, 127, 141
Uppfeldt, A., 288

Vair, C., 37, 131, 137, 143, 270
Valanné, E., 151, 158
Valera, L., 130
VanderMeulen, P. R., 108
Vane, J. R., 181
Vapaatalo, H., 279
Varni, J. W., 23, 32, 35, 56, 61, 63,
  80, 121, 123, 148, 155, 157, 207,
  212, 213, 215, 216, 217, 245, 251,
  270, 277, 300, 303
Vaughan, K. B., 159, 273, 298
Vaughan, R. C., 159, 273, 298
Venham, L., 98
Ventafridda, V., 130, 180
Vere, D., 176, 195
Verebely, K., 189
Vernon, D. T. A., 32, 218
Vesell, E. S., 178
Vidyasagar, D., 177
Vilkin, B., 90
Villamira, M. A., 130
Villoldo, A., 6
Vincent, C. A., 198, 199, 200
Violon, A., 23, 84, 85, 275
Visintainer, M. A., 32, 130
Vollman, R. F., 253
Volpe, J., 29
von Frey, M., 10, 76
Vrancken, M. A., 23
Vuorenkoski, V., 59, 151, 158

Wachter-Shikora, N. L., 288
Waechter, E. H., 171, 231, 248, 288
Wagner, J. M., 300
Wagner, M. M., 259, 260, 261, 265
Wahlstrom, A., 25, 161
Wain, H. J., 161
Wakeman, R. J., 270
Walker, L. J. S., 265, 271
Wall, P. D., 1, 2, 3, 4, 9, 10, 11, 12, 14,
  15, 17, 19, 20, 25, 26, 27, 60, 77, 78,
  174, 203, 293, 298, 312

Wallace, N. E., 65, 107, 108
Wallenstein, S. L., 119, 159
Waller, J. J., 4
Walsh, J., 81, 137, 289
Walsh, M. E., 35, 36, 41, 42, 43, 44,
  45, 46, 141
Walsh, T. D., 137
Ward, J. A., 44, 46, 51, 99, 143
Warden, G. D., 259
Waring, E. M., 85
Wasz-Höeckert, O., 151, 158
Waters, W. E., 274
Watkins, C. J., 4
Watkins, L. R., 200
Watzlawick, P., 227
Weakland, J., 227
Webster, S. K., 255
Weddell, G., 10, 11
Weeks, D. J., 121
Wegner, C., 44, 46, 51, 99, 143
Weighill, V. E., 28
Weis, O. F., 137
Weisenberg, M., 1, 11, 16, 24, 27, 89,
  90, 95
Weisz, A. Z., 95
Weisz, G. M., 85
Weitzenhoffer, A. M., 233
Welch, C. A., 259, 260
Werder, D. S., 207
Wert, A., 233
Werthmann, M. W., 29
Wesley, M., 64
Wesley, R. A., 194
Wessell, M. L., Sr., 298
Westbrook, T., 205
Wester, W. C., II, 235
Westerman, M. P., 199
Whalen, C. K., 73, 78, 79, 89, 94, 99
Whisler, W. W., 27
White, J. C., 17
White, R., 52
Widger, M., 295
Widholm, O., 254
Wiggins, J. S., 114, 119
Wikler, D., 27
Wilcox, K. T., 80
Wilkinson, V. A., 48
Willems, E. P., 78
Willer, J. C., 25
Williams, D. E., 73
Williams, D. T., 235

Williams, G. F., 61
Williams, K. O., 302
Williamson, D. A., 213, 281
Williamson, M. L., 29, 160
Williamson, P. S., 29, 160
Willis, R. J., 167
Wills, T. A., 52, 98, 99
Wilson, P. R., 11, 16, 24, 26
Winnicott, D. W., 107
Wisely, D. W., 259
Wiswell, T. E., 301
Witkin, H. A., 90
Wolberg, A. R., 226
Wolberg, L. R., 226
Wolf, S. R., 28
Wolf, Y., 95
Wolfer, J. A., 32, 130
Wolff, B. B., 2, 89, 112, 159, 180, 231
Wolff, V. A., 22, 89
Wolfle, T. L., 25
Wolpe, J., 246
Woodley, J., 271
Woodrow, K. M., 89
Woody, P. D., 87
Woolf, C. F., 16
Wortis, H., 14

Wright, B., 60
Wright, B. A., 302
Wright, G. Z., 32
Wright, J. E. C., 104
Wurtele, S. K., 219
Wynder, E. L., 110, 304

Yaffe, S. J., 183
Yalom, I. D., 225
Ylikorkala, O., 252
Youssef, A. E., 253
Yurcheson, R., 159, 161

Zachary, R. A., 219
Zajonc, R. B., 298
Zaskow, C., 29, 150, 151, 155, 158, 293
Zborowski, M., 89
Zeichner, A., 85, 221
Zeitlin, C., 280
Zeltzer, L., 30, 32, 65, 153, 156, 235
Ziegler, D. K., 273, 274
Zimin, R., 84, 275
Zimmerman, J. L., 228
Zubek, J. P., 88

Subject Index

Acupressure, 201–202
  procedure in, 201
    for dental pain, 202
    for headaches, 202
Acupuncture, 16, 197–201. *See also*
    Acupressure and Myotherapy
  analgesic effects, 199–201
    endorphin-mediated, 200
    neurophysiological, 199–200
    placebo controversy, 200–201
  with children, 197–198
  criticisms of, 199
    Hoku points, basis for, 199
    undifferentiated needling, 199
  and cultural learning, 87
  and gate control theory, 16
  theory of, 197
Acute pain, 18–19
  in children, 59–61
    anxiety in, source of, 60
  definition of, 18–19
  descriptors for, 60
  function of, 19
  management, adequacy of, 193–197
  physiological reactions to, 19,
    158–164
Adolescents
  coping by, and maternal behavior, 79
  and formal operations period, 39
  interview studies of, 36–37
  pain management for, 171–173
  pharmacotherapy for, 179–180
  primary dysmenorrhea in, 252–259
Analgesics, narcotic
  action of, 184
  agonist and antagonist, properties of,
    184, 186
  buprenorphine, 191
  categorization of, 184–186
  codeine, 190
  differences in, 186
  fentanyl, 189–190
  heroin, 18
  meperidine, 190–191

  methadone, 189
  morphine, 187–189
  oxycodone, 190
  patient-regulated, 187
  pentazocine, 191–192
  pharmacokinetics, and dosages of, 185
  in prescientific period, 8–9
  routes of administration, 186–187
  similarities in, 186
  weak, 190–192
Analgesics, nonnarcotic, 180–184
  acetaminophen, 182–183
  acetylsalicylic acid, 181–182
    Reye's syndrome, 181
    side effects, 181
  classification of, 180
  ibuprofen, 183
  mechanism of action, 181
  naproxen, 183
  tolmetin, 183–184
Aristotle, 8
Arthritis, 61–64
  adult reactions to, 63–64
  and family therapy, 63–64
  naproxen *vs.* aspirin in, 183
  pain descriptors in, 61
  pain reactivity in, 80
  types of pain in, 61–62
  understanding of, age differences in,
    62–63
Attention
  diversion, as coping strategy, 54,
    95–96
  and pain attenuation, 95–96
Avicenna, 9

Behavior observation procedures,
    148–158. *See also* Behavior
    rating scales; Global ratings;
    Pain-related behaviors, measures
    of.
  limitations of, 148–149
  strengths of, 148–149
  types of, 148

Behavior rating scales, 149–156
  Children's Hospital of Eastern Ontario
    Pain Scale (CHEOPS), 152–153
  Expressive Pain Interaction Coding
    System (EPICS), 156
  facial movement coding systems
    (Affex) (Max), 151–152
  format, limitations of, 149
  Infant Pain Behavior Rating Scale
    (IPBRS), 150–151
  Observational Scale of Behavioral
    Distress, oncology (OSBD),
    153–155
  Procedural Behavior Check List
    (PBCL), oncology, 153
  Procedural Behavior Rating Scale
    (PBRS), oncology, 153
Biofeedback, 203–206
  with children, 204
  factors in, 204–206
    active involvement, 205
    competence, sense of, 206
    control, role of, 205
    personality, 205
    therapist, effect of, 206
  for migraine, 204–206, 281–282
  procedure in, 203
  research on, criticism of, 203–204
  types of, 281
Bonica
  contributions of, 13
  and pain clinics, 25–26
  textbook on pain, 13
Burns, 26–27, 259–273
  categories of, 260–261
  coping strategies for, 60
  immediate phase, 26–27
  incidence of, 259
  medical care of, 260–270
  and operant conditioning, 213–214
  pain relief in, status of, 272
  phases in, 260–263
    acute, 261–263
    emergent, 260–262
    rehabilitation, 261, 263
  treatment of, 264–270
    expectancy, effect of, 266–267
    participation model, 267–270, 296
    medical, 264–270
    psychological, 270–272
    team, 264
    traditional, 264–266

Case studies
  headaches and parental response, 82
  cognitive factors in pain perception,
    174–175
  Kavanagh's burn model, 268–269
  migraine, self-hypnosis, 282
  operant conditioning, 212–214
  play therapy, 222, 223
  provocation ecology, 79, 102–103
  rarefaction ecology, 103, 109
  RAP, family systems therapy,
    227–228
  of thermography, 163
Catastrophizing, 297
  in adults, 297
  combatting, procedure for, 297
  rate of, 297
Childhood pain. See also Acute pain,
    Adolescents, Infants, Neonates
  acupuncture for, 197–198
  acute, 59–61
  analgesics for, use of, 43–44
  categories of, 56–57
  children's views of, 32–33, 35–74,
    146
    causality, 44–46
    developmental changes in, 35–39
    pain descriptors, 42–44, 50–51,
      58–73
    value of, 46–47
    what helps most, 51–52
    worst aspect of, 49
    worst pain ever, 39–40, 50–51
  chronic pain, 61–64
    special needs of child, 174–175
  communication of, 29–30, 32
  competency pain, 68–71
  coping strategies for, 52–55
  current concept of, 293–294
  definitions of, 40–42, 141
    developmental transitions in,
      40–42, 293–294, 296
  endorphins in, 299
  erroneous beliefs re, attack on, 29–30
  and ethical constraints, 29–31
    research options, 30–31
  experiences, common, in 57–58
  and helplessness, 93–94
  interest, lack of, in, 28
  interview studies of, 35–40
  and learning, role of, 29
  locus of control, 90

maladaptive pain usage, 47–49
management of, guidelines for 31–32,
    167–175
meaning of, 91–92
memory of, 39
  in adolescents, 73–74
  in children, 39–40
  in infants, 39
and myelinization, 28–29
needle procedures in, 50
pain games, 32
and pain in adulthood, implications for
    300–303
pharmacotherapy for, 175–178
Piagetian stages in, 38–39
  and causality, 44–46
  formal operations, explanatory
    power of, 39
  pain definitions in, 40–42
preparation for, 32, 294–295
psychophysiological, 58–59
psychotherapeutic drugs in, 192–193
as punishment, 38
reactivity in, 80–109
recall *vs.* learning controversy, 39
reaction of child to, 296
and recurrent abdominal pain (RAP),
    31
research on, 31–32, 296–299,
    310–311
  dissemination in, 312
and restlessness, 157–158
and tertiary gains, 82–83
textbooks on, 32
tolerance of, differences in, 75
treatment related, 64–68
  in leukemia, 64–67
  in orthodontistry, 67–68
vicarious experiences, 71–73
  and pain expectancies, 72–73
Children's Comprehensive Pain
    Questionnaire, 123–124, 277
Children's Hospital of Eastern Ontario
    Pain Scale, 152–153
Children's Hypnotic Susceptibility Scale,
    233
Chronic pain, 16, 19–20. *See also*
    Chronic pain syndrome
  in children, 32, 61–64
  and enmeshment, 61–62
    marginality, 302
    pain clinics, 310

and prevention, 303–304
  psychological overlay, 302–303
  and socialization, 303
  and spread phenomenon, 63
costs of, 18, 300–301
definition of, 19
disease model of, 17
endorphins, role in, 25
functions of, 19–20
group therapy for, 224–226
learning theory model of, 17
malingering, 27–28
as a medical entity, 18, 25–26
pain clinics, 26
patients, categories of, 20–21
Chronic pain syndrome, 13, 20–23
  childhood pain, as precursor of,
    300–304
  costs of, 23, 300–301
  intervention in, 22
  management of, 300
  models of, 22–23
Circumcision, 29
  costs of, 301
Competency pain, 68–71
  descriptors of, 69
  and mastery models, 71
  tension vs. postexertion, 68–69
  types of, 68–69
Control
  in biofeedback, 205
  and hardiness, 55
  vs. helplessness, 93–94
  locus of, 90
  need to feel, 107–108
  and self-pacing, 229–231
  techniques of, 93–94
Coping strategies, 52–55
  in acute pain, 60
  in arthritis, 55, 63
  for burns, 60
  categorization of, 52
  cognitive, 54–55, 238–246
    attention diversion, 54, 95–96,
      242–243
    context transformation, 244
    efficacy of, 248–249
    hardiness, 55
    imagery, 54, 244–246
    for migraine, 283
    self-instruction, 243–244
    stimulus transformation, 244–245

Coping strategies *(continued)*
  teaching of, general procedures for,
    239–242
  vs. coping style, 52, 55
  direct action, 53
  and intrusive procedures, 287
  thought-stopping, 246–248
Cultural learning, 87–88
  and needle procedures, 87–88
  of stoicism, 87

Dysmenorrhea, primary, 251–259
  categories of, 255
  maternal input in, 253–254
  medical evaluation of, 254–255
  onset of, 252–253
  ovulation controversy, 252–253
  patient reeducation in, 258–259
  prostaglandins, role of, 253, 256–257
  vs. secondary, 252
  treatment regimen, 256–259
    pharmacotherapy, 256–257
    psychological intervention in,
      257–259

Endorphins, 24–25
  in childhood autism, 299
  and gate-control theory, 25
  humor, role of, 298
  as pain measures, 161–162
  in RAP, 299
Ethics of pediatric pain research, 30–31
Expressive Pain Interaction Coding
    System (EPICS), 156
Facial movement coding systems (Affex)
    (Max), 151–152
Family therapy, 63–64, 227–229
Fit, concept of, 73–74
  and classroom ecology, 73, 78
  in migraine treatment, 295
  and mode of communication, 73
  in preparatory information, 294–295

Gate-control theory, 14–16
  controversy re, 26
  criticisms of, 15
  drive model, Wall, 26–27
  endorphins, 25
  factors influencing gate action, 14–15
  psychological factors, role of, 14

Global ratings, 156–157
Graphic ratings scales (GRS), 137–141
  and card sort procedures, 164–165
  derivatives of, 139–141
    face interval scales, 139–140
    Oucher, 140
    Poker Chip Tool, 140–141
  description of, 134, 137–138
  descriptors, meaning of, 138
  limitations of, 134–136, 138
  strengths, 134, 138

Headache. *See also* Migraine
  acupressure for, 201–202
  biofeedback for, 204–206
  chronic, 27
  continuous model of, 273
  descriptors, child *vs.* adult, 43
  dichotomous model of, 27, 273
  relaxation for, 207–209
  trepanning, 7–8
  typology controversy, 27
Health care, 300–301, 304
  circumcision, 301
  containment of, 300–301
  costs of, 300–301
Helplessness, learned, 93
Hospice, 17
Humor, 298–299
  as analgesic, potential of, 298–299
    endorphin role in, 298
    reactive component, diminution of,
      298
  in scoliosis treatment, 298
  as treatment, advantages of, 298
Hypnosis, 17, 232–238
  hypnotherapy, 234–237
    arm levitation in, 233
    for BDC, 270–271
    essential characteristics for,
      234–235
    eye fixation in, 233
    favorite story technique, 236
    and pain reduction, 235
    research on, 235
    with preschool children, 235–236
  hypnotizability, 232–233
    tests for, 233
  self-hypnosis, 237–238
    efficacy of, 238
    learning of, 237–238

for migraine, 282
resistance to, 237

Infant Pain Behavior Rating Scale
(IPBRS), 150–151
categories, sample of, 150
facial expression, pain, 151–152
pain cry, 151
strengths of, 151
Infants
facial expression, pain, 151–152
injections, changing reactions to, 39
pain in, 28–30
pain cry, 150–151
pharmacotherapy for, 176–178
International Association for the Study of
Pain (IASP)
definition of pain, 2–3
journal, 24
Interview studies, 35–40
of adolescents, 36–37
of children, 35–40
communication medium fit, 73
response variance in, sources of, 56
Intrusive procedures, 284–291
anticipatory anxiety re, 285–286
and erroneous beliefs, 285–286
loss of control and, 285
audiovisual materials in, 290–291
and cognitive modification, 289–290
coping skills for, 287
and prior information, 286–287
branching program for, 286
techniques for, improvement of,
287–288
Mizzy Gun, 288–289
thought-stopping and, 286–287

Kavanagh's burn treatment, 267–270,
296

Leukemia, 64–67
behavior rating scales, 153–155
behavioral distress, concept of, 153
pain descriptors in, 65–66
treatment procedures, painful, 64–67

Maladaptive pain usage, 27–28, 47–49
in adults, 27–28
in children, 47–49

malingering in, 48
secondary gains in, 47–48
McGill Pain Questionnaire, 124–126,
277
content validity, 115
and labor pains, 119
pain descriptors, children's, 42, 58, 69
use with children, 124
Medical school curriculum, 109–110
changes in, 109
pain pharmacotherapy instruction,
deficits in, 195
Migraine, 273–284
assessment of, 277
biofeedback for, 204–206, 213
diagnostic criteria, 276–277
dichotomous *vs.* continuous headache
model, 273
pharmacotherapy, 277–280
abortive medication, 278–279
palliative treatment, 279–280
prophylactic medication, 277–278
precipitating factors, 275–276
predisposing factors, 275
prevalence of, 274
psychological intervention, 280–284,
295
biofeedback, 281–282
cognitive coping strategies, 283
multicomponent treatment, 295
reassurance, 280–281
rebreathing, 283–284
relaxation, 295
self-hypnosis, 282
Models (live and symbolic)
challenge, 221
coping, 217–219
and cultural transmission, 87–88
familial, 84–85, 110
mastery, 71, 218–219
in hospital setting, 104
multiple, effect of, 85
of pain reactivity, 84–86, 298–299
avoidant behavior and, 86
parental, and absenteeism, 86
peer, 85–86
repugnant, 221
Models (theoretical and applied)
buffering, 52
for burn treatment, Kavanagh,
267–270, 296

Models (continued)
of chronic pain, 17, 22–23
disease, 17
fear-avoidance, 23
operant conditioning, 17, 22–23
psychoanalytic, 22
psychophysiological, 23
systems theory, 23
headache, dichotomous vs.
continuous, 273
pain clinics, 26
major comprehensive (Bonica), 26
modality-oriented, 26
symptom-oriented, 26
of pain reactivity, 76–79
of prevention, 303
radical behavioral, 70
social support, 52
Modeling procedures, 217–221
film, 217–221
and dental fears, 218–219
differential reaction to, 220–221
and hospital fears, 218–219
information, timing of, 219
prior experience, effect of, 218–219
Myotherapy, 202–203
with children, 202–203
trigger point, 202

Needle procedures
and cultural learning, 87–88
in leukemia treatment, 64–67
as worst pain ever, 50
Neonates, 296
pain reactivity, heterogeneity of, 296
maternal and other factors in, 296
Numerical rating scales (NRS), 141–145
description of, 134, 141
limitations, 134–136, 142
pain thermometer, 142–143
statistical limitations of, 142
strengths of, 134, 141–142
Nuprin Pain Report, 3–5, 90

Observational Scale of Behavioral
Distress, oncology (OSBD),
153–155
behavior categories in, 154–155
Operant conditioning, 211–217
for burn treatment, 213–214
criticisms of, 214, 216–217

essential requirements in, 211
and reinforcement of pain behavior,
212
schedules of reinforcement, 211
secondary gains in, RAP, 212
Orthodontistry, 67–68
adults' reports of, 67–68
pain descriptors in, 67
peak pain periods in, 67
prestigious model, effect of on, 86
Oucher, 140

Pain. See also Acute pain, Childhood
pain, Chronic pain
advances in, 6–7
readiness for, 17–18
Aristotelian view of, 8
childhood, 28–33
children's views of, 32–33, 35–74
clinics, 22
efficacy of, reviews, 22
complexity of, 1, 6, 69–70, 75
congenital analgesia, 1
and endorphins, 25
costs of, 18, 300–302
cultural transmission of, 87–88
definitions, 1–3, 40–42
drive model of, 26–27
etiological factors in, 1
experiences, range of, 3
functions of, 1
in infants, 29
learning controversy, 29
mechanisms, 4
multidimensionality of, 1, 13
in neonates, 29
pattern theory, contribution of, 12
phantom limb, 9, 11–12
prevalence of, 1, 3–4
by diagnostic category, 3–5
prevention of, 302–305
primary characteristics of, 21
radical behavioral model of, 70
research, funding of, 6, 24
retrospective reports of, 39–40,
67–68, 74
secondary problems in, 21
and suffering, unnecessary, 18
typologies, 9
understanding of, evolution of, 7–11

current scientific period, 13–28,
16–18, 23–28
early scientific period, 9–13
and multidisciplinary teams, 23–24
prescientific period, 8–9
primitive period, 7–8
progress in, 4–7
Pain assessment, 111–165. *See also*
Behavior observation,
Physiological measures,
Subjective assessment
approach to, indirect, 112
behavioral measures, 113, 148–158
controversy in, 111
physiological measures, 113, 158–163
reliability, 113–114
interrater, 114
test-retest, 113–114
standardization in, 113
status of, 112
of subjective component, 113, 116–148
validity, 114–115
concurrent, 115
construct, 115
content, 115
face, 115
Pain clinics, 22
for children, 310
focus of, 26
models of, 26
multidisciplinary teams in, 24
Pain diaries, 73, 126–127
Pain drawings, 127–131
limitations, 130
validity of, 130
Pain interview studies, 33, 35–37, 73
recall *vs.* learned response in, 39–40
type of question, 53, 56, 118–121
Pain management
classification system for, 175
and cognitive regression, 168
and control, need for, 172–173
guidelines for, general, 167–175
active involvement in, 170–171
adolescents, 173
chronic pain patients, 174–175
honesty, importance of, 167–168
joking, 170
predictability in, 169
preparatory information, 168
self-control in, 171–173

use of signals, 169
procedural refinements, 294–295
conceptual framework, for
pediatrician, 296
Pain reactivity
and attention, 95–96
and anxiety, state, 94–95
cognitive factors, role of, 174–175
differences in, intraindividual and
interindividual, 75–76
environmental nonsocial factors,
105–108
activity, purposeful, 108
comfort, 105–107
control, 107–108
environmental social factors, 76,
97–105
mother's absence, effect of,
100–101
mother's presence, effect of,
98–100
others, effect of, 104–105
pediatric personnel, effect of,
101–103
and meaning of pain, 91–92
predisposing factors in, 76
avoidant learning, 86
contingent social reinforcement,
81–83, 117
cultural learning, 87–88
demographic variables, 88–89
direct training, 80–81
diurnal variation, 90–91
familial models, 84–85
observational learning experiences,
83–86
peer models, 85–86
personality, 89–90
provocation *vs.* rarefaction
ecologies, 78–79, 82, 99,
102–103, 108–109
and self-efficacy, 96–97
sex differences in, in infancy, 88–89
situational factors in, 76
situation-specific child factors, 91–97
attention, role of, 95–96
helplessness *vs.* control, 93–94
meaning of pain, 91–92
self-efficacy, 96–97
state anxiety, 94–95
as state, 76

Pain reactivity *(continued)*
  theories of, 76–77
  as trait, 75
Pain-related behaviors, measures of,
    157–158
  restlessness, 157–158
  strengths and limitations, 157
Pain thermometer, 115, 142
Pain threshold, 28
  changes in, with age, 88–89
  and sensory deprivation, animals, 28
Pattern theory, 11–13
  common assumptions in, 11–12
  criticisms of, 12
  Goldscheider's formulation, 11
  sensory interaction theory, 12
  vs. specificity theory, 12–13
Pediatric Pain Inventory (PPI), 146–147
Pharmacotherapy of pain, 175–197. *See
    also* Narcotic analgesics,
    Nonnarcotic analgesics,
    Psychotherapeutic drugs
  adequacy of, in acute pain, 193–197
    attitudes and beliefs, role of,
      194–197
    pain reactivity, role of in children,
      195
  for adolescents, 179–180
  analgesic, ideal, critical properties of,
    175–176
  analgesics, classification of, 180
  analgesics, guidelines, 178
    addiction controversy, 195
  for burns, 264–265
  centrally acting analgesics, 179,
    184–192
  for dysmenorrhea, 256–257
  for infants and children, 176–178
    drugs, evaluation of, 177–178
    guidelines for, 178
    problems in, 177–178
  for intrusive procedures, 288
  for migraine, 277–280
    abortive, 278–279
    palliative, 279–280
    prophylactic, 277–288
  peripherally acting analgesics,
    179–184
  pharmacokinetic parameters,
    176–177
  prescientific, 8–9

Physiological measures, 158–164
  biochemical assessment, 161–162
  cardiac rate, 160
  global arousal pattern to pain, 159
  and outward demeanor, 159–160
  pain-specific, search for, 158–159
  palmar sweat index, 160–161
  thermography, 162–163
Placebos
  acupuncture as, 200–201
  in migraine treatment, 278
  operant conditioning as, 216–217
Poker Chip Tool, 140–141
Preparatory information, 32, 294–295
  child's choice of, 294
  and fit, 294–295
  Well Doll Clinic, 295
Prevention
  of chronic pain syndrome, 302–304
    predisposing factors in childhood,
      302–303
    primary and secondary programs,
      303
  intervention program for school years,
    303–310
    costs, 308
    lesson content, example of, 305
    long-term results, 307
    personnel involved, 304
    resistance to, 307–308
    short-term results, example,
      306–307
  school programs, health-related,
    303–304
Procedural Behavior Check List (PPCL),
    oncology, 153
Procedural Behavior Rating Scale
    (PBRS), oncology, 153
Projective tests, 145–147
  Eland Projective Tool, 145–146
  Pediatric Pain Inventory (PPI),
    146–147
  Scott cartoons, 145
Provocation ecology, 78–79, 82,
    99–100, 102–103, 108–109
Psychotherapeutic drugs, 192–193
  amitriptyline, 193
  imipramine, 193
Psychotherapy, 221–229
  family, 63–64, 227–229
  family systems, 227–229

procedure in, 228
psychosomatic illness, model of,
    228
group, 224–227
    for chronic problems, 225–226
    composition of, 224–225
    therapist's role in, 225
    vs. individual, 221
for painful procedures, 222–224
play, 222–224
    reports, programs of, 223–224
    strengths of, 222–223

Quieting reflex, 209–210
and classroom program, 209
procedure, 209

Rarefaction ecology, 78–79, 82,
    99–100, 102–103, 108–109
Rebreathing, migraine, 283–284
Recurrent abdominal pain (RAP), 31,
    58–59
endorphin hypothesis, 299
familial models in, 84
family systems therapy for, 227–228
and operant conditioning, 212–213
Relaxation
for migraine, 207–208
for primary dysmenorrhea, 257–258
school program for, 208–209
and self-control, 207
for tension headaches, 208–209

School programs, 303–310
for chronic pain syndrome, as
    prevention strategy, 304–310
health related, 304
on pain, 304–310
    content of, 305
    costs of, 309–310
    parents' role in, 305–306
    pediatric personnel, role in, 305
    resistance to, 307–309
    results of, 306–307
    school personnel, role in, 304–305
    scope of, 304–305
quieting reflex, 209–210
relaxation, 208–209
Self-pacing, 230–232
Social ecology theory, 77–80
and mother's presence, 98–99

and pediatric setting, 78–80
provocation ecologies, 78–79, 82,
    99–100, 102–103, 108–109
rarefaction ecologies, 78–79, 82,
    99–100, 102–103, 108–109
theoretical antecedents of, 76–78
Specificity theory, 10–11
criticisms of, 11
crucial assumption of, 10
Stanford Hypnotic Clinical Scale for
    Children, 233
Subjective assessment, 116–148
as estimates, 116
graphic rating scales (GRS), 137–141.
    See also Graphic rating scales
numerical rating scales (NRS),
    141–145. *See also* Numerical
    rating scales
pain color matching, 142–144
    Eland's scale, 144
    Nayman's scale, 144
pain diaries, 126–127
pain drawings, 127–131
    procedure for, 130
    validity of, 130
pain maps, 131–133
    validity of, 131, 133
projective tests, 145–147. *See also*
    Projective tests
questionnaires, 121–126
    Children's Comprehensive Pain
        Questionnaire (CCPQ), 123–124
    McGill Pain Questionnaire (MPQ),
        124–126
    Varni/Thompson Pediatric Pain
        Questionnaire (PPQ), 121–123
self-rating scales, strengths and
    limitations, 133–136
verbal self-report, 116–121
    of duration of pain, 120
    limitations of, 117
    maximizing quality of, 118–121
    strengths of, 117
    temporal pattern of pain, 120–121
    value of, controversy, 116–117
visual analogue scale (VAS), 133–137.
    See also Visual analogue scales

Talking through, 229–230
Theories of pain
Aristotle, 8

Theories of pain *(continued)*
  Galen, 8
  gate-control theory, 14–16
  pattern theory, 11–13
  specificity theory, 10–11
Thermography, 162–163
  case study of, 163
  principle of, 162–163
  procedure in, 163
Thought-stopping, 246–248
Treatment procedures
  analgesic drugs, 8–9
  behavioral management, 22
  medical, 17

psychologists, impact on, 17
Trepanning, 7–8

Varni/Thompson Pediatric Pain
      Questionnaire (PPQ), 121–123,
      277
Visual analogue scales (VAS), 133,
      136–137
  adult procedures, applications of, 164
  description of, 133, 134, 136
  limitations of, 134–136, 137
  practice session, 136
  reliability and validity of, 137
  strengths of, 134, 137